A Comprehensive Study of Metabolic Syndrome

A Comprehensive Study of Metabolic Syndrome

Editor: Damian Wayne

AMERICAN
MEDICAL PUBLISHERS
www.americanmedicalpublishers.com

AMERICAN
MEDICAL PUBLISHERS
www.americanmedicalpublishers.com

Cataloging-in-publication Data

A comprehensive study of metabolic syndrome / edited by Damian Wayne.
p. cm.
Includes bibliographical references and index.
ISBN 979-8-88740-262-8
1. Metabolic syndrome. 2. Metabolism--Disorders. 3. Insulin resistance. I. Wayne, Damian.
RC662.4 .C66 2023
616.399--dc23

American Medical Publishers,
41 Flatbush Avenue,
1st Floor, New York,
NY 11217, USA

ISBN 979-8-88740-262-8 (Hardback)

Contents

Preface

The world is advancing at a fast pace like never before. Therefore, the need is to keep up with the latest developments. This book was an idea that came to fruition when the specialists in the area realized the need to coordinate together and document essential themes in the subject. That's when I was requested to be the editor. Editing this book has been an honour as it brings together diverse authors researching on different streams of the field. The book collates essential materials contributed by veterans in the area which can be utilized by students and researchers alike.

Metabolic syndrome is referred to as the presence of at least three of the five medical conditions, including high blood sugar, abdominal obesity, low serum high-density lipoprotein (HDL), high blood pressure and high serum triglycerides. Ethnicity, a high-fat diet, aging, a history of frequent drinking and stress are some of the risk factors strongly linked to metabolic syndrome. The risk of acquiring type 2 diabetes and cardiovascular disease is correlated with metabolic syndrome. Its diagnosis involves measuring blood pressure, fat levels, waist circumference and fasting blood sugar. There are several ways of preventing and managing metabolic syndrome such as quitting smoking and other tobacco products, eating a balanced diet, being physically active, and maintaining a healthy weight. This book presents the complex condition of metabolic syndrome in the most comprehensible and easy-to-understand language. From theories to research to practical applications, case studies related to all contemporary topics of relevance to metabolic syndrome have been included in this book. Its extensive content provides the readers with a thorough understanding of this medical condition.

Each chapter is a sole-standing publication that reflects each author's interpretation. Thus, the book displays a multi-facetted picture of our current understanding of application, resources and aspects of the field. I would like to thank the contributors of this book and my family for their endless support.

Editor

1

Neural Mechanisms of Feeding Behavior and its Disorders

Hisao Nishijo and Taketoshi Ono

Abstract

There are two forms of feeding behavior. The hypothalamus and the lower brainstem monitor the internal environment of the body and are involved in the control of feeding behavior to maintain energy balance and homeostasis (homeostasis-dependent feeding behavior). On the other hand, humans and animals, when placed in an environment similar to modern society (e.g., cafeterias), where organisms can easily ingest highly preferred foods, consume more than necessary (homeostasis-independent feeding behavior). The emotion/reward system, including the amygdala and nucleus accumbens, is involved in this type of feeding behavior. These two control systems interact in the lateral hypothalamic area (LHA), where feeding behavior is controlled by systems with higher activity. In modern society, there is abundant information on food, and high-calorie foods such as snacks are readily available. Thus, in modern society, the homeostasis-independent control system easily surpasses the homeostasis-dependent control system, which results in obesity. Various feeding and eating disorders might be ascribed to dysregulations in the two control systems. In the future, more effective treatments for feeding and eating disorders can be developed by elucidating the mechanisms of these two control systems.

Keywords: feeding behaviors, hypothalamus, LHA, homeostasis, energy balance, reward, motivation

1. Introduction

Feeding behavior is a series of actions that includes food acquisition, food intake into the oral cavity, taste perception, chewing, and swallowing. Feeding behavior is affected by a number of factors such as the internal state of the body (hunger or satiety), the taste of the food as well as health, mood, as well as the atmosphere around an individual. Hunger and satiety, appetite, and food reward are the most important factors that regulate feeding behavior.

Both humans and animals engage in feeding behaviors to obtain pleasure (food reward: pleasure when ingesting food), and the desire for this food reward is driven by appetite. When a gastric tube was placed in an animal to discharge ingested food, the animal continued to eat to obtain a food reward; however, when the gastric tube was closed, the feeding stopped with the extension of the stomach [1]. This finding suggests that food reward is obtained by a series of feeding behaviors up to the swallowing stage, and the satiety that terminates feeding is dependent on the stomach extension and the subsequent digestive absorption processes. Thus, food reward is elicited by several events that occur before it passes through the esophagus:

the appearance and shape of the food, the taste and smell of the food, and the pleasure obtained by swallowing the food [1]. Food reward is therefore defined as the momentary value of a food at the time of ingestion, while "liking" is defined as pleasantness (tastiness) of food in the mouth [2]. The particular taste of food is the most important factor in eliciting the food reward obtained during ingestion. In contrast with this statement, it has recently been reported that infusing glucose or sucrose solution directly into the stomach via the feeding tube without passing through the oral cavity has a rewarding effect; however, the detailed neural circuits involved in the acquisition of visceral reward are unknown [3].

The brain forms appetite and controls feeding behavior by integrating several factors such as hunger, satiety, and the rewarding effects of food palatability. In other words, feelings of hunger and satiety are visceral sensations that reflect the energy balance in the body, but appetite is a type of desire for a specific behavior (feeding behavior) that leads to the ingestion of specific foods by integrating information including food rewards as well as visceral sensations.

Such feeding behavior is controlled by the neural networks, including the hypothalamus. Specific areas in the hypothalamus and lower brainstem lack the blood-brain barrier; hence, the neural membrane is in direct contact with the blood to monitor humoral information such as nutrients and various hormones released from the digestive system. In addition, the hypothalamus receives information from the digestive system (e.g., stomach extension, chemical nature of ingested

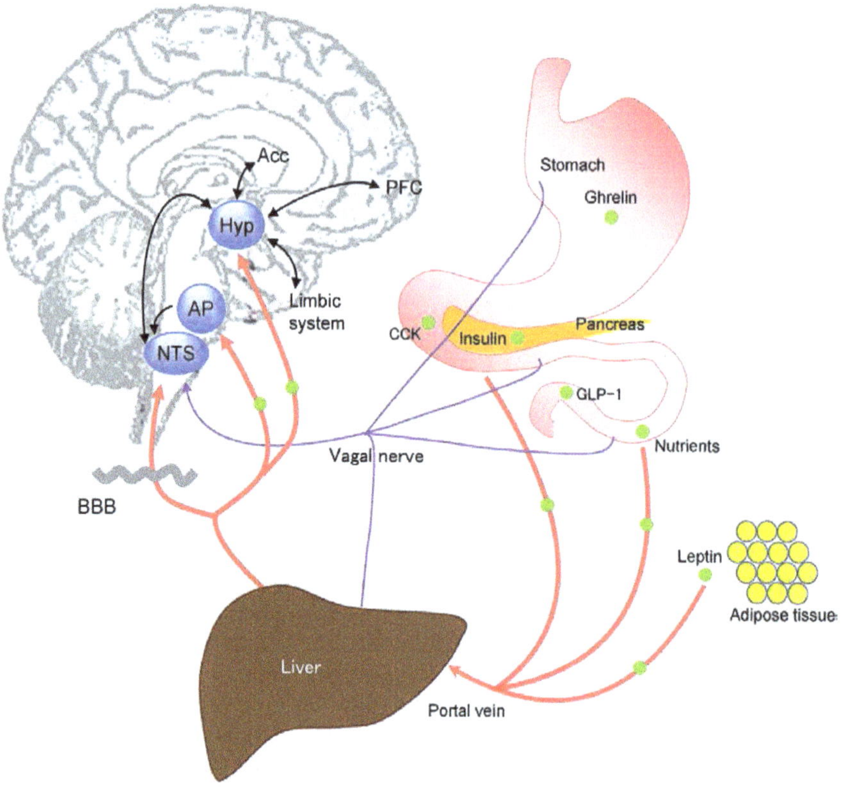

Figure 1.
Schematic diagram of the hypothalamic feeding control system that receives information on the internal energy balance (humoral factors in the blood and visceral information from the vagus nerve). The hypothalamic system also receives information from the emotion/reward system (limbic system, prefrontal cortex, and Acc). Hyp, hypothalamus; AP, area postrema; NTS, nucleus tractus solitarius; PFC, prefrontal cortex; Acc, nucleus accumbens; CCK, cholecystokinin; GLP-1, glucagon-like peptide 1; BBB, blood-brain barrier.

food in the digestive tract, and metabolic activity of the liver) via the autonomic nervous system and lower brain stem (**Figure 1**). Thus, the hypothalamus monitors the internal environment to control feeding behavior to maintain energy balance and homeostasis (homeostasis-dependent hypothalamic feeding control system). The arcuate nucleus in the hypothalamus plays a crucial role in this control system (**Figure 2**). In addition, the hypothalamus further receives information from the emotion/reward system: (1) information on food rewards and emotions from the nucleus accumbens and the limbic system and (2) higher cognitive information from the prefrontal (orbital) cortex (**Figure 1**). The hypothalamus, especially the lateral hypothalamic area (LHA), integrates these types of information to control feeding behavior [4, 5]. This review focuses on how the emotion/reward system affects feeding behavior.

2. Roles of the emotion/reward system in feeding behavior

2.1 Interaction between the hypothalamic feeding control system and the emotion/reward system

One of the important factors that control human and animal behavior, including feeding behavior, is reward (e.g., food and water required for survival, or conspecific individuals) and punishment (or disgust stimuli) (e.g., pain due to tissue damage, natural enemies, or carnivores that threaten their survival). These rewards and punishments are closely linked to emotions. Emotion is a psychophysical response to the rewarding and punishing stimuli itself or the omission (or suspension) of the rewarding or punishing stimulus [1]. For example, fear and joy are responses to punishing and rewarding stimuli, respectively, while anger and sense of security (relief) are responses to omission (or suspension) of reward-ing and punishing stimuli, respectively. These emotions play a motivating role in guiding specific behaviors, including feeding behavior. In other words, animals, including humans, pursue rewarding stimuli that give pleasure or joy (approaching behavior), and avoid punishing stimuli that cause discomfort, anger, fear, or sadness (avoidance or flight behavior) [6]. Based on their influence on behavior, rewarding stimuli are also known as positive reinforcers that strengthen behaviors to seek rewards, while punishing stimuli are also known as negative reinforcers that strengthen behaviors to avoid punishing stimuli. The emotion/reward system evaluates sensory inputs [evaluation of biological value (rewarding or punishing)] from the viewpoint of individual survival, and forms the motivation for a specific survival behavior.

Feeding behavior corresponds to an approaching behavior in which an organism approaches and obtains rewarding stimuli (food) from the viewpoint of emotional behavior. It has been suggested that the emotion/reward system affects the feeding control system in the hypothalamus via the LHA (**Figure 2**) [5, 7, 8]. Reward information is transmitted to the nucleus accumbens by dopaminergic projections from the ventral tegmental area, and is further transmitted to the LHA via the ventral medial part of the pallidum. Injection of various drugs into this pathway has been reported to cause overeating (promotion of feeding behavior) and suppression of feeding behavior [7]. On the other hand, emotional information (especially negative emotions) is transmitted from the amygdala to the LHA. In general, there is a trade-off between feeding behavior and fear-induced emotional behavior. Fear usually suppresses feeding behavior, but in a fasted state, fear or anxiety-induced emotional behavior is suppressed [9, 10]. Conversely, pleasant emotions promote feeding behavior (see below). Furthermore, the

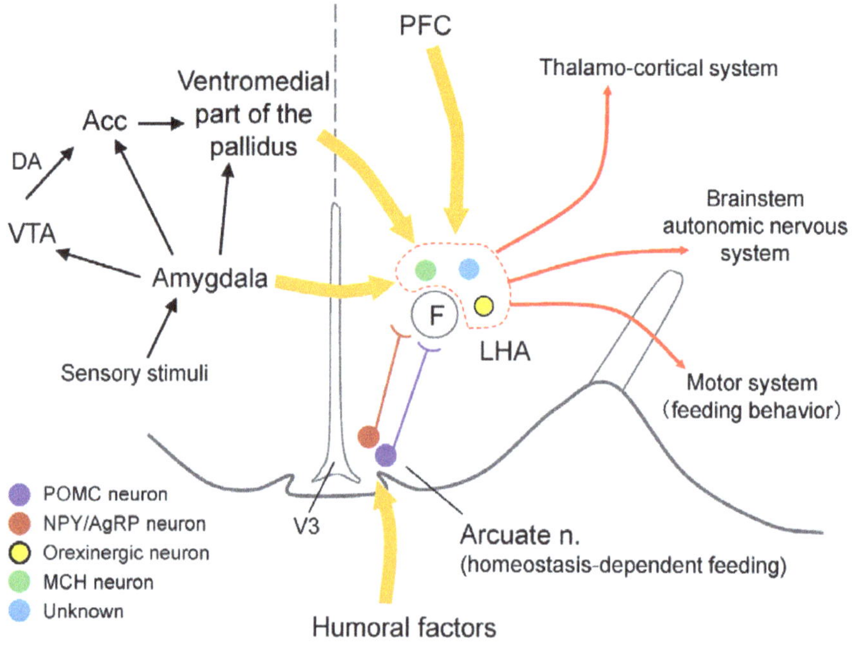

Figure2.
Interaction between the hypothalamic feeding control system and the emotion/reward system in the LHA. F: Fornix; LHA: Lateral hypothalamic area; V3: Third ventricle; PFC: Prefrontal cortex; DA: Dopamine; Acc: Nucleus accumbens; VTA: Ventral tegmental area; PFC: Prefrontal cortex.

prefrontal (orbital) cortex, which is a higher association area of olfaction and taste, sends not only cognitive information but also food information such as taste and smell to the LHA (see below).

2.2 Reward-related information processing in the nucleus accumbens

The nucleus accumbens plays a key role in the dopaminergic reward pathway and is implicated in overeating, leading to obesity. Two hypotheses have been proposed as the mechanisms that implicate the dopaminergic reward pathway in overeating and subsequently obesity [11]. The first hypothesis proposes that in obese subjects, responses to dopamine release during food intake (reward responses) are reduced. In line with this hypothesis, previous positron emission tomography (PET) studies have reported that dopamine D2 receptor utilization was reduced in obese subjects, which suggests a decrease in dopamine D2 receptor density. Thus, obese individuals may consume more food that causes dopamine release to compensate for the reduced reward response. A similar hypothesis (decreased dopamine D2 receptor utilization) has also been proposed as a mechanism for substance abuse. Furthermore, an animal study reported that when a chronic electrode was implanted in a specific brain region such as the medial forebrain bundle and an electric current (rewarding) was applied by a lever press, the animal preferred to press the lever [intracranial self-stimulation (ICSS) behavior]. However, in sup-port of this first hypothesis, injection of a dopamine D2 receptor antagonist into the nucleus accumbens suppressed ICSS behavior due to electrical stimulation of the medial forebrain bundle. The second hypothesis proposes that obese people are more sensitive to cue stimuli (such as food smell and visual appearance, or conditioned stimuli) that predict food availability, rather than food ingestion itself. A higher sensitivity to food cues lead to an increase in food intake, which in turn, gradually reduces the reward response when food is consumed. Thus, food intake is further increased by the individual to compensate for the reduced reward response. In support of the second hypothesis, in obese individuals as well as obesity-prone rats, responses to cues associated with food are enhanced in certain brain regions, including the nucleus accumbens [12, 13]. The nucleus accumbens is suggested to play a crucial role in incentive motivation: a process that translates expected reward derived from cues into behavioral manifestation for food acquisition [14]. A functional magnetic resonance imaging (fMRI) study on alcohol-dependent patients reported that activity in the ventral striatum, including the nucleus accumbens, increased in response to visual cues associated with alcohol [15]. It must be noted that obese individuals might have already experienced high-reward foods such as high fat or high calorie foods. Therefore, it is difficult to clarify which hypotheti-cal mechanism causes a decrease in the reward response [11]. However, a human genetic study reported that obese subjects had a genetic polymorphism, called *Taq1A*, with decreased dopamine D2 receptor density [16]. These findings suggest that there are multiple underlying mechanisms for obesity.

A study analyzed neuronal responses in the ventral striatum, including the nucleus accumbens during discrimination of foods from nonfoods in a lever-press feeding task, in monkeys (unpublished data). This task consisted of three phases: (1) a visual recognition phase during which various objects including food and nonfood were presented to the monkey by opening an opaque shutter in front of an object, (2) a lever-press phase during which the monkey pressed the lever by a pre-determined number of times if food was presented, and (3) an ingestion phase dur-ing which the monkey could take food after the last lever press opened a transparent shutter in front of the object [17–19]. In this task, white and red cylinders were associated with drops of juice and water, respectively. A predetermined number of lever presses opened a valve to deliver a drop of juice and water, respectively. When a brown cylinder was presented, the monkey had to press the lever a predetermined number of times to avoid electric shock. An example of a ventral striatum neuron in the monkey that selectively responded to rewarding objects has been shown in **Figure 3A**. This neuron responded to the rewarding objects, including orange and white cylinders associated with juice and water, but not to the brown cylinder and aversive syringe associated with electric shock. It should be noted that the responses to the rewarding objects were not related to simple lever-pressing movements, since the neuron did not respond to the brown cylinder even though the monkey pressed the lever. The response magnitudes of this neuron to various objects have been shown in **Figure 3B**. The results showed that this neuron was highly responsive to the monkeys' favorite (highly rewarding) objects. The existence of this type of neu-ron in the ventral striatum suggests that the ventral striatum is involved in incentive motivation for rewarding objects.

Previous studies have suggested that dopamine release in the ventral striatum is involved in the motivation for appetitive behaviors. Tonic (slow) increases in dopamine levels were shown to be involved in motivation [20, 21]. A positive correlation between reward-seeking behavior and dopamine levels was also reported [21]. Another study analyzed the activity of medium spiny neurons (MSNs), the major output neurons in the nucleus accumbens that receive dopaminergic projections [22] in the rat nucleus accumbens [23]. In this study, water-deprived rats were trained with an operant conditioning task in which the licking of a spout was associated with intragastric glucose (glucose group) or water (water group) infusion. After training, it was observed that rats in the glucose group were more vigorous in licking the spout in the absence of intragastric infusion. The inter-spike interval variability of MSNs, which reflects dopamine release in the striatum, was higher in the glucose group than in the water group [23]. These findings suggest that dopamine release in the nucleus accumbens plays a crucial role in motivation.

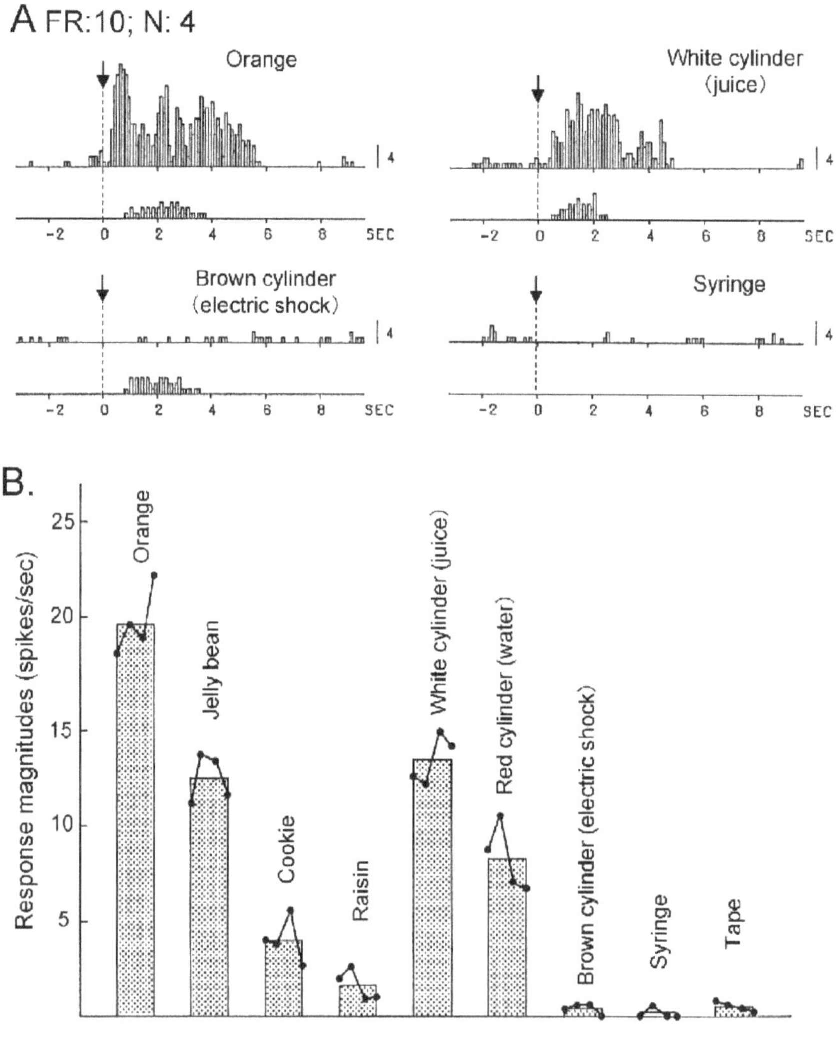

Figure 3.
Response of a monkey ventral striatal neuron to various objects. (A) Responses of a ventral striatal neuron to various objects. Upper histogram: Summed histogram of neuronal activity (bin width, 100 ms bin); lower histogram: Summed histograms of lever-press signals. Zero on time axis: Onset of object presentation. Calibration shown at the right of each histogram (4 spikes/bin). FR, number of lever presses; N, number of trials. (B) Average response magnitudes for various objects. Closed circle, response magnitude in each trial.

However, the actual roles of dopamine and other neurotransmitters in motivation (wanting) and hedonic pleasure (liking) is still under debate [24–26].

2.3 Food valuation in the amygdala

Food is a rewarding object that induces pleasant emotions. The amygdala is involved in evaluating the biological (motivational) values of objects such as food. The activity of amygdala neurons has been reported to correlate with the biological value of sensory stimuli in monkeys as well as humans [17–19, 27, 28]. Therefore, it can be said that humans select an object with a high reward value based on value evaluation in the amygdala [27]. Thus, when the reward value of food decreases (devaluation), approaching behavior to the conditioned stimulus associated with that food also decreases. For example, the injection of lithium after eating causes discomfort, which reduces the reward value of the food to induce appetitive behaviors. However, it has been reported that basolateral amygdala lesions in rats abolished these changes in behaviors after devaluation [29]. Similarly, in another study, monkeys were trained to form an association between two pairs of specific objects with specific foods. They were then allowed to eat only one of the foods to satisfaction (i.e., devaluation of one of the foods) after which it was observed that the monkeys chose the specific object associated with the other food (food-specific satiety) when given the option. However, lesions to the amygdala or surgical discon-nection of neural fibers between the amygdala and orbital cortex reduced such behavioral changes associated with devaluation [30, 31]. Also, in a human fMRI study, devaluation of a specific food after eating it reduced brain hemodynamic responses to the odor of that specific food in the amygdala and orbital cortex [32]. These findings suggest that the amygdala receives information about the internal state of the body from the hypothalamus and evaluates the expected reward. Since stimulation of the amygdala increases dopamine release in the nucleus accumbens [33], value information from the amygdala may modulate dopamine release in the nucleus accumbens. This further suggests that an interaction between the amygdala and the nucleus accumbens is crucial in behavioral alterations in devaluation or food-specific satiety.

Some previous studies have shown that recordings from the amygdala neurons of monkeys were made during performance of the same lever-press feeding task (as shown in **Figure 3**) [17–19]. About one-fourth of the recorded amygdala neurons responded differentially to various rewarding and aversive objects with biological value (differential neurons). An example of such differential neurons has been shown in **Figure 4A**. These neurons responded strongly to orange, which was highly preferred (**Figure 4Aa**) in the visual discrimination and ingestion phases, but had a weak response to raisin, which was less preferred (**Figure 4Af**). The neuron had no response to tape, which had no biological value (**Figure 4Ag**). The neurons also responded to an aversive spider model (**Figure 4Ad**) and a brown column associated with electric shock (**Figure 4Ae**). Furthermore, this neuron responded more strongly to the preferred white cylinder associated with juice compared with the less preferred red cylinder associated with water, in the visual discrimination and ingestion phases (**Figure 4Ab, c**). These results suggest that the activity of the amygdala neuron reflects the biological values of objects. Similar types of amygdala neurons have been reported in a human study [27]. In this study, recordings from the amygdala neurons of a patient were made, while the patient rated specific foods displayed on a monitor by bidding. It was observed that the activities of some amygdala neurons positively correlated with food evaluation (bid price).

In the same studies done by Nishijo et al. [17–19], the monkeys drank 80 mL of water after the initial recording, which reduced the values of the red cylinder. The same neuron in **Figure 4A** was again tested with the white and red cylinders. **Figure 4B** shows altered neuronal responses in the amygdala after drinking. Although the neuron responded similarly to the white cylinder in the visual discrimination and ingestion phases, its responses to the red cylinder were attenuated (**Figure 4B**). These findings suggest that neuronal activity in the amygdala changes online based on the biological significance of objects.

2.4 Comprehensive food valuation in the frontal orbital cortex

Delicious food is highly rewarding. Both humans and animals consume foods with high reward values. Several factors can affect the expected reward value of a specific food when cues associated with that food are presented. Several factors can also affect food reward when food is ingested. Factors that can affect the expected reward value and food reward includes the following: (1) sensory factors derived

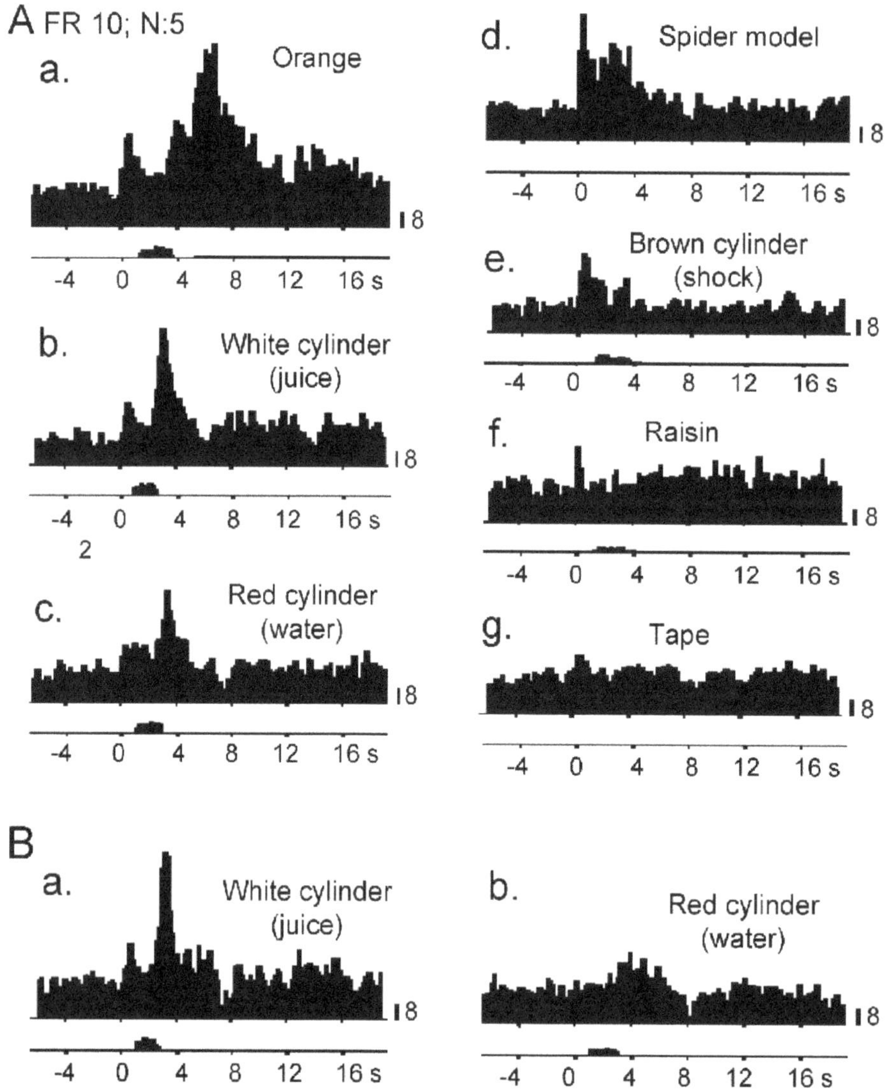

Figure 4.
Changes in responsiveness of amygdala neurons in a monkey before and after drinking. (A) Responses of an amygdala neuron to various objects with and without biological significance. (B) Changes in neuronal responses to the white and red cylinders after drinking 80 mL of water. Upper and lower histograms indicate summed histograms of neuronal activity and lever-press signals (bin width, 200 ms), respectively. Calibration is shown on the right of each histogram (8 spikes/bin). FR, number of lever presses; N, number of trials. A zero on the time scale indicates stimulus onset.

from foods such as taste and smell, (2) internal states such as hunger and satiety, (3) previous experience of ingesting foods, (4) cognitive factors, and (5) temporal factors such as immediate availability of foods [11, 34]. The orbital cortex receives multisensory inputs, such as visual and auditory inputs, and also functions as a secondary taste and olfactory area. This brain region also receives inputs from the somatosensory cortex and is involved in processing food texture in the oral cavity. Thus, the orbital cortex receives all food-related sensory inputs and is involved in the valuation of food reward. Second, the orbital cortex receives information on the internal states and other visceral information from the hypothalamus and amygdala and is involved in food-specific satiety (see above). It has been shown in monkeys that lesions of the orbital cortex as well as the amygdala impair food-specific satiety [35]. In humans, frontotemporal dementia with atrophy of the ventral frontal lobe leads to overeating even with awareness of satiety [36, 37]. Third, knowledge about specific foods or previous experience of eating certain foods may affect the reward values of it [34, 38]. Humans simulate the expected reward of foods using this cognitive information. For example, a famous food brand or food at a famous restaurant may have a high expected reward value. Fourth, the expected reward value of food decreases as the time for acquiring food (or food reward) increases (temporal discounting). For example, healthy foods that lead to longevity and slimming seem to be highly rewarding, but it takes a long time for the effects to be observed. Due to temporal discounting, the expected reward value of heathy foods may decrease. In contrast, junk food, which can provide an immediate reward when ingested, has a higher reward value than healthy

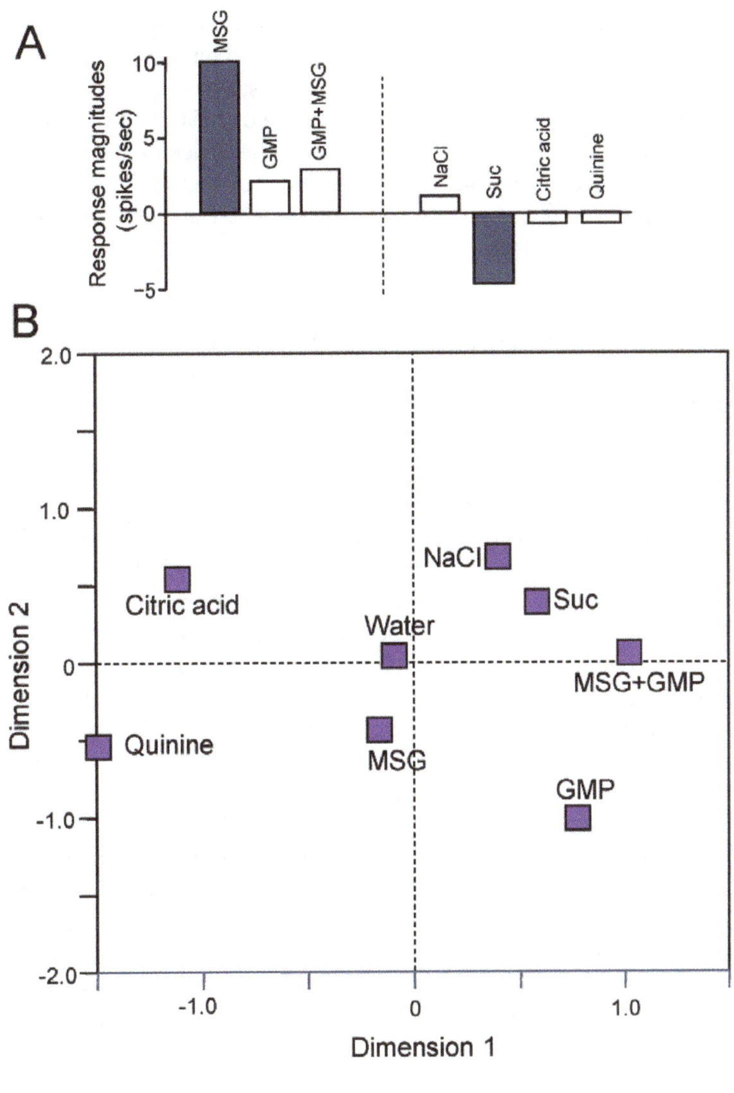

Figure 5.
Representation of taste solutions in the orbital cortex of rats. (A) An example of a response profile of a taste neuron to four basic and umami tastes. MSG, 0.1 M monosodium glutamate; GMP, 0.5 mM guanylic acid. Filled bars indicate significant taste responses (2.5 SD above or below the water response). The top bars indicate excitatory responses, and the down bars indicate inhibitory responses. (B) Distribution of taste solutions and water in a two-dimensional space.

foods. The orbital cortex is suggested to comprehensively evaluate and integrate this food-related multiple sensory, visceral, and cognitive information, and is involved in the final decision of food selection based on these factors [34, 39].

Human fMRI studies have reported that activity in the orbital cortex correlates with the subjective pleasantness of liquid foods, including umami solutions [40, 41]. To investigate the representation of taste solutions in the orbital cortex, a study analyzed neuronal responses to various taste solutions in the rat orbital cortex after infusing the solutions into the oral cavity of awake rats through implanted chronic intraoral cannulae (unpublished data). **Figure 5A** shows an example of the neuronal activity recorded from the rat orbital cortex during ingestion of various taste solutions including monosodium glutamate (MSG). This neuron responded to 0.1 M MSG, but not to 0.1 M sodium chloride (NaCl). The neuron had an inhibi-tory response to sucrose solution. **Figure 5B** shows a representation of these taste solutions resulting from a multidimensional scaling analysis of response patterns of 21 orbital cortical taste neurons. Each taste solution is arranged almost in a straight line from the left, where the most aversive quinine and citric acid are located. On the right side, there are rewarding solutions including sucrose, GMP (0.5 mM guanylic acid, a kind of umami), and MSG + GMP (mixture of MSG and GMP). In addition, the MSG and water are located in the center of the space. These orders are fairly consistent with the orders of the rats' preference for taste solutions. These results suggest that the rat orbital cortical neurons represent reward values based on sensory information derived from food.

3. Eating disorders in neuropsychiatric disorders

3.1 Feeding and eating disorders

Feeding and eating disorders are classified into several subtypes including anorexia nervosa, bulimia nervosa, binge-eating disorder, and others. Patients with anorexia nervosa show reduced dietary intake, weight loss, increased activity, hypo-thermia, and often present with symptoms of compulsive behavior. Since patients with anorexia nervosa have a fear of food or its intake, they restrict themselves from eating. The arcuate nucleus of the hypothalamus contains two groups of neurons that reciprocally regulate feeding behavior in response to blood hormones [42]. One is a group of neurons that produce neuropeptide Y and agouti-related peptide (NPY/AgRP neurons), which promotes feeding behavior. The other group of neurons produces α -melanocyte-stimulating hormone (α -MSH), which suppresses feeding behavior. Since α-MSH is a neurotransmitter produced by processing the precursor protein proopiomelanocortin (POMC), α-MSH-producing neurons are called POMC neurons. The hunger state that occurs due to this restriction of food intake leads to excessive NPY/AgRP neuronal activity, which in turn suppresses the activity of POMC neurons. A recent study using chemogenetic methods showed that selective enhancement of NPY/AgRP neuronal activity in mice increases behav-ioral activity and repetitive behaviors, which is similar to the compulsive behavior exhibited in human anorexia nervosa [43]. Furthermore, since POMC neurons promote oxytocin production in the paraventricular and supraoptic nuclei in the hypothalamus [44, 45], the reduction of POMC neuronal activity in fasting states may reduce oxytocin production and lead to the development of autistic traits. Reduced oxytocin production and autistic traits are also traits that are hallmarks of anorexia nervosa [46].

Bulimia nervosa is characterized by the repetition of eating large amounts of food in a short period of time (binge eating). To prevent weight gain, patients restrict their diet, vomiting, and abuse laxatives. Clinical studies have reported that there are reduced levels of dopamine metabolites in the cerebrospinal fluid of bulimia patients. Administration of alpha-methyl-para-tyrosine (AMPT), an inhibitor of tyrosine hydroxylase (the rate-limiting enzyme in catecholamine synthesis), causes binge eating to reoccur in patients who have remitted binge eating [47]. Therefore, it can be suggested that the dopamine release (which reflects food reward when ingesting food) is reduced in bulimia nervosa; thus, patients overeat to compensate for a shortage of dopamine. It has also been reported that patients with anorexia nervosa and bulimia nervosa are more likely to have autoantibodies to α-MSH and adrenocorticotropic hormone (ACTH) in their blood, suggesting that these autoantibodies may disrupt the functions of hypothalamic neurons in the feeding control system [48]. Taken together, it is likely that patients with feeding and eating disorders have some deficits in the feeding control system of the hypo-thalamus and/or the emotion/reward system.

3.2 Eating disorders in autism

In recent years, the prevalence of autism spectrum disorder has increased: 1 in 68 children have autism in the United States. It has been suggested that the orbital cortex and amygdala are involved in the development of autism [49]. These brain regions play important roles in information processing and in assessing food reward for taste (see above). Thus, it can be suggested that autism might present with some eating disorders. In line with this, patients with autism spectrum disorders have been shown to prefer eating limited kinds of foods (less than five foods at the lowest) [50], and their ability to identify sweetness, sourness, and bitterness is reduced [51].

It has been suggested that environmental pollution is partly involved in increasing the prevalence of brain development disorders, including autism. According to a study investigating the brain development of infants in dioxin-contaminated areas in Vietnam, the concentration of dioxins (particularly 2,3,7,8-tetrachlorodibenzo-p-dioxin, TCDD) in the breast milk of mothers at 1 month of age was significantly correlated with that in autistic traits of children at 3 years of age [52]. In another study, a single dose of TCDD was administered to pregnant female rats. Analyses of the offspring indicated that there were disorders of social behaviors and alteration of synaptic activity as well as altered levels and/or activity of calcium ion (Ca^{2+})/calmodulin-dependent protein kinase IIα (CaMKIIα) in the amygdala and orbital cortex [53]. As shown in human patients, deficits of parvalbumin-positive neurons were also observed in the offspring of the rats [54]. These epidemiological and experimental reports suggest that rats that are administered TCDD during the fetal period can be used as animal models of autism.

Parvalbumin-positive neurons are known to be sensitive to endoplasmic reticulum (ER) stress, while TCDD has been suggested to cause ER stress. Furthermore, POMC neurons are parvalbumin-positive neurons [55], suggesting that they are impaired by TDCC. It has also been reported that TDCC reduces parvalbumin-positive neurons in the amygdala [54]. These findings suggest that parvalbumin-positive neuronal damage is caused by TDCC, and that TCDD may induce abnormal eating. Consequently, a clinical study reported that patients with anorexia nervosa, bulimia nervosa, and binge-eating disorder showed more symptoms of subthreshold autism compared with healthy controls [56]. In order to examine the effects of TCDD on feeding behavior, TCDD was administered to pregnant female rats and the intake of amino acid solutions of the pups was investigated after weaning [57]. The pups could freely take in eight kinds of solutions (histidine, sodium glutamate, glycine, arginine, lysine hydrochloride, threonine, salt, and distilled water). **Figure 6** shows

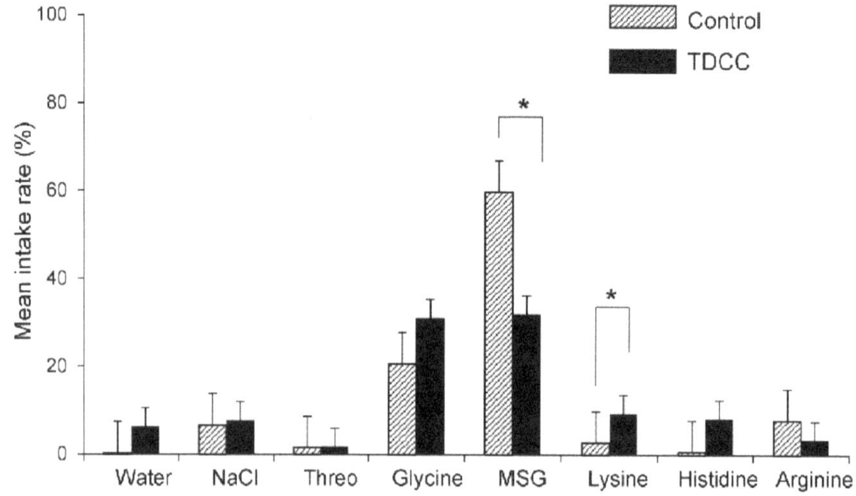

Figure 6.

Effects of fetal TCDD exposure on amino acid intake behavior. Average intake rates of eight solutions (0.05 M histidine, 0.15 M MSG, 0.5 M glycine, 0.05 M arginine, 0.2 M lysine hydrochloride, 0.4 M threonine, 0.15 M salt, and distilled water) from 29 to 35 days after birth are shown. The ordinate indicates the intake rate (percentage of each solution in total liquid consumption). In the TCDD-administered group, the intake of lysine solution increased significantly and that of MSG decreased significantly compared with the control group. TCDD, tetrachlorodibenzo-p-dioxin.

the mean intake rate of each solution (the ratio of each solution to the total liquid consumption) between 29 and 34 days after birth. The control group took almost no lysine solution, while the TCDD-treated group took more lysine than the control group. Conversely, the intake of MSG solution was significantly reduced in the TCDD-treated group compared with that in the control group. These findings suggest that abnormalities in the hypothalamus, orbital cortex, and amygdala caused by TCDD administration may induce these eating disorders. Future studies in human autistic patients are required to draw valid conclusions.

4. Conclusions

The hypothalamus and the lower brain stem monitor the internal state of the body and control feeding behavior to maintain energy balance and homeostasis (homeostasis-dependent feeding behavior). A disruption in this system could lead to obesity. For a review of how molecular mechanisms of the central nervous system (CNS) regulate energy homeostasis in the hypothalamus and mechanisms of obesity due to their dysregulation, see Timper and Brüning (2017) [42]. On the other hand, when humans and animals are placed in a similar cafeteria-style environment, ingestion of unnecessary high-preference food occurs, which leads to becoming obese (homeostasis-independent eating behavior, or hedonic feeding). Hedonic feeding behaviors are controlled by an emotion/reward system. Both systems interact in the LHA (**Figure 2**), and feeding behavior is governed by the system with higher activ-ity. In modern society, even when the energy balance of a body is positive, feeding behavior may be elicited by decision-making information in the cerebral cortex. Furthermore, there is an overflow of information about food in modern society, and high-calorie foods such as snacks can be easily obtained. A recent study reported that after watching TV food commercials, children became more dependent on tastiness rather than health benefits when choosing foods. Those TV commercials were suggested to have activated the ventromedial prefrontal cortex involved in reward valuation [58]. Thus, in a modern society, the homeostasis-independent con-trol system of feeding behavior easily surpasses the homeostasis-dependent control system of feeding behavior, which leads to obesity. In addition, various feeding and eating disorders are also presumed to be caused by disorders of both control sys-tems. We hope that the elucidation of the mechanisms of these two control systems will lead to the development of more effective treatments for feeding and eating disorders.

Author details

Hisao Nishijo* and Taketoshi Ono
System Emotional Science, Faculty of Medicine, University of Toyama, Sugitani, Toyama, Japan

*Address all correspondence to: nishijo@med.u-toyama.ac.jp

References

[1] Rolls ET. The Brain and Emotion. Oxford: Oxford Univ Press; 1999

[2] Rogers PJ, Hardman CA. Food reward. What it is and how to measure it. Appetite. 2015;**90**:1-15

[3] Bodnar RJ. Conditioned flavor preferences in animals: Merging pharmacology, brain sites and genetic variance. Appetite. 2018;**122**:17-25

[4] Kim KS, Seeley RJ, Sandoval DA. Signaling from the periphery to the brain that regulates energy homeostasis. Nature Reviews. Neuroscience. 2018;**19**(4):185-196

[5] Petrovich GD. Lateral hypothalamus as a motivation-cognition interface in the control of feeding behavior. Frontiers in Systems Neuroscience. 2018;**12**:14

[6] Lowe R, Ziemke R. The feeling of action tendencies: On the emotional regulation of goal-directed behavior. Frontiers in Psychology. 2011;**2**:346

[7] Kelley AE, Baldo BA, Pratt WE, Will MJ. Corticostriatal-hypothalamic circuitry and food motivation: Integration of energy, action and reward. Physiology & Behavior. 2005;**86**(5):773-795

[8] Qualls-Creekmore E, Münzberg H. Modulation of feeding and associated behaviors by lateral hypothalamic circuits. Endocrinology. 2018;**159**(11):3631-3642

[9] Verma D, Wood J, Lach G, Herzog H, Sperk G, Tasan R. Hunger promotes fear extinction by activation of an amygdala microcircuit. Neuropsychopharmacology. 2016;**41**(2):431-439

[10] Cassidy RM, Lu Y, Jere M, Tian JB, Xu Y, Mangieri LR, et al. A lateral hypothalamus to basal forebrain neurocircuit promotes feeding by suppressing responses to anxiogenic environmental cues. Science Advances. 2019;**5**(3):eaav1640

[11] Farr OM, Li CS, Mantzoros CS. Central nervous system regulation of eating: Insights from human brain imaging. Metabolism. 2016;**65**(5):699-713

[12] Stoeckel LE, Weller RE, Cook EW III, Twieg DB, Knowlton RC, Cox JE. Widespread reward-system activation in obese women in response to pictures of high-calorie foods. NeuroImage. 2008;**41**(2):636-647

[13] Derman RC, Ferrario CR. Enhanced incentive motivation in obesity-prone rats is mediated by NAc core CP-AMPARs. Neuropharmacology. 2018;**131**:326-336

[14] Berridge KC. Motivation concepts in behavioral neuroscience. Physiology & Behavior. 2004;**81**(2):179-209

[15] Sjoerds Z, van den Brink W, Beekman AT, Penninx BW, Veltman DJ. Cue reactivity is associated with duration and severity of alcohol dependence: An FMRI study. PLoS One. 2014;**9**(1):e84560

[16] Davis CA, Levitan RD, Reid C, Carter JC, Kaplan AS, Patte KA, et al. Dopamine for "wanting" and opioids for "liking": A comparison of obese adults with and without binge eating. Obesity. 2009;**17**(6):1220-1225

[17] Nishijo H, Ono T, Nakamura K, Kawabata M, Yamatani K. Neuron activity in and adjacent to the dorsal amygdala of monkey during operant feeding behavior. Brain Research Bulletin. 1986;**17**(6):847-854

[18] Nishijo H, Ono T, Nishino H. Topographic distribution of

modality-specific amygdalar neurons in alert monkey. The Journal of Neuroscience. 1988;**8**:3556-3569

[19] Nishijo H, Ono T, Nishino H. Single neuron responses in amygdala of alert monkey during complex sensory stimulation with affective significance. The Journal of Neuroscience. 1988;**8**:3570-3583

[20] Niv Y, Daw ND, Joel D, Dayan P. Tonic dopamine: Opportunity costs and the control of response vigor. Psychopharmacology. 2007;**191**:507-520

[21] Hamid AA, Pettibone JR, Mabrouk OS, Hetrick VL, Schmidt R, Vander Weele CM, et al. Mesolimbic dopamine signals the value of work. Nature Neuroscience. 2016;**19**:117-126

[22] Gerfen CR, Surmeier DJ. Modulation of striatal projection systems by dopamine. Annual Review of Neuroscience. 2011;**34**:441-466

[23] Patrono E, Matsumoto J, Nishimaru H, Takamura Y, Chinzorig IC, Ono T, et al. Rewarding effects of operant dry-licking behavior on neuronal firing in the nucleus accumbens core. Frontiers in Pharmacology. 2017;**8**:536

[24] Berridge KC. The debate over dopamine's role in reward: The case for incentive salience. Psychopharmacology. 2007;**191**(3):391-431

[25] Peciña S. Opioid reward 'liking' and 'wanting' in the nucleus accumbens. Physiology & Behavior. 2008;**94**(5):675-680

[26] Berridge KC, Robinson TE. Liking, wanting, and the incentive-sensitization theory of addiction. The American Psychologist. 2016;**71**(8):670-679

[27] Jenison RL, Rangel A, Oya H, Kawasaki H, Howard MA. Value encoding in single neurons in the human amygdala during decision making. The Journal of Neuroscience. 2011;**31**(1):331-338

[28] Mormann F, Bausch M, Knieling S, Fried I. Neurons in the human left amygdala automatically encode subjective value irrespective of task. Cerebral Cortex. 2019;**29**(1):265-272

[29] Hatfield T, Han J-S, Conley M, Gallagher M, Holland P. Neurotoxic lesions of basolateral, but not central, amygdala interfere with Pavlovian second-order conditioning and reinforcer devaluation effects. The Journal of Neuroscience. 1996;**16**:5256-5265

[30] Málková L, Gaffan D, Murray EA. Excitotoxic lesions of the amygdala fail to produce impairments in visual learning for auditory secondary reinforcement but interfere with reinforcer devaluation effects in rhesus monkeys. The Journal of Neuroscience. 1997;**17**:6011-6020

[31] Baxter MG, Parker A, Lindner CCC, Izquierdo AD, Murray EA. Control of response selection by reinforcer value requires interaction of amygdala and orbital prefrontal cortex. The Journal of Neuroscience. 2000;**20**:4311-4319

[32] Gottfried JA, O'Doherty J, Dolan RJ. Encoding predictive reward value in human amygdala and orbitofrontal cortex. Science. 2003;**301**(5636):1104-1107

[33] Jackson ME, Moghaddam B. Amygdala regulation of nucleus accumbens dopamine output is governed by the prefrontal cortex. The Journal of Neuroscience. 2001;**21**(2):676-681

[34] Zald DH. Orbitofrontal cortex contributions to food selection and decision making. Annals of Behavioral Medicine. 2009; **38** (Suppl1):S18-S24

[35] Izquierdo A, Suda RK, Murray EA. Bilateral orbital prefrontal cortex lesions in rhesus monkeys disrupt choices guided by both reward value and reward contingency. The Journal of Neuroscience. 2004;**24**:7540-7548

[36] Woolley JD, Gorno-Tempini ML, Seeley WW, et al. Binge eating is associated with right orbitofrontal-insular-striatal atrophy in frontotemporal dementia. Neurology. 2007;**69**:1424-1433

[37] Whitwell JL, Sampson EL, Loy CT, et al. VBM signatures of abnormal eating behaviours in frontotemporal lobar degeneration. NeuroImage. 2007;**35**:207-213

[38] Higgs S. Cognitive processing of food rewards. Appetite. 2016;**104**:10-17

[39] Small DM, Bender G, Veldhuizen MG, Rudenga K, Nachtigal D, Felsted J. The role of the human orbitofrontal cortex in taste and flavor processing. Annals of the New York Academy of Sciences. 2007;**1121**:136-151

[40] Kringelbach ML, O'Doherty J, Rolls ET, Andrews C. Activation of the human orbitofrontal cortex to a liquid food stimulus is correlated with its subjective pleasantness. Cerebral Cortex. 2003;**13**(10):1064-1071

[41] McCabe C, Rolls ET. Umami: A delicious flavor formed by convergence of taste and olfactory pathways in the human brain. The European Journal of Neuroscience. 2007;**25**:1855-1864

[42] Timper K, Brüning JC. Hypothalamic circuits regulating appetite and energy homeostasis: Pathways to obesity. Disease Models & Mechanisms. 2017;**10**(6):679-689

[43] Dietrich MO, Zimmer MR, Bober J, Horvath TL. Hypothalamic Agrp neurons drive stereotypic behaviors beyond feeding. Cell. 2015;**160**(6):1222-1232

[44] Sabatier N, Caquineau C, Dayanithi G, Bull P, Douglas AJ, Guan XM, et al. Alpha-melanocyte-stimulating hormone stimulates oxytocin release from the dendrites of hypothalamic neurons while inhibiting oxytocin release from their terminals in the neurohypophysis. The Journal of Neuroscience. 2003a;**23**:10351-10358

[45] Sabatier N, Caquineau C, Douglas AJ, Leng G. Oxytocin released from magnocellular dendrites: A potential modulator of alpha-melanocyte-stimulating hormone behavioral actions? Annals of the New York Academy of Sciences. 2003b;**994**:218-224

[46] Baron-Cohen S, Jaffa T, Davies S, Auyeung B, Allison C, Wheelwright S. Do girls with anorexia nervosa have elevated autistic traits? Molecular Autism. 2013;**4**(1):24

[47] Grob S, Stern J, Gamper L, Moergeli H, Milos G, Schnyder U, et al. Behavioral responses to catecholamine depletion in unmedicated, remitted subjects with bulimia nervosa and healthy subjects. Biological Psychiatry. 2015;**77**(7):661-667

[48] Fetissov SO, Hallman J, Oreland L, Af Klinteberg B, Grenbäck E, Hulting AL, et al. Autoantibodies against alpha - MSH, ACTH, and LHRH in anorexia and bulimia nervosa patients. Proceedings of the National Academy of Sciences of the United States of America. 2002;**99**(26):17155-17160

[49] Bachevalier L, Loveland KA. The orbitofrontal–amygdala circuit and self-regulation of social – Emotional behavior in autism. Neuroscience and Biobehavioral Reviews. 2006;**30**:97-117

[50] Cermak SA, Curtin C, Bandini LG. Food selectivity and sensory sensitivity

in children with autism spectrum disorders. Journal of the American Dietetic Association. 2010;**110**:238-246

[51] Tavassoli T, Baron-Cohen S. Taste identification in adults with autism spectrum conditions. Journal of Autism and Developmental Disorders. 2012;**42**(7):1419-1424

[52] Nishijo M, Pham TT, Nguyen ATN, Tran NN, Nakagawa H, Hoang LV, et al. 2,3,7,8-tetrachlorodibenzo-p-dioxin in breast milk increases autistic traits of 3-year-old children in Vietnam. Molecular Psychiatry. 2014a;**19**:1220-1226

[53] Nguyen ATN, Nishijo M, Hori E, Nguyen NM, Pham TT, Fukunaga K, et al. Influence of maternal exposure to 2,3,7,8-tetrachlorodibenzo-p-dioxin on socioemotional behaviors in offspring rats. Environmental Health Insights. 2013a;**7**:1-14

[54] Nguyen MN, Nishijo M, Nguyen AT, Bor A, Nakamura T, Hori E, et al. Effects of maternal exposure to 2,3,7,8-tetrachlorodibenzo-p-dioxin on parvalbumin- and calbindin-immunoreactive neurons in the limbic system and superior colliculus in rat offspring. Toxicology. 2013b;**314**(1):125-134

[55] Sotonyi P, Gao Q , Bechmann I, Horvath TL. Estrogen promotes parvalbumin expression in arcuate nucleus POMC neurons. Reproductive Sciences. 2010;**17**(12):1077-1080

[56] Dell'Osso L, Carpita B, Gesi C, Cremone IM, Corsi M, Massimetti E, et al. Subthreshold autism spectrum disorder in patients with eating disorders. Comprehensive Psychiatry. 2018;**81**:66-72

[57] Nishijo M, Tran NN, Nakagawa H, Torii K, Kondo T, Nishijo H. Effects of prenatal 2,3,7,8-tetrachlorodibenzo-p-dioxin exposure on development of taste preference in rat offspring. Journal of Addiction Research and Therapy. 2014b;**5**:173

[58] Bruce AS, Pruitt SW, Ha OR, Cherry JBC, Smith TR, Bruce JM, et al. The influence of televised food commercials on children's food choices: Evidence from ventromedial prefrontal cortex activations. The Journal of Pediatrics. 2016;**177**:27-32

2

Metabolic Syndrome and Pathogenesis of Obesity-Related Adverse Outcomes in Pregnancy

Motoi Sugimura

Abstract

Obese women with metabolic syndrome are at increased risk for cardio-thrombo-metabolic dysfunction that leads to pregnancy-related venous thromboembolism (VTE), hypertensive disorders of pregnancy (HDP), and gestational diabetes mellitus (GDM). Indeed, maternal death secondary to a pregnancy-related VTE has an enormous impact on the childbearing population. Recent research has provided evidence that elucidates the pathogenesis of adverse outcomes in obese pregnant women with metabolic syndrome. The chronic inflammation elicited by dysregulated infiltration of macrophages into adipose tissue and increased thrombin generation by inflammatory cytokines with activation of the tissue factor pathway may play important roles in the pathogenesis; however, a simple question has yet to be answered. Specifically, "why does prepregnancy obesity increase the risk of pregnancy-related VTE in association with a high estrogenic and prothrombo-genic state?" The present review of the extant literature has focused on further understanding obesity-related adverse outcomes in pregnancy by elucidating the underlying pathogenesis of metabolic syndrome.

Keywords: obesity, metabolic syndrome, pregnancy-related venous thromboembolism, hypertensive disorders of pregnancy, gestational diabetes mellitus, inflammatory cytokines, thrombin formation, estrogen

1. Introduction

Epidemiologic studies in North America and Europe have shown that obesity increases the risk of venous thromboembolism (VTE) during pregnancy and the puerperium [1, 2], as well as postpartum hemorrhage [3]. Furthermore, women with prepregnancy obesity are also at increased risk of hypertensive disorders of pregnancy (HDP) [4, 5], including preeclampsia [6]. HDP is associated with placental abruption, which may lead to severe obstetric complications with dissemi-nated intravascular coagulation (DIC) [7].

Recent research has shown that HDP and gestational diabetes mellitus (GDM) increase the risk of hypertension and diabetes mellitus (DM) later in life [8]. Conversely, maternal malnutrition during pregnancy because of inadequate dietary intake increases the risk of fetal growth restriction and low-birth-weight infants; it is increasingly evident that offspring are at increased risk of developing hyper-tension and DM as well [9]. Indeed, addressing nutrition and weight gain before pregnancy are an important part of perinatal care [10].

Thus, prepregnancy body weight and changes in weight gain during pregnancy may be indicators of maternal nutritional status, reflecting the balance between caloric intake and basal metabolism and exercise caloric expenditure [11].

Although hypertension and DM in obese patients with metabolic syndrome [12] are worrisome with respect to future health issues and increased mortality rate, pregnancy-related VTE has a greater and more direct impact on families among the childbearing population. Based on the annual report of the trends in maternal deaths and maternal mortality rates by cause of death from the Japan Ministry of Health, Labor, and Welfare in 2017 [13], the number of maternal deaths in Japan has decreased over time; however, 70% of maternal deaths are caused by hemorrhage, pulmonary embolism (including pulmonary thromboembolism and amniotic fluid embolism), and HDP. The percentage of maternal mortalities by cause of death has remained essentially unchanged over the past two decades, as shown in **Figure 1**. Increasing maternal age [14] due to changes in social lifestyle, advances in assisted reproductive medicine, and increased cesarean section rates may also be important factors in maternal deaths in Japan and developed countries worldwide [15]. Changes

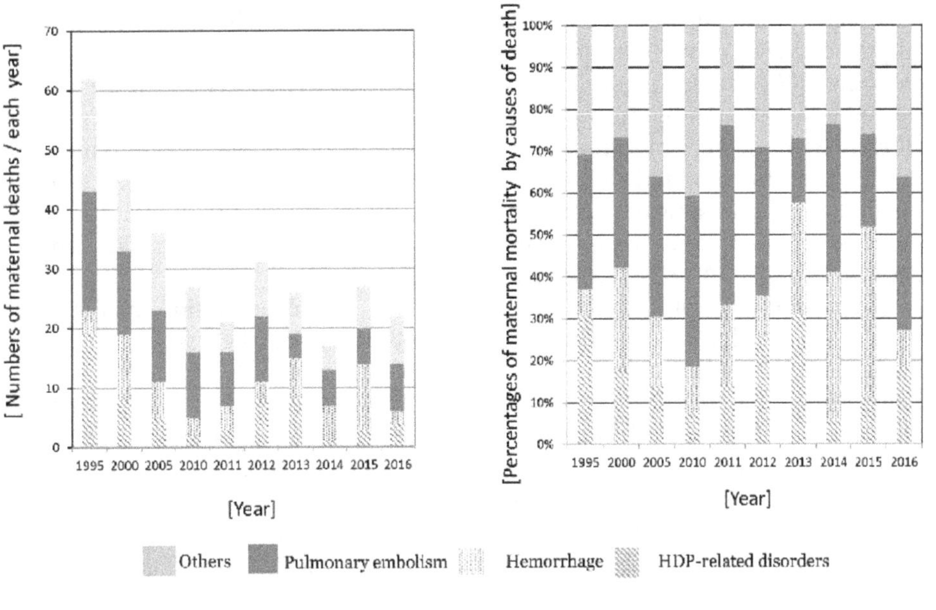

Figure 1.
Trends in maternal deaths and maternal mortality rates (per 100,000 total births) by causes of death in Japan.

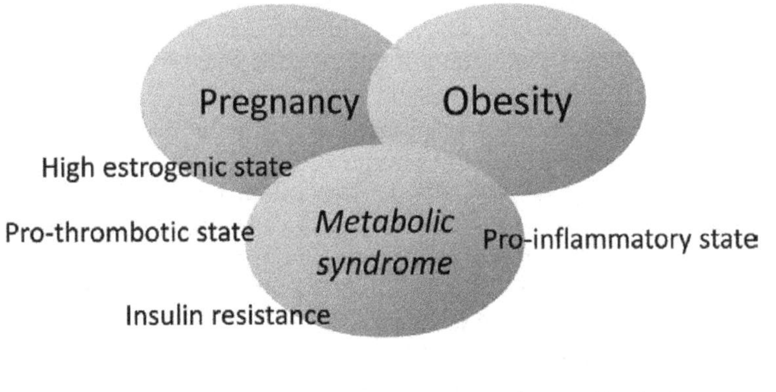

Figure 2.
Pathogenesis of obesity-related adverse outcomes in pregnancy with a similar background to metabolic syndrome. Key words are pro-inflammatory state with insulin resistance and a prothrombotic state with a high estrogenic state in obese pregnant women.

in dietary habits and a sedentary modern lifestyle are partly responsible for prepregnancy obesity, which is followed by obesity-related adverse outcomes in pregnancy.

A growing number of epidemiologic observations on obesity in pregnancy have linked basic research findings [16] with the pathogenesis of obesity-related adverse outcomes in pregnancy with a similar background to metabolic syndrome [12, 17], as shown in **Figure 2**.

2. Obesity-related adverse outcomes in pregnancy

2.1 Pathogenesis of obesity-related adverse outcomes in pregnancy with a background of metabolic syndrome

In recent years, visceral fat has been regarded as one of the endocrine organs [18]. Visceral fat plays an important role in the pathogenesis of local and systemic chronic inflammation in obese patients [19]. A large number of studies have demonstrated a relationship between obesity and the pathophysiology underlying metabolic syndrome, specifically involving dysfunction of adipocytes with reduced adiponectin and innate immune cells with subsequent production of inflammatory cytokines [16]. Inflammatory cytokines induce tissue factor (TF) and enhanced thrombin generation by up-regulation of TF expression on various types of cells (**Figure 3**). Enhanced thrombin generation consecutively leads to inflammation, thrombus formation, and vascular damage due to activation of the cell signaling system via protein-activated receptors (PARs) [20] with TF as a receptor [21]. The induction of cytokines and thrombin generation interacts with the crosstalk between coagulation and inflammation [22, 23].

Adipose tissue formed by adipocytes with fat accumulation increases the level of triglycerides and decreases the adiponectin level. The tissue also activates immunocompetent cells, such as macrophages and mast cells, which produce and release pro-inflammatory cytokines (TNF-α, IL-6, IFN-ϒ, and IL-1β) [24]. The induction of TF on the cell surface of adipocytes and macrophages accelerates the prothrombotic state accompanied by thrombin generation. With respect to the high estrogenic state in pregnancy, prothrombotic conditions are likely to be induced in obese women because of the additional effects of dietary, social, environmental, and genetic factors which increase the risk of pregnancy-related VTE, although the precise mechanisms are still uncertain.

The most recent hypothesis regarding the pathogenesis of HDP suggests that impaired trophoblastic invasion into the inner myometrial portion of the spiral arteries causes the vessels to retain musculoelastic properties, thereby inducing hypoperfusion and hypoxia [25]. The subsequent release of inflammatory cytokines [26] promotes the excess production of soluble fms-like tyrosine kinase 1 (sFLT1) [27], which binds to VEGF as a decoy instead of VEGFR. The cytokines may also enhance maternal inflammatory responses and systemic endothelial dysfunction, leading to maternal symptom [28]. The resulting inflammatory cytokines induce TF, which subsequently initiates the TF-dependent coagulation pathway as the receptor for coagulation factors VIIa/VII [29]. In a vicious cycle, activation of the coagulation system and thrombin formation in the placental intervillous space enhances the production of sFLT1s through G protein-coupled protease-activated receptors [30] and causes further ischemic damage to trophoblastic cells in a hypercoagulable state [31, 32], as shown in **Figure 4**.

As one of the current hypotheses of the pathogenesis in pregnancy-related VTE and HDP, these observations provide the probable relationship between the high estrogenic state of pregnancy and prothrombotic conditions caused by chronic

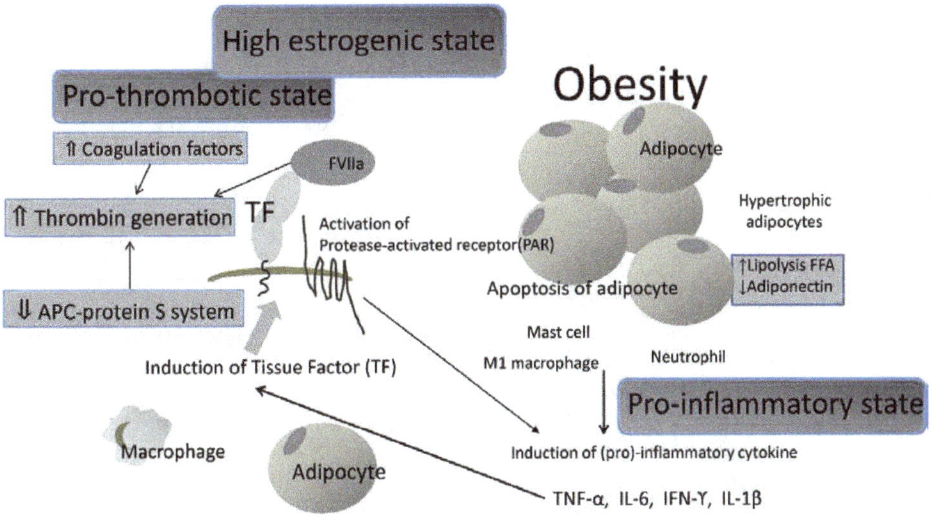

Figure 3.
Enhanced thrombin generation by tissue factor (TF) with activation of protease-activated receptor (PAR). The increased coagulation factors and reduced sensitivity to activated protein C in pregnancy accelerate the enhanced thrombin generation on tissue factor (TF) induced by (pro)-inflammatory cytokines (TNF-α, IL-6, IFN-Υ, and IL-1β). The formed thrombin induces (pro)-inflammatory cytokines via activation of the protease-activated receptor (PAR).

inflammation due to the obesity with metabolic syndrome, although there is a lack of high-quality evidence (**Figure 5**).

2.2 Epidemiologic aspects of obesity-related adverse outcomes in pregnancy

Prepregnancy body mass index (BMI), weight changes during pregnancy, and perinatal prognosis are the epidemiologic aspects of obesity-related adverse outcomes in pregnancy.

Although various academic societies have recommended guidelines for optimal weight gain and nutrition during pregnancy, the basic concept for the management of maternal nutrition has changed over time based on epidemiologic data. From the view of adverse maternal outcomes in North America in the first half of the twentieth century, a weight gain of 9.1 kg throughout pregnancy was recommended to prevent HDP and operative deliveries, such as cesarean section and forceps deliver-ies, because of macrosomic fetuses.

By the 1970s, at least 11.4 kg of weight gain during pregnancy was recommended to prevent spontaneous preterm births, fetal growth restriction, and adverse neona-tal outcomes [33]. In the 1990s, the BMI classification was introduced as a means to establish optimal weight gain based on body weight and surface area. A weight gain of 11.5–16 kg was recommended in pregnant women with a normal prepregnancy BMI (19.8–26 kg/m^2) [17].

During pregnancy, it is preferable to increase caloric intake by approximately 390 kcal per day with small variations in addition to the daily caloric intake during non-pregnancy [34]. Insufficient calorie intake leads to increased proteolysis and the lack of nutrition for fetal growth. Strict limitation of weight gain during pregnancy may increase the risk of preterm birth and fetal growth restriction [33], which is why an 11–16 kg weight gain is recommended for women with a normal prepregnancy BMI in North America [35]. Maternal weight gain with excessive calorie intake increases the risk of dystocia with macrosomic fetuses. Recent research has also suggested that maternal obesity increases the risk of childhood obesity [36] and the risk of autism spectrum [37].

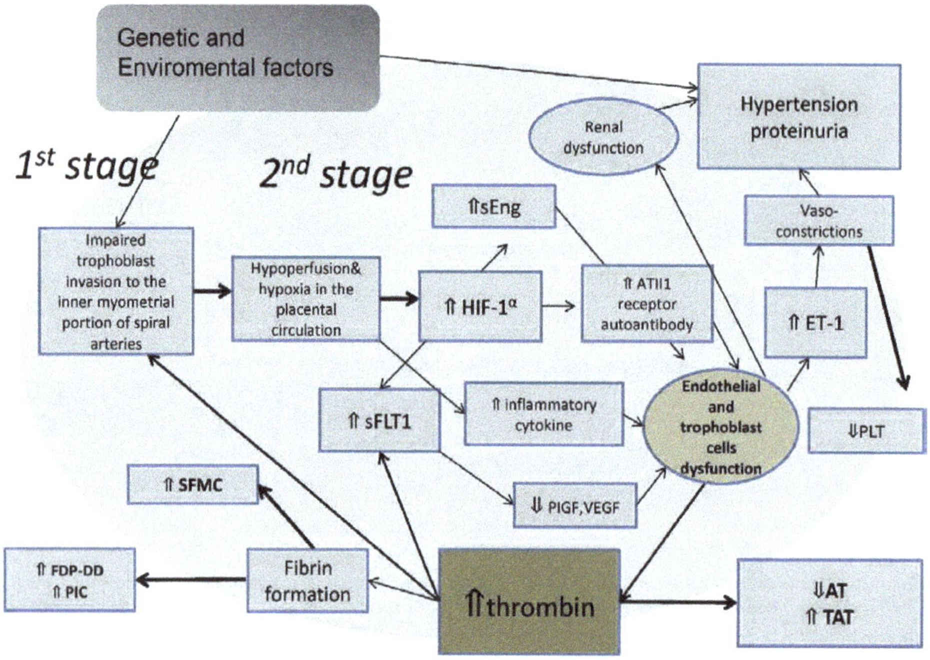

Figure4.
Pathogenesis of hypertensive disorders of pregnancy (HDP). The important role of thrombin generation in the "two-stage disorder" theory for the pathogenesis of HDP. sEng: soluble endoglin, HIF-1$^{\alpha}$: hypoxia-induced factor, ET: endothelin, AT: angiotensin, sFLT1: soluble FLT1, PlGF: placental growth factor, VEGF: vascular endothelial growth factor, AT: antithrombin, TAT: thrombin-antithrombin complex, SFMC: soluble fibrin-monomer complex, PIC: plasmin-α 2-plasmin inhibitor complex.

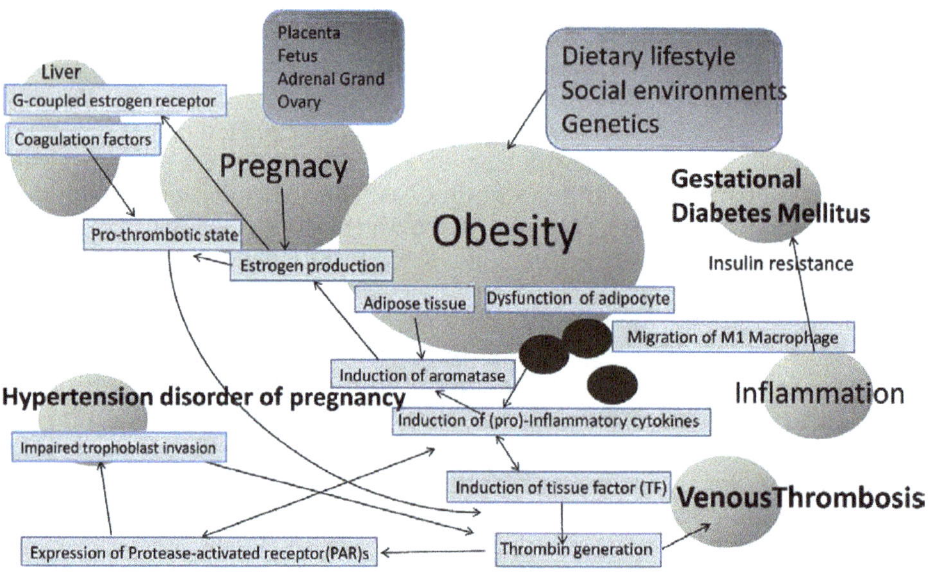

Figure5.
Pathogenesis of obesity-related adverse outcomes in pregnancy. The critical role of the induction of pro-inflammatory cytokines by dysfunction of adipocytes with fat accumulation initiates the thrombin generation of tissue factor (TF) in various cells. The prothrombotic state with estrogen-induced hypercoagulability plays a role in the pathogenesis of venous thrombosis and hypertensive disorders of pregnancy.

The Institute of Medicine (IOM) guidelines in 2009 recommended that weight gain during pregnancy should be 0.3 kg/week for women who are overweight before pregnancy (25–29.9 kg/m^2) and 0.18 kg/week for women who are obese

(>30 kg/m^2) after the second trimester [38]. In addition, the IOM recommended an 11.3–15.8 kg weight gain during pregnancy for women with a normal prepregnancy BMI (18.5–24.9 kg/m^2), 6.8–11.3 kg for women who are overweight before pregnancy, and 4.9–9.0 kg for women who are obese before pregnancy. In 2015, the American College of Obstetricians and Gynecologists (ACOG) recommended a similar proposal in an ACOG Practice Bulletin [10]; however, it has been shown that women who are overweight and obese before pregnancy with inappropriate weight gain and loss during pregnancy are at increased risk for fetal growth restriction [39] due to pathologic placental changes [40].

In recent years, although underweight pregnant women with a prepregnancy BMI ≤18.5 kg/m^2 have a reduced risk of HDP compared with obese pregnant women, a decrease in newborn birth weight in underweight pregnant women is associated with future health problems [41]. With respect to fetal programming, future health issues in adulthood should focus on the relationship between an increased risk for essential hypertension and DM [42] and low birthweight infants. Barker's hypothesis in the 1980s [43] was based on epidemiologic observations of malnutrition during pregnancy in World War II and underweight children with an increased risk for hypertension (ischemic heart disease) and DM in adulthood.

Malnutrition is a significant problem in the developing countries. There is a relatively high prevalence of women of childbearing age who are obese worldwide [44]. During pregnancy, obesity with metabolic syndrome shares an underlying pathogenesis of cardio-thrombo-metabolic dysfunction and further worsens the health status. Specifically, pregnancy-related VTE and sudden maternal death have a greater impact [45] on the family and society compared with HDP and GDM.

2.3 Pregnancy-related VTE in the UK and North America

In Europe, especially in the United Kingdom, with a background of heritable thrombotic predisposition, medical journals have reported clinical cases of maternal deaths due to VTE since the 1860s [46, 47]. National policy in the UK has provided guidance to reduce maternal mortality from pregnancy-related VTE [45, 48]. Epidemiologic and clinical studies have focused on pregnancy-related VTE [49] and showed the relationship between VTE and prepregnant obesity in pregnant women [50]. Multivariate analysis of prepregnant obese patients compared with non-obese patients as controls demonstrated that the adjusted odds ratio (aOR) is 1.93 (95% CI, 1.10–3.39) for VTE in the moderately obese group and 4.32 (95% CI, 1.26–14.84) for VTE in the highly obese group, as shown in 2008 [49].

Studies focusing on prepregnancy BMI and immobilization in the hospital showed a further increased risk of VTE during pregnancy and postpartum [49]. The aOR for VTE in pregnant women with a prepregnancy BMI >25 kg/m^2 is 1.8 (95% CI, 1.3–2.4). During immobilization with bed rest, the aOR for VTE increases to 62.3 (95% CI, 11.5–337.6) in patients with a BMI >25 kg/m^2 [49]. The aOR for VTE in patients with a prepregnancy BMI >25 kg/m^2 is 2.4 (95% CI, 1.7–3.3) during the postpartum period. The aOR is 40.1 (95% CI, 8.0–201.5) in a similar condition [49]. These epidemiologic data have supported the guidelines for the prevention and reduction in the risk of pregnancy-related VTE in the UK [51, 52] and North America [53].

The Royal College of Obstetricians and Gynecologists published data in 2015 that indicated 60% of women who died of pulmonary thromboembolism (PE) between 2003 and 2008 were obese with a BMI ≥30 kg/m^2. The prevalence of obesity with a similar BMI at 16–44 years of age in the population was 20% in the UK [52]. Pregnancy is a risk factor for VTE, and the risk increases in proportion to the degree of obesity. Obese pregnant women had a higher aOR for PE (aOR, 14.9; 95% CI, 3.0–74.8) than for deep vein thrombosis (DVT) (aOR, 4.4; 95% CI, 1.6–11.9). The risk for pregnancy-related VTE is minimal in overweight pregnant women who had a prepregnancy BMI of 25–29.9 kg/m^2; however, the guidance in the UK states that VTE risk in overweight women is extremely common, affecting nearly 50% in the childbearing population [52].

Obesity with a BMI of 3040 kg/m^2 alone is classified as a lower risk category for VTE according to the guidelines [52]. However, pregnant women with a BMI of 30–40 kg/m^2 are classified as having an intermediate risk if they have two or more additional risk factors, including elective cesarean section, prolonged labor (>24 h), and operative delivery. These risk factors are more likely encountered in daily clini-cal situations compared with a history of VTE.

The American College of Chest Physicians has also proposed similar guidelines to prevent pregnancy-associated VTE in obese pregnant women based on epidemio-logic risk [51, 53]. Specifically, the American College of Chest Physicians showed that the occurrence of VTE is 3% among all women in the puerperium and the OR increases to >6 compared with women with a normal prepregnancy BMI if obese pregnant women with a prepregnancy BMI ≥30 kg/m^2 are combined with those with other risk factors in women undergoing emergency cesarean section [53]Epidemiologic observations have suggested that obesity and pregnancy are related to the prothrombotic state. The pathophysiology of metabolic syndrome may, in part, provide insight into understanding the increased hypercoagulable status with obese women in pregnancy with a high estrogenic state.

2.4 Obesity and estrogen

Estrogens are a type of sex steroid hormone. The endogenous estrogens are classified into estrone (E1), estradiol (E2), estriol (E3), and esterol (E4) [54]. Estrogens were initially thought to be female hormones; however, it has recently been shown that estrogens are involved not only in female physiologic functions but also in male reproductive physiologic functions. Recent studies have explored the bioactivity of estrogen in the neuroendocrine [55], vascular [56], musculoskeletal [57], and immune systems. Estrogen is associated with the pathogenesis of infertility, obesity [58], osteoporosis, endometriosis [59], and various types of cancers [60]. Estrogen crosses the cell membrane and binds to estrogen receptor (ER) α and ERβ in the cell as a ligand and estrogen receptors (mERs) on the cell membrane as ligands. Then, estrogen regulates the expression of gene products by binding to a specific DNA sequence, the hormone response element [61].

In pregnancy, the placenta and fetal adrenal cortex are the main estrogen production sites. E3 is produced through the maternal liver, placenta, and fetal adrenal gland, although E2 is mainly produced by ovarian granulosa and capsular cells in women of reproductive age. By contrast, estrogen is produced in testicular stromal Sertoli cells in men [62]. The physiologic hormonal bioactivity is the highest in E2 and then decreases in the order of E1 and E3.

Epidemiologic observations have shown that obesity increases the risk of estrogen-dependent breast [63] and endometrial cancer [64].

As described above, apoptotic cell death of adipocytes in adipose tissue by overstored fat in obese patients induces the migration of macrophages to the tissues [19, 65]. Consequently, chronic inflammation caused by pro-inflammatory cytokines, such as TNFα and IL-8, leads to activation of the NF-κB signaling system and increased aromatase activity in various cells, including adipocytes, thus resulting in estrogen production [66]. Although the abnormal regulation of aromatase activity in adipose stromal cells in response to various inflammatory mediators involves a complex signaling pathway, visceral fat, which contributes to obesity, plays an important role in the local and systematic production of estrogen [67]. The enhanced production of estrogen can be associated with the upregulated production of coagulation factors that may lead to the induction of a prothrombotic state.

2.5 Estrogen and prothrombotic state

As described above, it is widely accepted that the risk of VTE is increased during pregnancy and the puerperium. The hypercoagulable state with elevated maternal estrogen levels during pregnancy is, in part, one of the explanations for the pathogenesis, although the mechanism has not been fully elucidated.

Maternal estrogen levels during pregnancy increase enormously over the course of pregnancy, reaching concentrations approximately 100–500 times higher than non-pregnant levels [68]. Ninety percent of urinary estrogens are the conjugated form of E3, which has a 500- to 1000-fold higher concentration compared with non-pregnant women. The rapid increase in maternal estrogen levels is mainly due to the enhanced production of estrogen from the ovaries until the seventh week of gestation. Thereafter, the main origin of estrogen production shifts from the ovary to the fetal placental tissues [69].

LDL cholesterol is the main source of dehydroepiandrosterone sulfate (DHEA-S) in the fetal adrenal gland [69]. The 16α-hydroxylase converts a part of DHEA-S to 16OH-DHEA-S in the fetal liver, and the sulfatase and aromatase in the placenta convert the substrates to E2 and E3, which is followed by the secretion of E2 and E3 into the maternal blood [70]. Therefore, the fetal placental system gives rise to higher estrogen status, especially at the end of pregnancy.

By contrast, the high estrogen levels in pregnancy show abrupt reductions during the postpartum period because of the delivery of the placenta and fetus; the placenta is the main organ of estrogen production. Epidemiologic observations demonstrate that the risk of developing VTE during the puerperium is the highest within 1 week after delivery and then the risk of VTE decreases gradu-ally 2 weeks after delivery. From the intrapartum to the postpartum period, the high levels of inflammatory cytokines associated with the onset of labor change dramatically [71]. Because of the changes in the levels of coagulation factors, endothelial injury, and stasis of blood flow [72], which are related to the onset of VTE, it is difficult to evaluate how estrogen-related coagulation factors are involved in the pathogenesis of VTE.

In 1961 [73], a patient with oral contraceptive (OC)-related VTE presented after taking an OC. Initially, the pathogenesis of VTE was understood to be simply due to dehydration caused by vomiting after taking the OC. Recently, upregulated production of coagulation factors by ethinyl E2 (EE2), a synthetic E2 that is less metabolized in the digestive system, is seen as a potential cause of VTE [74]. There is a significant correlation between the amount of EE2 contained in OCs and the increased risk of developing a VTE in an estrogen-dependent manner, which has led to the development of OCs containing ultra-low-dose estrogen (<50 μg) [75].

The current formulation of combined OCs (COCs) is a fourth-generation COC, which is defined as those containing a new type of progestin. However, different risks of VTE have been presented in COCs with different types of progestins instead of a low-dose estrogen (<50 μg) [76].

Some reports have suggested significant differences between second-generation COCs and third-generation COCs in the level of various coagulation factors [77]. These reports have speculated that the different progestins in COCs may be associated with the increased risk of OC-related VTE because of changes in coagulation. Prothrombin and factor VII levels are significantly increased in third-generation COCs compared with that of second-generation COCs. Furthermore, the activated protein C resistance by the aPTT method and the endogenous thrombin potential (ETP) method has been shown to be greater in third-generation COCs compared with that of second-generation COCs. These observations may indicate the probable relationship between female hormones and a thrombophilic tendency [77].

The second- and third-generation COCs have a different type of synthetic progestin. Although the mechanisms are not fully understood and are controversial [78], some studies have indicated that a small statistical difference exists in the risk of developing VTE [76].

Interestingly, unlike EE2, the endogenous estrogen 17β-E2 is rapidly metabolized by 17β dehydroxysteroid dehydrogenase [79] to E1 with less estrogenic activity. A COC containing a low dose of 17β-E2 has a relatively little effect on changes in the levels of coagulation factors [80]. Therefore, a COC containing 17β-E2 has been approved in Europe as a novel COC [81].

However, it is unclear how much of the endogenous estrogen (E2 and E3) in pregnant women magnifies the risk of pregnancy-related VTE compared with that of non-pregnant women. The changes in coagulation factors by female hormones do not provide strong evidence with the understanding of the mechanisms in the developing of VTE so far.

The changes in various markers of coagulation and fibrinolysis during the postpartum period of pregnancy have shown a significant increase in the levels of fibrinogen, FV, FVII, FVIII, and FX after pregnancy compared with that of non-pregnancy [82].

Focusing on the inhibitory coagulation factor, protein S, which acts as a coenzyme in the activated protein C system, is significantly reduced during pregnancy [83]. In fact, 17β estradiol acts on ER-mediated suppression of the protein Sα gene (PROS1) mRNA and antigen production in a hepatocellular carcinoma-derived cultured cell line (HepG2) in an *in vitro* experimental system [84]. The experiment in a cultured cell line suggests that the increased estrogen during pregnancy can suppress protein S production. In addition, a report describes that a decrease in free protein S level due to an increase in C4b-binding protein during pregnancy is also associated with a decrease in protein S during pregnancy [85]. The changes in the various coagulation-fibrinolysis-related factors quickly return to the prepregnancy state during the postpartum period.

To confirm the hypothesis that the maternal high estrogenic conditions in pregnancy are related to the onset of the pregnancy-related VTE, previous research provided data on the changes in thrombin generation in an experiment with animals treated with exogenous estrogen [86] and the *ex vivo* determinants of thrombin potential reflecting prothrombotic conditions in pregnant women [87].

A variety of thrombin generation tests for evaluating the hypercoagulable state have been proposed for clinical samples derived from patients [88]. An *ex vivo* clotting assay has been the classical method, such as the aPTT and PT methods [88]. These clotting time assays initiate the coagulation reaction by adding a coagulation-inducing substance, thromboplastin, into sample plasma and estimate the thrombin activity based on the fibrin clot formation time.

By contrast, as an alternative standardized method to evaluate the production of thrombin, the thrombin generation test by the endogenous thrombin potential (ETP)-based method was presented [89]. In this method, the extrinsic coagula-tion cascade is activated in the presence of calcium ions by adding standardized phospholipids containing recombinant tissue factor into samples. The amount of thrombin generated is calculated from continuous measurement of the changes in fluorescence emission (or coloring) of the synthetic substrate. The activity measured over time and integrated is defined as ETP.

In aPTT- and PT-based methods, by measuring the time to fibrin clot formation, these reactions terminate at the time of clot formation; however, thrombin continues to be formed after the termination of clot formation and the activity is maintained in the fibrin clot as the trapped form in α-2 macroglobulin. Compared with the thrombin activity measured by the PT-based method, the activity by the ETP-based method can reveal the approximate value of coagulation ability in *ex vivo* samples [89].

An animal experiment has shown that thrombin generation is upregulated in high estrogenic conditions [86]. The ETP-based assay detected changes in thrombin generation in non-pregnant rats treated with exogenous estrogen compared to controls to examine the direct effect of estrogen on the thrombin generation. A peak of ETP was observed on day 21 of administration compared to the control group. ETP in the administration group showed a significant increase as compared to that of the control group and returned to a similar level as the control group. By contrast, the conventional method did not show a difference in coagulation ability between the rats treated with estrogen and control. This animal experiment may simply indicate that estrogen induces a hypercoagulable state [86].

Other studies have demonstrated changes in thrombin generation, which is measured by an ETP-based method because the conventional method detects a small difference between thrombin generation in pregnant and non-pregnant women. Those studies showed that thrombin generation is significantly enhanced in late pregnancy and on day 1 postpartum compared to non-pregnancy. This obser-vation indicates more directly that the hypercoagulable state can be induced during pregnancy and the puerperium [87].

The prothrombotic state is regulated by the balance between coagulation and inhibitory factors. This concept has focused on the resistance to the inhibitory regulation of thrombin generation by activated protein C (APC) in studies of OC users [77, 90] because the reduced activity of APC can be associated with an increase in the risk of pregnancy-related VTE.

Like the COC studies, a clinical case report [91] and previous research have shown a significant decrease in sensitivity to APC [87] during the postpartum period. Decreased sensitivity to APC during pregnancy in clinical samples is partially dependent on reduced protein S levels; however, it is difficult to conclude that resistance to APC in pregnancy and the puerperium is associated with the development of pregnancy-related VTE. Although the phenomena of APC resistance may be relevant [87], the sample size measured in the study is too small to judge the impact of the mechanisms in VTE during pregnancy and the puerperium.

3. Conclusions

Epidemiologic observations have demonstrated that prepregnant obese women with underlying mechanisms of metabolic syndrome are at increased risk of pregnancy-related adverse outcomes of VTE, HDP, and GDM. Above all, maternal death by pregnancy-related VTE has an impact of great magnitude in the childbearing population. The mechanisms underlying the pathogenesis of VTE remain poorly understood although the overlapping connections among obesity, high estrogen levels, and prothrombotic status are essential keys for expanding knowledge.

Author details

Motoi Sugimura
Department of Obstetrics, Gynecology and Family Medicine, Hamamatsu University School of Medicine, Hamamatsu, Japan

*Address all correspondence to: msugimu@hama-med.ac.jp

References

[1] Hibbard JU, Gilbert S, Landon MB, Hauth JC, Leveno KJ, Spong CY, et al. Trial of labor or repeat cesarean delivery in women with morbid obesity and previous cesarean delivery. Obstetrics and Gynecology. 2006;**108**:125-133. DOI: 10.1097/01.AOG.0000223871.69852.31

[2] Heit JA, Spencer FA, White RH. The epidemiology of venous thromboembolism. Journal of Thrombosis and Thrombolysis. 2016;**41**:3-14. DOI: 10.1007/s11239-015-1311-6

[3] Butwick AJ, Abreo A, Bateman BT, Lee HC, El-Sayed YY, Stephansson O, et al. Effect of maternal body mass index on postpartum hemorrhage. Anesthesiology. 2018;**128**:774-783. DOI: 10.1097/ALN.0000000000002082

[4] Anderson NH, LM MC, Fyfe EM, Chan EH, Taylor RS, Stewart AW, et al. The impact of maternal body mass index on the phenotype of pre-eclampsia: A prospective cohort study. BJOG. 2012;**119**:589-595. DOI: 10.1111/j.1471-0528.2012.03278.x

[5] Gasse C, Boutin A, et al. Body mass index and the risk of hypertensive disorders of pregnancy: The great obstetrical syndromes (GOS) study. The Journal of Maternal-Fetal & Neonatal Medicine. 2017;**13**:1-6

[6] Brown MA, Magee LA, Kenny LC, Karumanchi SA, McCarthy FP, Saito S, et al. The hypertensive disorders of pregnancy: ISSHP classification, diagnosis & management recommendations for international practice. Pregnancy Hypertension. 2018;**13**:291-310. DOI: 10.1016/j.preghy.2018.05.004

[7] Miranda M, Ambrosio B, Gomes R, Matos T, Santos I, Nazaré A. Severe hypertensive complications in pregnancy—Two years study (2011-2012). Pregnancy Hypertension. 2013;**3**:98-99. DOI: 10.1016/j.preghy.2013.04.111

[8] Catalano PM, Shankar K. Obesity and pregnancy: Mechanisms of short term and long term adverse consequences for mother and child. BMJ. 2017;**8**:356-372. DOI: 10.1136/bmj.j1

[9] Calkins K, Devaskar SU. Fetal origins of adult disease. Current Problems in Pediatric and Adolescent Health Care. 2011;**41**:158-176. DOI: 10.1016/j.cppeds.2011.01.001

[10] American College of Obstetricians and Gynecologists. Obesity in pregnancy. Practice bulletin no. 156. Obstetrics and Gynecology. 2015;**126**:e112-e126

[11] Mousa A, Naqash A, Lim S. Macronutrient and micronutrient intake during pregnancy: An overview of recent evidence. Nutrients. 2019;**11**: 443-463. DOI: 10.3390/nu11020443

[12] Grundy SM, Brewer HB Jr, Cleeman JI, Smith SC Jr, Lenfant C. Definition of metabolic syndrome: Report of the National Heart, Lung, and Blood Institute/American Heart Association conference on scientific issues related to definition. Circulation. 2004;**109**:433-438. DOI: 10.1161/01.CIR.0000111245.75752.C6

[13] Ministry of Health Labour and Welfare of Japan. Trends in maternal deaths and maternal mortality rates (per 100,000 total births) by causes of death. Annual Vital Statistics Report. 2017;**1**:5-38

[14] Davis NL, Hoyert DL, Goodman DA, Hirai AH, Callaghan WM. Contribution of maternal age and pregnancy checkbox on maternal mortality

ratios in the United States, 1978-2012. American Journal of Obstetrics and Gynecology. 2017;**217**:352.e1-352.e7. DOI: 10.1016/j.ajog.2016.10.011

[15] GBD 2015 Maternal Mortality Collaborators. Global, regional, and national levels of maternal mortality, 1990-2015: A systematic analysis for the global burden of disease study 2015. Lancet. 2016;**388**(10053):1775-1812. DOI: 10.1016/S0140-6736(16)31470-2

[16] Saltiel AR, Olefsky JM. Inflammatory mechanisms linking obesity and metabolic disease. The Journal of Clinical Investigation. 2017;**127**:1-4. DOI: 10.1172/JCI92035

[17] Grieger JA, Bianco-Miotto T, Grzeskowiak LE, Leemaqz SY, Poston L, McCowan LM, et al. Metabolic syndrome in pregnancy and risk for adverse pregnancy outcomes: A prospective cohort of nulliparous women. PLoS Medicine. 2018;**15**:e1002710. DOI: 10.1371/journal.pmed.1002710

[18] Kershaw EE, Flier JS. Adipose tissue as an endocrine organ. The Journal of Clinical Endocrinology and Metabolism. 2004;**89**:2548-2556. DOI: 10.1210/jc.2004-0395

[19] Kuroda M, Sakaue H. Adipocyte death and chronic inflammation in obesity. The Journal of Medical Investigation. 2017;**64**:193-196. DOI: 10.2152/jmi.64.193

[20] Coughlin SR. Protease-activated receptors in hemostasis, thrombosis and vascular biology. Journal of Thrombosis and Haemostasis. 2005;**3**:1800-1814. DOI: 10.1111/j.1538-7836.2005.01377.x

[21] Samad F, Ruf W. Inflammation, obesity, and thrombosis. Blood. 2013;**122**:3415-3422. DOI: 10.1182/blood-2013-05-427708

[22] Esmon CT. The interactions between inflammation and coagulation. British Journal of Haematology. 2005;**131**:417-430. DOI: 10.1111/j.1365-2141.2005.05753.x

[23] Zelaya H, Rothmeier AS, Ruf W. Tissue factor at the crossroad of coagulation and cell signaling. Journal of Thrombosis and Haemostasis. 2018;**16**:1941-1952. DOI: 10.1111/jth.14246

[24] Maurizi G, Guardia DL, Maurizi A, Poloni A. Adipocytes properties and crosstalk with immune system in obesity-related inflammation. Journal of Cellular Physiology. 2018;**233**:88-97. DOI: 10.1002/jcp.25855

[25] Nevo O, Soleymanlou N, Wu Y, Xu J, Kingdom J, Many A, et al. Increased expression of sFlt-1 in in vivo and in vitro models of human placental hypoxia is mediated by HIF-1. American Journal of Physiology. Regulatory, Integrative and Comparative Physiology. 2006;**291**:R1085-R1R93. DOI: 10.1152/ajpregu.00794.2005

[26] Cindrova-Davies T, Sanders DA, Burton GJ, Charnock-Jones DS. Soluble FLT1 sensitizes endothelial cells to inflammatory cytokines by antagonizing VEGF receptor-mediated signaling. Cardiovascular Research. 2011;**89**:671-679. DOI: 10.1093/cvr/cvq346

[27] Maynard SE, Min JY, Merchan J, Lim KH, Li J, Mondal S, et al. Excess placental soluble FMS-like tyrosine kinase 1 (sFlt1) may contribute to endothelial dysfunction, hypertension, and proteinuria in preeclampsia. The Journal of Clinical Investigation. 2003;**111**:649-658. DOI: 10.1172/JCI17189

[28] Myatt L, Webster RP. Vascular biology of preeclampsia. Journal of Thrombosis and Haemostasis. 2009;**7**:375-384. DOI: 10.1111/j.1538-7836.2008.03259.x

[29] Bevilacqua MP, Pober JS, Majeau GR, Cotran RS, Gimbrone MA Jr. Interleukin 1 (IL-1) induces biosynthesis and cell surface expression of procoagulant activity in human vascular endothelial cells. The Journal of Experimental Medicine. 1984;**160**:618-623. DOI: 10.1084/jem.160.2.618

[30] Zhao Y, Koga K, Osuga Y, Nagai M, Izumi G, Takamura M, et al. Thrombin enhances soluble Fms-like tyrosine kinase 1 expression in trophoblasts; possible involvement in the pathogenesis of preeclampsia. Fertility and Sterility. 2012;**98**:917-921. DOI: 10.1016/j.fertnstert.2012.06.038

[31] Sugimura M, Kobayashi T, Shu F, Kanayama N, Terao T. Annexin V inhibits phosphatidylserine-induced intrauterine growth restriction in mice. Placenta. 1999;**20**:555-560. DOI: 10.1055/s-2005-872438

[32] Sugimura M, Ohashi R, Kobayashi T, Kanayama N. Intraplacental coagulation in intrauterine growth restriction: Cause or result? Seminars in Thrombosis and Hemostasis. 2001;**27**:107-113. DOI: 10.1055/s-2001-14068

[33] Ehrenberg HM, Dierkar L, Milluzzi C, Mercer BM. Low maternal weight, failure to thrive in pregnancy, and adverse pregnancy outcomes. American Journal of Obstetrics and Gynecology. 2003;**189**:1726-1730. DOI: 10.1016/s0002-9378(03)00860-3

[34] Most J, Dervis S, Haman F, Adamo KB, Redman LM. Energy intake requirements in pregnancy. Nutrients. 2019;**11**:1812-1830. DOI: 10.3390/nu11081812

[35] Food and Nutrition Board of the Institute of Medicine. Dietary Reference Intake. Washington, DC, USA: National Academy of Sciences; 2004

[36] Catalano PM, Farrell K, Thomas A, Huston-Presley L, Mencin P, Hauguel de Mouzon S, et al. Perinatal risk factors for childhood obesity and metabolic dysregulation. The American Journal of Clinical Nutrition. 2009;**90**:1303-1313. DOI: 10.3945/ajcn.2008.27416

[37] Krakowiak P, Walker CK, Bremer AA, Baker AS, Ozonoff S, Hansen LH, et al. Maternal metabolic conditions and risk for autism and other neurodevelopmental disorders. Pediatrics. 2012;**129**:e1121-e1128. DOI: 10.1542/peds.2011-2583

[38] Institute of Medicine. Weight Gain During Pregnancy: Reexamining the Guidelines. Washington, DC, USA: National Academies Press; 2009

[39] American College of Obstetricians and Gynecologists. Weight gain during pregnancy. ACOG Committee opinion no. 548. Obstetrics and Gynecology. 2013;**121**:210-212

[40] Brett KE, Ferraro ZM, Yockell-Lelievre J, Gruslin A, Adamo KB. Maternal-fetal nutrient transport in pregnancy pathologies: The role of the placenta. International Journal of Molecular Sciences. 2014;**15**:16153-16185. DOI: 10.3390/ijms150916153

[41] Segedal LR, Øverby NC, Bere E, Torstveit MK, Lohne-Seiler H, Småstuen M, et al. Lifestyle intervention to limit gestational weight gain: The Norwegian fit for delivery randomized controlled trial. BJOG. 2017;**124**:97-109. DOI: 10.1111/1471-0528.13862

[42] Fowden AL, Giussani DA, Forhead AJ. Endocrine and metabolic programming during intrauterine development. Early Human Development. 2005;**81**:723-734. DOI: 10.1016/j.earlhumdev.2005.06.007

[43] Barker DJ, Winter PD, Osmond C, Margetts B, Simmonds SJ. Weight in infancy and death from ischaemic heart disease. Lancet. 1989;**2**:577-580. DOI: 10.1016/s0140-6736(89)90710-1

[44] Goldstein RF, Abell SK, Ranasinha S, Misso ML, Boyle JA, Harrison CL, et al. Gestational weight gain across continents and ethnicity: Systematic review and meta-analysis of maternal and infant outcomes in more than one million women. BMC Medicine. 2018;**16**:153-168. DOI: 10.1186/s12916-018-1128-1

[45] Guimicheva B, Czuprynska J, Arya R. The prevention of pregnancy-related venous thromboembolism. British Journal of Haematology. 2015;**168**:163-174. DOI: 10.1111/bjh.13159

[46] Robert L. Case of pulmonary phlebitis. Medico-Chirurgical Transactions. 1835;**19**:44-47

[47] Playfair WS. Observation on a case of sudden death after delivery from embolism of the pulmonary artery. British Medical Journal. 1869;**1**:282-283. DOI: 10.1136/bmj.1.430.282

[48] Royal College of Obstetricians and Gynecologists. Why Mothers Die: Confidential Enquiries into Maternal Deaths in the United Kingdom. London, UK: The RCOG Press at Royal College of Obstetricians and Gynaecologists; 2000

[49] Jacobsen AF, Skjeldestad FE, Sandset PM. Ante- and postnatal risk factors of venous thrombosis: A hospital-based case-control study. Journal of Thrombosis and Haemostasis. 2008;**6**:905-912. DOI: 10.1111/j.1538-7836.2008.02961.x

[50] Robinson HE, O'Connell CM, Joseph KS, McLeod NL. Maternal outcomes in pregnancies complicated by obesity. Obstetrics and Gynecology. 2005;**106**:1357-1364. DOI: 10.1097/01.AOG.0000188387.88032.41

[51] Royal College of Obstetrician and Gynaecologist. Thromboprophylaxis during pregnancy, labour and after vaginal delivery (reducing the risk of thrombosis and embolism during pregnancy and the puerperium). In: Green-Top Guideline No. 37a. 2009. pp. 1-35

[52] Royal College of Obstetrician and Gynaecologist. Reducing the risk of thrombosis and embolism during pregnancy and the puerperium. In: Green-Top Guideline No. 37a. London, UK: Royal College of Obstetricians and Gynaecologists; 2015. pp. 1-40. Available from: https://www.rcog.org.uk/globalassets/documents/guidelines/gtg-37a.pdf

[53] American College of Chest Physicians Evidence-Based Clinical Practice Guidelines (9th Edition). Venous thromboembolism, thrombophilia, antithrombotic therapy, and pregnancy. Chest. 2012;**141**:e691S-e736S

[54] Tata JR. One hundred years of hormones. EMBO Reports. 2005;**6**:490-496. DOI: 10.1038/sj.embor.7400444

[55] Xu Y, Nedungadi TP, Zhu L, Sobhani N, Irani BG, Davis KE, et al. Distinct hypothalamic neurons mediate estrogenic effects on energy homeostasis and reproduction. Cell Metabolism. 2011;**14**:453-465. DOI: 10.1016/j.cmet.2011.08.009

[56] Usselman CW, Stachenfeld NS, Bender JR. The molecular actions of oestrogen in the regulation of vascular health. Experimental Physiology. 2016;**101**(3):356-361. DOI: 10.1113/EP085148

[57] Chidi-Ogbolu N, Baar K. Effect of estrogen on musculoskeletal performance and injury risk. Frontiers in Physiology. 2019;**9**:1834-1845. DOI: 10.3389/fphys.2018.01834

[58] Heine PA, Taylor JA, Iwamoto GA, Lubahn DB, Cooke PS. Increased adipose tissue in male and female estrogen receptor-alpha knockout mice.

Proceedings of the National Academy of Sciences of the United States of America. 2000;**97**:12729-12734. DOI: 10.1073/pnas.97.23.12729

[59] Vercellini P, Viganò P, Somigliana E, Fedele L. Endometriosis: Pathogenesis and treatment. Nature Reviews. Endocrinology. 2014;**10**:261-275. DOI: 10.1038/nrendo.2013.255

[60] Hamilton KJ, Hewitt SC, Arao Y, Korach KS. Estrogen hormone biology. Current Topics in Developmental Biology. 2017;**125**:109-146. DOI: 10.1016/bs.ctdb.2016.12.005

[61] Fuentes N, Silveyra P. Estrogen receptor signaling mechanisms. Advances in Protein Chemistry and Structural Biology. 2019;**116**:135-170. DOI: 10.1016/bs.apcsb.2019.01.001

[62] Dorrington JH, Armstrong DT. Follicle-stimulating hormone stimulates estradiol-17beta synthesis in cultured Sertoli cells. Proceedings of the National Academy of Sciences of the United States of America. 1975;**72**:2677-2681. DOI: 10.1073/pnas.72.7.2677

[63] Zahid H, Simpson ER, Brown KA. Inflammation, dysregulated metabolism and aromatase in obesity and breast cancer. Current Opinion in Pharmacology. 2016;**31**:90-96. DOI: 10.1016/j.coph.2016.11.003

[64] Brown SB, Hankinson SE. Endogenous estrogens and the risk of breast, endometrial, and ovarian cancers. Steroids. 2015;**99**:8-10. DOI: 10.1016/j.steroids.2014.12.013

[65] Thomas D, Apovian C. Macrophage functions in lean and obese adipose tissue. Metabolism. 2017;**72**:120-143. DOI: 10.1016/j.metabol.2017.04.005

[66] Labrie F, Bélanger A, Luu-The V, Labrie C, Simard J, Cusan L, et al. DHEA and the intracrine formation of androgens and estrogens in peripheral target tissues: Its role during aging. Steroids. 1998;**63**:322-328. DOI: 10.1016/s0039-128x(98)00007-5

[67] Nelson LR, Bulun SE. Estrogen production and action. Journal of the American Academy of Dermatology. 2001;**45**(Suppl 3):S116-S124. DOI: 10.1067/mjd.2001.117432

[68] Siiteri PK, MaCDonald PC. Placental estrogen biosynthesis during human pregnancy. The Journal of Clinical Endocrinology and Metabolism. 1966;**26**:751-761. DOI: 10.1210/jcem-26-7-751

[69] Pepe GJ, Albrecht ED. Actions of placental and fetal adrenal steroid hormones in primate pregnancy. Endocrine Reviews. 1995;**16**(5):608-648. DOI: 10.1210/edrv-16-5-608

[70] Gurpide E, Schwers J, Welch MT, Vande Wiele RL, Lieberman S. Fetal and maternal metabolism of estradiol during pregnancy. The Journal of Clinical Endocrinology and Metabolism. 1966;**26**:1355-1365. DOI: 10.1210/jcem-26-12-1355

[71] Gomez-Lopez N, StLouis D, Lehr MA, Sanchez-Rodriguez EN, Arenas-Hernandez M. Immune cells in term and preterm labor. Cellular & Molecular Immunology. 2014;**11**:571-581. DOI: 10.1038/cmi.2014.46

[72] Blann AD, Lip GY. Virchow's triad revisited: The importance of soluble coagulation factors, the endothelium, and platelets. Thrombosis Research. 2001;**101**:321-327. DOI: 10.1016/s0049-3848(00)00419-9

[73] Jordan WM. Pulmonary embolism. Lancet. 1961;**7212**:1146-1147

[74] Sitruk-Ware R. Hormonal contraception and thrombosis. Fertility and Sterility. 2016;**106**:1289-1294. DOI: 10.1016/j.fertnstert.2016.08.039

[75] Roach RE, Helmerhorst FM, Lijfering WM, Stijnen T, Algra A, Dekkers OM. Combined oral contraceptives: The risk of myocardial infarction and ischemic stroke. The Cochrane Database of Systematic Reviews. 2015;**8**:CD011054. DOI: 10.1002/14651858.CD011054.pub2

[76] ESHRE Capri Workshop Group. Venous thromboembolism in women: A specific reproductive health risk. Human Reproduction Update. 2013;**9**:471-482. DOI: 10.1093/humupd/dmt028

[77] Tchaikovski SN, Rosing J. Mechanisms of estrogen-induced venous thromboembolism. Thrombosis Research. 2000;**126**:5-11. DOI: 10.1016/j. thromres.2010.01.045

[78] Middeldorp S, Meijers JC, van den Ende AE, van Enk A, Bouma BN, Tans G, et al. Effects on coagulation of levonorgestrel- and desogestrel-containing low dose oral contraceptives: A crossover study. Thrombosis and Haemostasis. 2000;**84**:4-8

[79] Goebelsmann U, Mashchak CA, Mishell DR Jr. Comparison of hepatic impact of oral and vaginal administration of ethinyl estradiol. American Journal of Obstetrics and Gynecology. 1985;**151**:868-877. DOI: 10.1016/0002-9378(85)90664-7

[80] Klipping C, Duijkers I, Parke S, Mellinger U, Serrani M, Junge W. Hemostatic effects of a novel estradiol-based oral contraceptive: An open-label, randomized, crossover study of estradiol valerate/dienogest versus ethinylestradiol/levonorgestrel. Drugs in R&D. 2011;**11**:159-170. DOI: 10.2165/11591200-000000000-00000

[81] Agren UM, Anttila M, Mäenpää-Liukko K, Rantala ML, Rautiainen H, Sommer WF, et al. Effects of a monophasic combined oral contraceptive containing nomegestrol acetate and 17b-oestradiol compared with one containing levonorgestrel and ethinylestradiol on haemostasis, lipids and carbohydrate metabolism. The European Journal of Contraception & Reproductive Health Care. 2011;**16**:444-457. DOI: 10.3109/13625187.2011.604450

[82] Hellgren M. Hemostasis during normal pregnancy and puerperium. Seminars in Thrombosis and Hemostasis. 2003;**29**:125-130. DOI: 10.1055/s-2003-38897

[83] Brenner B. Haemostatic changes in pregnancy. Thrombosis Research. 2004;**114**:409-414. DOI: 10.1016/j. thromres.2004.08.004

[84] Suzuki A, Sanda N, Miyawaki Y, Fujimori Y, Yamada T, Takagi A, et al. Down-regulation of PROS1 gene expression by 17-estradiol via estrogen receptor (ER)-Sp1 interaction recruiting receptor-interacting protein 140 and the corepressor-HDAC3 complex. The Journal of Biological Chemistry. 2010;**285**:13444-13453. DOI: 10.1074/jbc.M109.062430

[85] Dahlbäck B. Interaction between vitamin K-dependent protein S and the complement protein, C4b-binding protein. A link between coagulation and the complement system. Seminars in Thrombosis and Hemostasis. 1984;**10**:139-148. DOI: 10.1055/s-2007-1004416

[86] Ohashi R, Sugimura M, Kanayama N. Estrogen administration enhances thrombin generation in rats. Thrombosis Research. 2003;**112**:325-328. DOI: 10.1016/j.thromres.2003.11.014

[87] Hirai K, Sugimura M, Ohashi R, Suzuki K, Itoh H, Sugihara K, et al. A rapid activated protein C sensitivity test as a diagnostic marker for a suspected venous thromboembolism in pregnancy and puerperium. Gynecologic and

Obstetric Investigation. 2011;**72**:55-62. DOI: 10.1159/000322880

[88] Winter WE, Flax SD, Harris NS. Coagulation testing in the core laboratory. Laboratoriums Medizin. 2017;**48**:295-313. DOI: 10.1093/labmed/lmx050

[89] Hemker HC, Willems GM, Béguin S. A computer assisted method to obtain the prothrombin activation velocity in whole plasma independent of thrombin decay processes. Thrombosis and Haemostasis. 1986;**56**:9-17

[90] Trigg DE, Wood MG, Kouides PA, Kadir RA. Hormonal influences on hemostasis in women. Seminars in Thrombosis and Hemostasis. 2011;**37**:77-86. DOI: 10.1055/s-0030-1270074

[91] Sugimura M, Kobayashi T, Kanayama N, Terao T. Detection of marked reduction of sensitivity to activated protein C prior to the onset of thrombosis during puerperium as detected by endogenous thrombin potential-based assay. Thrombosis and Haemostasis. 1999;**82**:1364-1365

3

Neural Control of Homeostatic Feeding and Food Selection

Yasuhiko Minokoshi

Abstract

Neural regulation of feeding is key to the control of body energy balance. Recent studies have identified multiple neural circuits that contribute to the control of homeostatic or hedonic feeding, with these circuits acting cooperatively to regulate feeding overall. Neuropeptide Y (NPY)-agouti-related peptide (AgRP) neurons and pro-opiomelanocortin (POMC) neurons in the arcuate nucleus of the hypothala-mus appear to be primary and reciprocal regulators of homeostatic food intake. However, the central mechanisms underlying the regulation of nutrient intake remain largely unknown. 5′-Adenosine monophosphate-activated protein kinase (AMPK) is an important molecule in the regulation of energy metabolism. We recently showed that AMPK-regulated corticotrophin-releasing hormone (CRH) neurons in the paraventricular nucleus of the hypothalamus regulate the selection of carbohydrate over a more palatable diet. Here, I address key recent findings that have shed light on the homeostatic regulation of feeding including total calorie and macronutrient intake.

Keywords: homeostatic feeding, hedonic feeding, hypothalamus, AMPK, macronutrient, carbohydrate selection

1. Introduction

Feeding is one of the most important motivated behaviors for maintenance of body energy balance. Although obesity has become a pandemic in the modern world, young individuals are able to maintain their body weight over a long period, suggesting that body energy balance, at least at a young age, is precisely regulated.

Regulation of feeding is generally divided into homeostatic and nonhomeostatic mechanisms [1]. The hypothalamus and brain stem play important roles in homeostatic regulation (**Figure 1**). Nonhomeostatic regulation relates to "hedonic" feeding that manifests as hyperphagia for palatable diets rather than to the control of body energy balance. The reward system including dopaminergic neurons in the ventral tegmental area is associated with hedonic feeding. Homeostatic and nonhomeostatic systems are coordinately regulated under physiological and pathological conditions.

The recent introduction of new technologies including optogenetic and pharmacogenetic methods has led to the identification of neural circuits for the regulation of homeostatic feeding in the hypothalamus and other brain areas. In addition to hormones such as leptin, ghrelin, cholecystokinin (CCK), and glucagon-like peptide-1 (GLP-1), less well-known hormones such as asprosin and growth and differentiation factor 15 (GDF15) have also recently been implicated in the central regulation of homeostatic and hedonic feeding [2, 3].

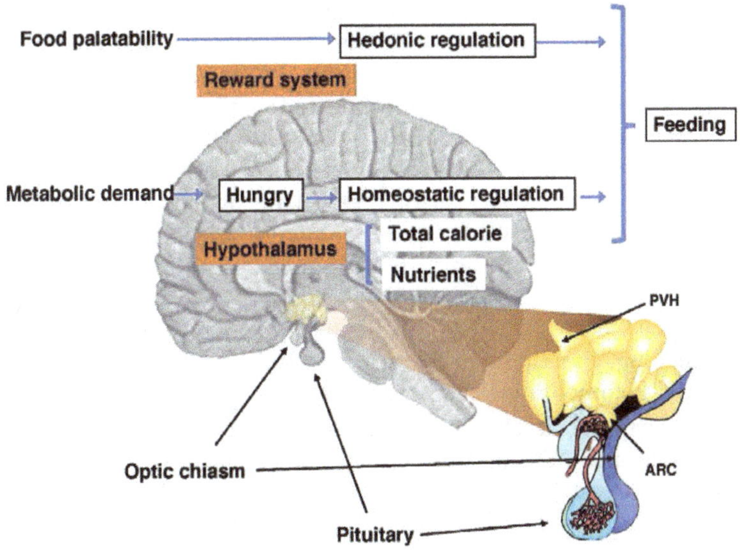

Figure1.
Homeostatic and hedonic regulation of feeding. Feeding is regulated by homeostatic and hedonic mechanisms in the brain. The hypothalamus contributes to homeostatic regulation, and the reward system in the brain contributes to hedonic regulation.

In this chapter, I will review regulatory mechanisms for homeostatic feeding in the hypothalamus, with a focus on the role of neuropeptide Y (NPY) and agouti-related peptide (AgRP) containing neurons in the arcuate nucleus of the hypothalamus (ARC). I will also address the role of novel regulatory hormones including asprosin and GDF15 in feeding. With regard to the molecular mechanisms of energy sensing in the hypothalamus, I will describe the role of 5′-adenosine monophosphate (AMP)—activated protein kinase (AMPK)—a metabolic sensor and regulator of intermediate metabolism, autophagy, and mitochondrial function—in feeding regulation [4–7].

In addition to the regulation of total calorie intake with regard to whole-body energy balance, macronutrient intake plays an important role in cardiometabolic health, aging, and longevity [8, 9] and is regulated by the brain. We recently showed that AMPK-regulated neurons in the paraventricular nucleus of the hypothalamus (PVH) that express corticotropin-releasing hormone (CRH) are necessary and sufficient for the fasting-induced selection of carbohydrate over a basally preferred diet such as a high-fat diet (HFD) in mice [10]. Such consumption of a high-carbohydrate diet (HCD) after fasting resulted in a rapid reversal of the fasting-induced increase in the plasma concentration of ketone bodies. Whereas intake of an HFD can also improve ketone body metabolism, this occurs at a slower rate. These observations indi-cate that, when offered a choice of diets, rodents select an HCD as a means to achieve a rapid normalization of ketone and glucose metabolism during refeeding after fasting. I will thus also describe in more detail in this chapter our recent study regarding the role of AMPK-regulated CRH neurons of the PVH in carbohydrate selection.

2. Neural circuits for homeostatic regulation of feeding

2.1 NPY/AgRP and POMC neurons in the ARC

The ARC contains neurons that express both NPY and AgRP as well as neurons that express pro-opiomelanocortin (POMC), with both of these types of neuron having been shown to contribute to the monitoring of body energy balance and to the regulation of feeding [11] (**Figure 2**). The ARC does not have an effective blood-brain barrier and possesses a specific transport system for the uptake of hormones such as leptin into the brain [12]. In addition to the neuropeptides NPY and AgRP, NPY/AgRP neurons release the inhibitory neurotransmitter γ-aminobutyric acid (GABA), with all three of these agents contributing to the induction of feeding. AgRP is an endogenous antagonist of the melanocortin 4 receptor (MC4R) and melanocortin 3 receptor (MC3R). AgRP and α-melanocyte-stimulating hormone (α-MSH) regulates feeding in a reciprocal manner by acting at MC4R and MC3R [11]. Mammals express five different NPY receptors, of which Y1 and Y5 regulate feeding [11]. Injection of NPY or GABA into the brain of mice induces a marked increase in feeding, but these effects are less long-lasting than is that of AgRP, persisting for ~3 h compared with ~24 h for AgRP.

α-MSH is produced by cleavage of the precursor protein POMC [11]. POMC neurons thus release α-MSH and thereby inhibit food intake through activation of MC4R and, to a lesser extent, that of MC3R [11]. Loss of POMC or MC4R gives rise to pronounced obesity in both humans and mice, with mutations of the MC4R gene being the most common monogenic cause of human obesity [13]. The POMC gene encodes various proteins and peptides including adrenocorticotropic hormone (ACTH) and endorphin as well as α -MSH, and mutations of the POMC gene or of genes for the POMC-processing enzymes convertase 1 and 2 give rise to adrenal insufficiency and red hair pigmentation as well as early-onset obesity in humans [13].

In contrast to the obesity associated with ablation of POMC or MC4R genes, mice lacking the NPY, AgRP, or both genes as well as those in which NPY/AgRP neurons were ablated by forced expression of diphtheria toxin during the neonatal

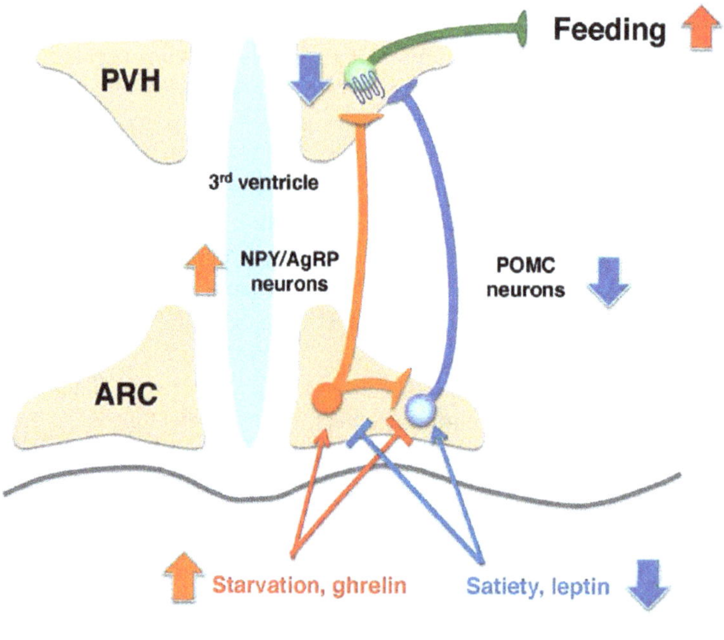

Figure2.
Reciprocal regulation of NPY/AgRP neurons and POMC neurons of the ARC in the control of food intake. Food deprivation and ghrelin activate NPY/AgRP neurons and inhibit POMC neurons in the ARC. In contrast, satiety and leptin activate POMC neurons and inhibit NPY/AgRP neurons in this nucleus. Activation of NPY/AgRP neurons and inhibition of POMC neurons result in inhibition of neurons in the PVH that suppress feeding, leading to an increase in food intake.

period were found to be able to maintain a normal body weight. However, ablation of NPY/AgRP neurons by diphtheria toxin during adulthood was shown to give rise to severe anorexia [14]. NPY/AgRP neurons are thus now recognized as key neurons in the regulation of food intake. The maintenance of a normal body weight after ablation of NPY/AgRP neurons during the neonatal period appears to reflect a compensatory rearrangement of neural circuits in the brain. Indeed, activation of certain other neuronal types has recently been found to induce hyperphagia to an extent similar to that triggered by activation of NPY/AgRP neurons. For example, somatostatin-expressing neurons in the tuberal nucleus of the hypothalamus increase food intake by releasing GABA and thereby inhibiting neurons in the PVH or the bed nucleus of the stria terminalis (BNST) [15]. In addition, GABAergic neurons in the zona incerta that project to the paraventricular nucleus of the thalamus also increase food intake [16]. However, in contrast to that of NPY/AgRP neurons, ablation of either of these two types of neuron during adulthood does not result in anorexia.

Activation of NPY/AgRP neurons in the ARC increases operant behaviors such as the pressing of a lever to get food. It also increased food intake even when mice were fed a noncaloric flavored diet [17, 18]. Furthermore, when mice were equipped with an optical fiber that allowed them to activate these NPY/AgRP neurons, they did so [19]. These observations suggest that activation of NPY/AgRP neurons increases the motivation for feeding. However, the optogenetic activation of NPY/AgRP neurons appears to induce different behaviors depending on whether mice are anticipating the presentation of food or not. Food reward is necessary to increase the self-stimulation of NPY/AgRP neurons. A conditioned place preference test also revealed that mice avoid the place where NPY/AgRP neurons are stimulated in the absence of food reward [20].

Recent studies have shown that the activity of NPY/AgRP neurons in the ARC rapidly decreases after the onset of feeding [17–20]. Infusion of a liquid meal into the stomach was also found to reduce the activity of these neurons, as was the injection into the brain of feeding-suppressive hormones or neurotransmitters such as serotonin, CCK, and peptide YY (PYY). Anticipatory stimuli for food such as its smell induce a transient decrease in the activity of NPY/AgRP neurons. These changes in neuronal activity appear to be correlated with the reward value of food, and they suggest that NPY/AgRP neurons in the ARC are regulated by higher brain systems such as the reward system.

2.2 Hormonal regulation of NPY/AgRP neurons in the ARC

2.2.1 Leptin, ghrelin, insulin, GLP-1, and CCK

The activities of NPY/AgRP neurons and POMC neurons are regulated not only by nutrients such as glucose but also by hormones. Leptin and ghrelin control the activity of both of these types of neuron by eliciting intracellular signaling (**Figure 3**) [11, 21, 22]. Insulin also contributes to suppression of feeding by acting at the insulin receptor expressed in these neurons [23]. Nutrient signals in the gut and liver are also indirectly transmitted to NPY/AgRP and POMC neurons via afferent nerves in the vagus nerve trunk [21, 22]. Indeed, the gastrointestinal hormones ghrelin, CCK, GLP-1, and PYY have been shown to regulate NPY/AgRP neurons and POMC neurons directly by acting at receptors expressed in these neurons as well as indirectly through the afferent nerve fibers in the vagus nerve (**Figure 3**).

Leptin is an adipocyte hormone that reciprocally regulates the activities of NPY/AgRP neurons and POMC neurons [11]. The plasma leptin concentration is correlated with the amount of adipose tissue in the body. Ablation of the leptin receptor

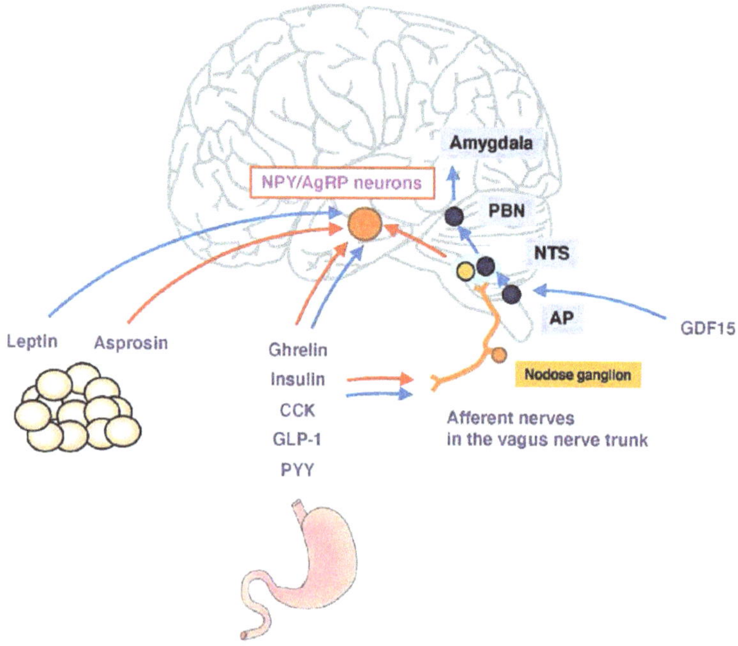

Figure3.
Hormonal regulation of NPY/AgRP neurons in the ARC and of food intake. The adipocyte-derived hormones leptin and asprosin directly regulate the activity of NPY/AgRP neurons in the ARC. Gastrointestinal hormones also regulate the activity of these neurons by direct effects as well as indirectly through afferent nerves in the vagus trunk and the NTS pathway. GDF15 inhibits feeding through the AP-NTS-PBN neural pathway.

in NPY/AgRP neurons or POMC neurons of mice during the fetal or neonatal period was found to have little effect on body weight and food intake, suggesting that these neurons might not play an important role in the regulation of whole-body energy balance by leptin. However, it was subsequently found that ablation of the leptin receptor in NPY/AgRP neurons of adult mice gives rise to obesity and diabetes simi-lar to those of ob/ob (leptin-deficient) and db/db (leptin receptor-deficient) mice [24]. NPY/AgRP neurons are thus indeed an important target for leptin-induced suppression of food intake.

Lipodystrophy is a congenital or acquired disease characterized by a reduction in the amount of adipose tissue in the body [25]. Some individuals with large reductions in the amount of adipose tissue have an increased appetite and develop type 2 diabetes associated with severe insulin resistance. However, leptin treatment was found to normalize food intake and the metabolic abnormalities of such individuals [25], and leptin is now the most effective medicine for patients with lipodystrophy. Given that injection of only a small amount of leptin into the brain is sufficient to inhibit food intake and to ameliorate metabolic abnormalities in lipodystrophy model mice, such effects of leptin are likely mediated by leptin receptors in the brain. The ventromedial nucleus of the hypothalamus (VMH) as well as ARC appears to be targets in the antidiabetic action of leptin (see Section 2.3.2).

Functional magnetic resonance imaging has been applied to examine the brain of lipodystrophy patients before and after feeding and with and without leptin treatment [26]. Control subjects showed a strong response of the reward system including the striatum when presented with photographs of palatable food after food deprivation, but the response rapidly declined after they were allowed to eat. In contrast, lipodystrophy patients continued to show increased activity in the striatum after feeding, whereas administration of leptin greatly improved the brain response to food. Unfortunately, such imaging, even with the most advanced machines, is not able to reliably detect changes in neuronal activity in the hypothalamus. Indeed, NPY/AgRP neurons and POMC neurons are reciprocally regulated in the ARC, which itself constitutes only a small proportion of the hypothalamus, making it difficult to study such changes in neuronal activity. However, given that individuals with a mutation of the POMC gene manifest hyperphagia and obesity similar to those of mutant mice, NPY/AgRP neurons and POMC neurons play an important role in feeding behavior and metabolic control in humans as well as rodents.

Ghrelin is a peptide released from the stomach and has a unique structure in that it is octanoylated at its third amino acid residue (serine) [22], with this acylation being essential for the orexigenic and metabolic effects of ghrelin. Ghrelin induces feeding by actions in the brain, including the activation of NPY/AgRP neurons and suppression of POMC neurons in the ARC. Until the discovery of asprosin, ghrelin was the only orexigenic peripheral hormone known. In humans, the plasma level of ghrelin increases immediately before breakfast, lunch, and dinner and declines after feeding. Fasting and anorexia nervosa are associated with an increased circulating concentration of ghrelin. Although ghrelin markedly stimulates feeding, its physi-ological function remains unknown because feeding and energy metabolism are largely unaffected in ghrelin knockout mice. It may contribute to the alert system for promotion of feeding at scheduled times such as breakfast, lunch, and dinner.

2.2.2 Asprosin

Asprosin was recently identified as an orexigenic hormone that is released from adipose tissue and which activates NPY/AgRP neurons in the ARC [2]. The name asprosin is derived from the Greek word for white (aspros) because the hormone is produced by white adipose tissue. Asprosin is a protein hormone composed of 140 amino acids, with a molecular mass of ~30 kDa.

Asprosin was discovered as a result of the study of Marfan lipodystrophy syndrome, which is caused by mutation of the profibrillin 1 gene (*FBN1*) and is characterized by congenital lipodystrophy and a neonatal progeroid appearance as well as by severe anorexia and leanness. It differs from the lipodystrophy associated with severe insulin resistance, type 2 diabetes, and hyperphagia, suggesting that leptin is not involved. Asprosin was found to be encoded by the 3′-terminal region of *FBN1*, and the protease furin produces asprosin and fibrillin by cleaving profibrillin 1.

Asprosin stimulates gluconeogenesis in the liver [27]. Similar to that of ghrelin, the plasma level of asprosin increases during fasting and decreases after refeeding. Whereas food intake and body weight remain largely unaltered in ghrelin knockout mice, however, they are both reduced in asprosin knockout mice.

2.2.3 GDF15

GDF15 is a member of the transforming growth factor-β family of proteins and exists in blood [3]. The amount of GDF15 mRNA is highest in adipose tis-sue, followed by skeletal muscle and bone marrow, and the GDF15 receptor, glial cell-derived neurotrophic factor receptor like (GFRAL), is expressed in the area postrema (AP), another brain area with a minimally effective blood-brain barrier. GDF15 activates GFRAL in the AP and thereby reduces food intake via the nucleus tractus solitarius (NTS)-parabrachial nucleus (PBN) pathway. GDF15 is likely a physiological regulator of feeding, given that both GDF15 and GFRAL knockout mice have an increased body weight. Furthermore, GDF15 may play a role in cancer or in stress-induced anorexia because its plasma level is increased in animal models of cancer or under conditions of severe stress.

2.3 Downstream neurons regulated by NPY/AgRP neurons

NPY/AgRP neurons and POMC neurons in the ARC are connected to many brain areas. In particular, connections between these neurons and the PVH, lateral nucleus of the hypothalamus (LH), dorsomedial nucleus of the hypothalamus (DMH), VMH, BNST, and PBN are important neural pathways for regulation of food intake and metabolism (**Figure 4**). Optogenetic activation of projections of NPY/AgRP neurons to the PVH, LH, and BNST has been shown to increase food intake [28]. In addition, the PBN has been found to be necessary for maintenance of a normal level of food intake [29]. I will address the role of the PVH, VMH, LH, and PBN in the regulation of food intake.

2.3.1 PVH

The PVH is an important area in the control of feeding. It contains many secondary neurons that are regulated by NPY/AgRP neurons and POMC neurons in the ARC [1, 11, 21]. Given that NPY, AgRP, and GABA—neurotransmitters or neuromodulators released from NPY/AgRP neurons—all act at inhibitory receptors, activation of NPY/AgRP neurons stimulates feeding via suppression of these secondary neurons. NPY/AgRP neurons were found to increase food intake via MC4R-expressing neurons in the PVH [30], and more recent studies showed that oxytocin- or GLP-1 receptor-expressing neurons in the PVH induce feeding through PBN neurons [31, 32].

2.3.2 VMH

The VMH is known as the satiety center. Indeed, activation of VMH neurons expressing the transcription factor SF1 (steroidogenic factor 1) reduces food intake and increases energy expenditure in mice [33]. VMH neurons including some SF1 neurons express MC4R or MC3R, suggesting that NPY/AgRP neurons and POMC neurons in the ARC regulate VMH neurons. We recently showed that activation of SF1-expressing neurons in the VMH by DREADD (designer receptors exclusively activated by designer drugs) technology not only reduces food intake and increases energy expenditure but also increases glucose uptake in certain peripheral tis-sues including interscapular brown adipose tissue, skeletal muscle, and the heart [33]. We have also shown that leptin increases insulin sensitivity in peripheral tissues as well as glucose utilization by the whole body through the VMH [34, 35]. Furthermore, we revealed that the hypothalamic neuropeptide orexin activates VMH neurons and thereby increases both insulin sensitivity and glucose utilization in skeletal muscle, with the orexin-VMH system being activated by taste stimulation and feeding [36]. These observations suggest that the orexin-VMH system preferentially increases glucose uptake in skeletal muscle during feeding. However, the physiological role of VMH neurons remains elusive, with further investiga-tion being necessary to explore their contribution to the regulation of whole-body energy metabolism.

2.3.3 LH

The LH is known as the feeding center given that some neurons of this area contribute to the control of feeding. Activation of orexin neurons and melanin-concentrating hormone (MCH) neurons of the LH and perifornical area thus increases food intake [37], and NPY/AgRP neurons and POMC neurons in the ARC

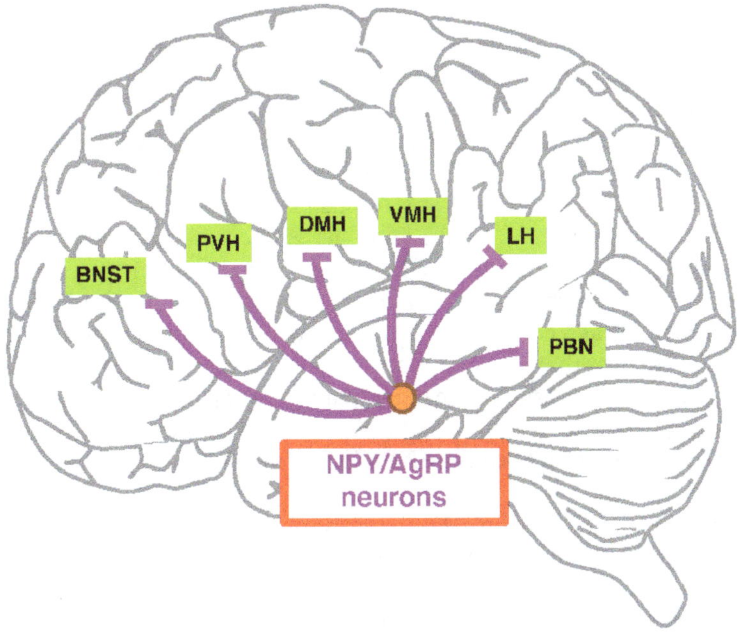

Figure 4.
Neurons downstream of NPY/AgRP neurons in the ARC. NPY/AgRP neurons in the ARC send axons to multiple brain areas. Optogenetic stimulation of NPY/AgRP neurons in the ARC that innervate the BNST, PVH, or LH induces a robust feeding response. Neurons that express melanocortin receptors in the VMH regulate metabolism in peripheral tissues. Tonic inhibition of PBN neurons by NPY/AgRP neurons is necessary for maintenance of a normal feeding level.

regulate the activity of these neurons. Orexin neurons and MCH neurons have multiple functions including regulation of both the sleep-wake cycle and motivated behaviors [38].

In addition to orexin neurons and MCH neurons, some glutamatergic and GABAergic neurons in the LH were found to regulate feeding [38], with activation of GABAergic neurons increasing food intake and that of glutamatergic neurons inhibiting it.

The LH is a unique hypothalamic area in that it interacts with the reward system including dopaminergic neurons in the ventral tegmental area that connect to the nucleus accumbens and striatum [38]. Both glutamatergic and GABAergic neurons in the LH regulate the reward system.

We recently showed that glutamatergic neurons of the LH regulate sweet and bitter taste sensitivities in response to changes in whole-body energy levels [39]. We found that fasting-induced activation of NPY/AgRP neurons in the ARC of mice increases the sensitivity to sweet taste and inhibits that to bitter taste through inhibition of distinct glutamatergic neurons in the LH.

2.3.4 PBN

Feeding can be suppressed via two mechanisms. One is mediated by satiety signals to regulate the physiological feeding cycle, and the other is mediated by anorexic signals such as abdominal pain or cancer cachexia. The PBN contributes to both mechanisms [29, 40–42]. As mentioned above (Section 2.2.3), GDF15-induced anorexia is mediated by the PBN. Neural signals from the gut associated with suppression of food intake are mediated by afferent nerve fibers in the vagus nerve, the NTS, and then the PBN. Recent studies have revealed that anorexic signals are mediated by calcitonin gene-related peptide (CGRP) expressing neurons in the PBN, whereas satiety signals are mediated by non-CGRP neurons in the PBN [29, 40–42].

NPY/AgRP neurons in the ARC constitutively inhibit CGRP neurons in the PBN through a GABAergic signal [29]. Ablation of these NPY/AgRP neurons in adult mice thus activates the CGRP neurons and halts feeding, thereby leading to starvation and death. Injection of GABA into the PBN, however, allows the mice to resume feeding and to survive. Furthermore, forced feeding of the mice with a liquid meal via a stomach tube for 1 week results in the recovery of food intake to normal levels, likely as a consequence of the rearrangement of neural circuits in the PBN. Neural circuits that converge on the PBN were recently found to encode competing danger signals such as fear and pain [40, 41].

2.4 Upstream neurons that regulate NPY/AgRP neurons

As described above (Section 2.1), the activity of NPY/AgRP neurons in the ARC is rapidly suppressed not only by actual feeding but also by food values, suggesting that these neurons are regulated by upstream neurons in the brain as well as by nutrient signals transmitted via the NTS and afferent nerves in the vagus nerve (**Figure 5**). Thyrotropin-releasing hormone (TRH)- or pituitary adenylate cyclase-activating polypeptide (PACAP)-expressing glutamatergic neurons in the PVH have been shown to activate NPY/AgRP neurons in the ARC and to increase food intake [11]. In contrast, GABAergic neurons in the DMH inhibit NPY/AgRP neurons [11]. POMC neurons in the ARC are also activated by glutamatergic neurons in the VMH [43].

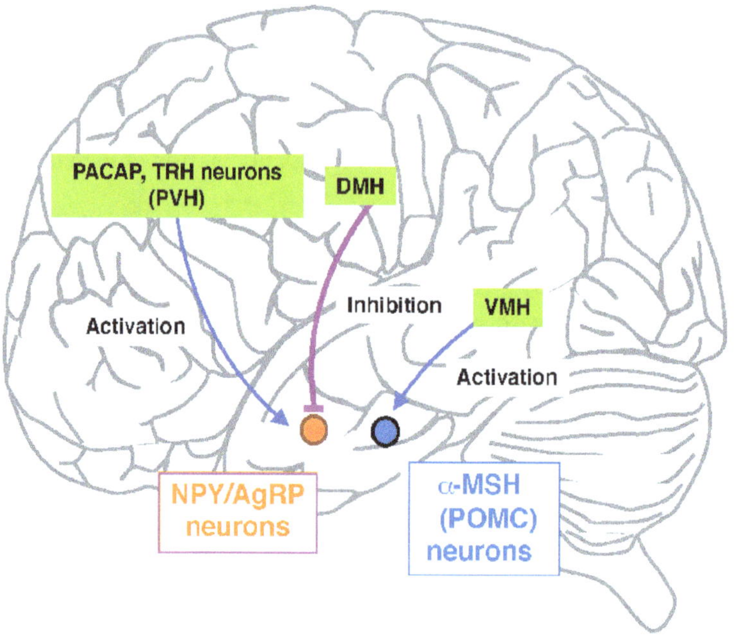

Figure5.
Neurons upstream of NPY/AgRP neurons in the ARC. TRH- or PACAP-expressing glutamatergic neurons in the PVH activate NPY/AgRP neurons in the ARC and increase food intake. In contrast, GABAergic neurons in the DMH inhibit NPY/AgRP neurons. POMC neurons in the ARC are also activated by glutamatergic neurons in the VMH.

3. Role of the metabolic sensor AMPK in feeding regulation

3.1 Regulation of total calorie intake by AMPK

AMPK is a serine-threonine kinase that is evolutionarily conserved from yeast to mammals. It is a heterotrimeric protein consisting of an α catalytic subunit as well as β and γ regulatory subunits (**Figure 6**) [4, 5], and it is activated through an allosteric effect of AMP and through phosphorylation of a threonine residue (at position 172) of the α subunit by AMPK kinases such as liver kinase B1 (LKB1) and Ca^{2+}- and calmodulin-dependent protein kinase (CaMKK) [4]. Furthermore, glucose deprivation directly activates AMPK via the glycolytic pathway [5, 44]. CaMKK is activated by an increase in the intracellular Ca^{2+} concentration induced by hormones or neurotransmitters, whereas LKB1 is activated by an increase in AMP levels and glucose deprivation. AMPK thus acts as a metabolic sensor that integrates multiple metabolic signals including hormones, neurotransmitters, nutrients, and energy charge.

Activation of AMPK suppresses 5′-adenosine triphosphate (ATP)-consuming anabolic pathways and activates ATP-producing catabolic pathways [4, 5]. For example, AMPK inhibits fatty acid synthesis, whereas it activates fatty acid oxidation. Activation of AMPK stimulates fatty acid oxidation, at least in part, by phosphorylation of acetyl coenzyme A (CoA) carboxylase (ACC), a decrease in the amount of malonyl-CoA, and activation of carnitine palmitoyltransferase 1 (CPT1) in mitochondria. We have previously shown that leptin increases fatty acid oxidation by activating AMPK in skeletal muscle both via the hypothalamus-sympathetic nervous system and through direct activation of the leptin receptor in skeletal muscle (**Figure 7**) [6].

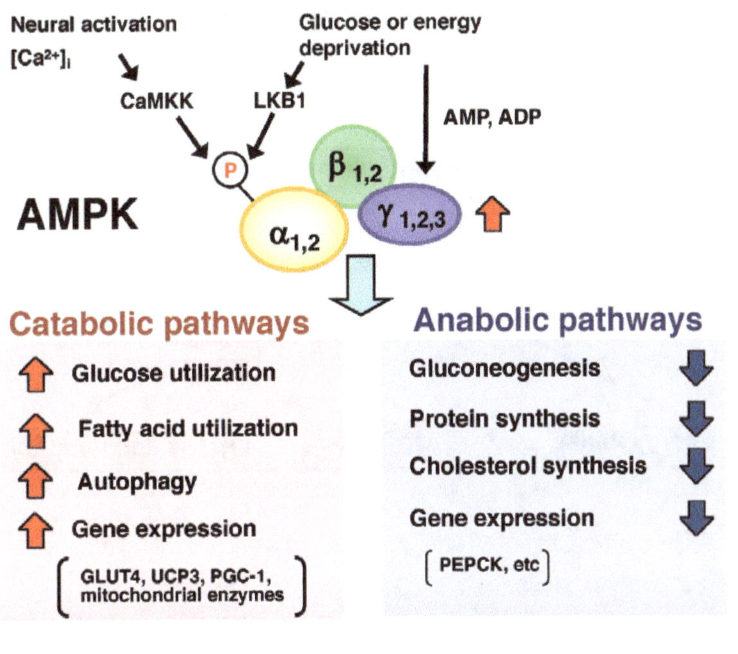

Figure 6.
Metabolic actions of AMPK. AMPK is a heterotrimeric protein consisting of an α (α1 or α2) catalytic subunit as well as β (β1 or β2) and γ (γ1 to γ3) regulatory subunits. It is activated by an allosteric effect of AMP on the γ subunit and through phosphorylation of the α subunit (at threonine-172) by AMPK kinases such as LKB1 and CaMKK. Activation of AMPK stimulates catabolic pathways and inhibits anabolic pathways of metabolism. Abbreviations not defined in text: ADP, 5′-adenosine diphosphate; GLUT4, glucose transporter 4; UCP3, uncoupling protein 3; PGC-1, peroxisome proliferator-activated receptor γ coactivator-1; PEPCK, phosphoenolpyruvate carboxykinase.

In addition to its metabolic actions in the periphery, AMPK in the hypothalamus regulates food intake [7, 44–49]. We found that leptin, glucose, a melanocortin receptor agonist or antagonist, and fasting-refeeding all reduced AMPK activity in several hypothalamic nuclei of mice [7]. A change in hypothalamic AMPK activity was sufficient to alter food intake and body weight (**Figure 7**). Other orexigenic and anorexigenic agents were also found to affect hypothalamic AMPK activity [45]. Downstream targets of AMPK, including ACC/malonyl-CoA and mammalian tar-get of rapamycin (mTOR) pathways, were also found to contribute to regulation of food intake [45]. Suppression of AMPK in the ARC is mediated by the phosphoryla-tion of AMPK via p70S6 kinase [46].

AMPK is necessary for activation of NPY/AgRP neurons in the ARC [47–50]. It is also necessary for activation of upstream neurons that activate NPY/AgRP neurons [51]. AMPK thus plays an important role in the activation of NPY/AgRP neurons and the regulation of food intake.

3.2 Regulation of carbohydrate selection by AMPK in the hypothalamus

3.2.1 Fasting increases carbohydrate preference in mice

Preferential consumption of high-fat foods among multiple palatable diets has increased worldwide and given rise to a high prevalence of metabolic syndrome, coronary heart disease, diabetes, and cancer [52]. The availability of highly palatable diets such as high-fat and high-sucrose diets promotes overfeeding in humans, with social stress often inducing "carbohydrate craving" [53, 54]. Although macronutrient components are associated with cardiometabolic health, aging, and longevity [55], the mechanisms for macronutrient intake have remained elusive.

The consumption of protein and essential amino acids is tightly controlled in animals. Previous studies revealed that forced feeding of animals with a low-protein diet increases total calorie intake, because of compensatory feeding for essential

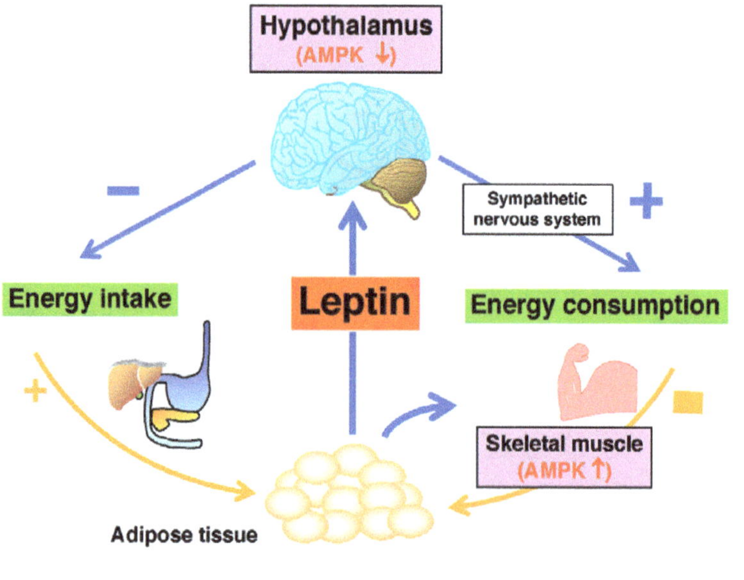

Figure 7.
Role of AMPK in leptin-induced suppression of feeding and activation of fatty acid oxidation in skeletal muscle. Leptin increases fatty acid oxidation in skeletal muscle through activation of AMPK both directly via the leptin receptor expressed in this tissue as well as indirectly through the hypothalamus-sympathetic nervous system. Leptin also inhibits food intake through suppression of AMPK in the hypothalamus.

amino acid intake [56]. In contrast, rodents reject diets that lack even a single essential amino acid [57]. They sense such a deficiency within the first hour of feeding [58–60], and this sensing of essential amino acids is independent of taste and smell [59, 61]. Although the regulation of essential amino acid intake had been thought to involve the action of the kinase GCN2 (general control nonderepressible 2) in the piriform cortex [58, 60], the mechanism remains unclear, given that GCN2 knockout mice were recently found to be still capable of sensing a deficiency of essential amino acids [62].

Selection of an HCD increases under certain physiological and pathological conditions [10, 63, 64]. In humans, carbohydrate craving is often induced by stressful life events and mood disturbances [53, 54]. Rodents increase selection of an HCD and reduce that of an HFD during 24-h refeeding after fasting [10]. Injection of NPY or dynorphin A into the brain of mice increases selection of carbohydrate and fat, respectively [64, 65]. Furthermore, pharmacological agents that induce gluco-privic cues promote carbohydrate intake [66]. Feeding with a low-carbohydrate diet also results in an increase in total calorie consumption as a compensatory response to maintain carbohydrate intake [56]. These observations suggest that animals including rodents as well as humans have a "carbohydrate-specific appetite" that increases carbohydrate intake over a basally preferable diet such as an HFD.

The regulation of macronutrient intake is relatively weaker than that of water intake in water-deprived animals [67]. Intake of carbohydrate versus fat is strongly influenced by the basal preference of animals and other factors [56]. Indeed, most natural sources of carbohydrate have little sweet taste, and most rodents choose a basally preferred HFD over an HCD. Therefore, macronutrient selection is affected by feeding paradigms. The presentation of a single diet (single-diet approach) often leads to the incorrect conclusions in studies of macronutrient selection [9]. This disadvantage is particularly important if the amount of a specific nutrient in the diet is suboptimal. The single-diet approach revealed that 24-h fasting increased intake of an HFD (and of total calories) to a greater extent than that of an HCD [10]. In contrast, when mice were presented with both a highly palatable HFD and HCD simultaneously in the two-diet choice approach during refeeding after a 24-h fast, they reduced their intake of the HFD and increased that of the HCD [10]. Total calorie intake did not change between that in the two-diet choice and single-diet approaches.

The increase in HFD and total calorie intake that was apparent during refeeding after fasting with the single-diet approach is likely due to a compensatory response to increase carbohydrate intake. We found that refeeding with the HCD alone after fasting rapidly decreased the plasma concentration of ketone bodies than that with the HFD alone [10]. Furthermore, when the fasted mice were pair-fed with the same number of calories of the HFD as they consumed when presented with the HCD, the plasma level of ketone bodies did not decrease. Plasma ketone body levels were then negatively correlated with the amount of carbohydrate intake in this experiment [10]. These results suggested that mice increase carbohydrate intake in the two-diet choice approach during refeeding after fasting as a means to rapidly improve whole body metabolism [68].

3.2.2 AMPK-regulated CRH neurons control carbohydrate selection

We recently showed that specific hypothalamic neurons increase selection of carbohydrate over fat in mice [10]. We thus found that a subset of CRH-positive neurons in the PVH that are regulated by AMPK regulate the selection of carbohydrate over a basally preferred HFD during refeeding for 24 h after food deprivation (**Figure 8**).

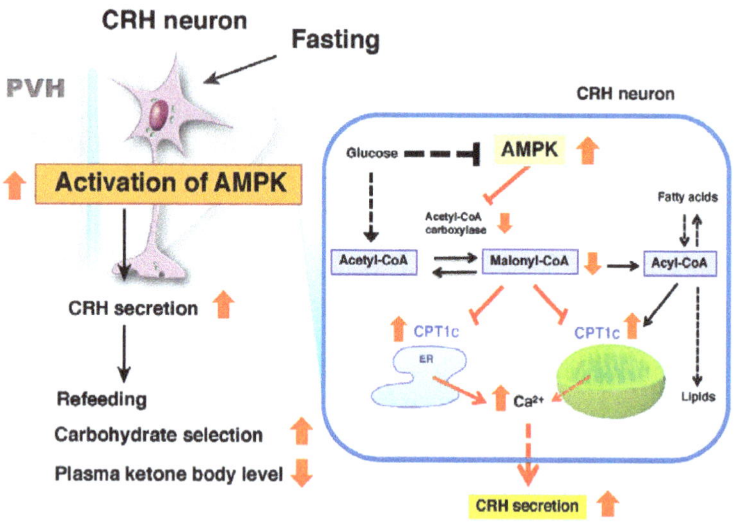

Figure8.
AMPK-regulated CRH neurons constitute a subpopulation of CRH neurons in the PVH that increases selection of an HCD over an HFD in a manner dependent on CPT1c. AMPK-regulated CRH neurons in the PVH are preferentially activated by fasting in a manner dependent on the AMPK-CPT1c axis. Activation of these neurons is sufficient and necessary for fasting-induced selection of an HCD over an HFD. The activated AMPK phosphorylates and thereby inhibits the activity of ACC, resulting in a reduction in the amount of malonyl-CoA and consequent increase in CPT1c activity. CPT1c, which is expressed in the ER and mitochondria, mediates an increase in the intracellular free Ca^{2+} concentration that results in neuronal activation and thereby promotes carbohydrate selection. Carbohydrate feeding after fasting results in a lowering of plasma ketone body levels.

As mentioned above (Section 3.1), AMPK in the ARC plays an important role in food intake. However, AMPK activity in the PVH was also found to change during fasting and refeeding in mice [7, 10]. The activation of AMPK in the PVH was suppressed by refeeding with lab chow or an HCD for 3 h. In contrast, sup-pression of AMPK activity in the PVH was small after refeeding with an HFD. Immunohistofluorescence analysis showed that 24 h-fasting increased the level of AMPK phosphorylation preferentially in CRH neurons present in the rostral region of the PVH, and it decreased after refeeding with lab chow or an HCD for 3 h [10]. These results suggested that AMPK activity in a subset of CRH neurons in the PVH is likely associated with carbohydrate feeding.

To examine the role of AMPK in PVH neurons in the regulation of food intake, we expressed an active (CA) form of the kinase [69] in PVH neurons of C57BL/6 J mice with the use of a lentivirus containing the synapsin gene promoter [10]. When the CA-AMPK mice were fed on lab chow, they increased body weight as a result of increased food intake. In contrast, when CA-AMPK mice were fed an HFD, they did not show hyperphagia or develop obesity. We performed a two-diet choice experiment with an HCD and an HFD that contained equal amounts of protein, micronutrients, and other constituents [10]. CA-AMPK mice chose the HCD, whereas control mice chose the HFD, with total calorie intake being similar for both groups of mice. Similar results were obtained with different combinations of diets derived from different nutrient sources. These observations suggested that AMPK in PVH neurons increases selection of an HCD over a basally preferable diet, such as an HFD.

We examined whether activation of AMPK in the PVH is necessary for the fasting-induced increase in HCD selection [10]. Decrease of AMPK expression in the PVH by expression of a short hairpin RNA (shRNA) specific for AMPK with the use of an adeno-associated virus suppressed the fasting-induced increase in

HCD selection and decrease in HFD selection in the two-diet choice approach. Intracerebroventricular (i.c.v.) injection of glucose, which inhibits AMPK activity in the PVH [7], also suppressed the fasting-induced increase in HCD selection without affecting total calorie intake. These results thus suggested that AMPK in the PVH is required for the fasting-induced increase in HCD selection.

We examined primarily responsible neurons in the PVH for regulation of selection between an HCD and an HFD by injecting various neuropeptides or cytokines that are expressed in the PVH into either the PVH or the lateral ventricle. Among the agents tested, injection of only CRH into the PVH increased selection of an HCD and reduced that of an HFD in the two-diet choice approach [10]. In contrast, injection of a CRH receptor 1 (corticotropin-releasing factor receptor 1, CRFR1) antagonist into the PVH suppressed the fasting-induced increase in HCD selection and decrease in HFD selection. CRFR1 is expressed at a high level in the PVH [70], and CRFR1-expressing neurons in this nucleus include glutamatergic and GABAergic neurons and do not express CRH, vasopressin, oxytocin, or TRH [70, 71]. CRFR1-expressing neurons in the PVH control brain areas that regulate food intake and sweet taste sensing [39, 68, 70, 72].

Suppression of CRH expression in the PVH with a specific shRNA inhibited the fasting-induced increase in HCD selection and decrease in HFD selection. Furthermore, it also blunted the effect of CA-AMPK expression in PVH neurons on HCD selection. Examination of the effects of activation and inhibition of CRH neurons in the PVH with the use of DREADD technology on selection between an HFD and an HCD in the two-diet choice approach also showed that these neurons are sufficient and necessary for the fasting-induced increase in carbohydrate selection [10].

Food selection has been reported to be affected by plasma corticosterone level [73]. We examined whether AMPK-regulated CRH neurons in the PVH might influ-ence HCD selection through change in plasma corticosterone level [10]. Expression of CA-AMPK in PVH neurons did not affect plasma corticosterone levels, although it increased selection of an HCD. In contrast, activation of CRH neurons in the PVH by DREADD technology increased the plasma corticosterone level, whereas inhibi-tion of these neurons by the same approach suppressed the fasting-induced increase in this parameter. Plasma corticosterone is thus unlikely to be a primary mediator of the change in food selection, although it might be necessary to control food intake [73]. AMPK-regulated CRH neurons in the rostral portion of the PVH appear to be distinct from the CRH neurons that regulate the hypothalamic-pituitary-adrenal axis.

CRH is known to be an anorexic neuropeptide. The i.c.v. injection of CRH thus attenuates total calorie intake in mice in the two-diet choice approach with an HCD and an HFD [10]. Activation of CRH neurons in the PVH with DREADD technology also decreased total calorie intake for the initial 3-h feeding but did not change after the 24-h feeding. In contrast, injection of CRH in the PVH did not change total calorie intake in mice in the two-diet choice approach. Thus, a subset of CRH neu-rons in the rostral part of the PVH that regulates CRFR1 neurons in the PVH may regulate selection of an HCD and an HFD, whereas another group of CRH neurons in this nucleus inhibits total calorie intake.

Diuretic hormone 44 (Dh44), the *Drosophila* ortholog of mammalian CRH, regulates the selection of nutritive sugars such as D-glucose, but not to that of nonnutritive sugars such as L-glucose [74]. Fasted wild-type flies initially choose the sweeter L-glucose before switching to D-glucose during refeeding in a two-diet choice paradigm. By contrast, Dh44 mutants choose the sweeter L-glucose but fail to increase the preference for D-glucose. Dh44 neurons do not regulate total consumption of food. Thus, CRH-dependent carbohydrate selection is likely conserved from insects to rodents.

We next examined whether AMPK and its downstream target CPT1c, the neuronal isoform of CPT1, in CRH neurons of the PVH regulate selection of an HCD versus an HFD in the two-diet choice approach [10]. Expression of CA-AMPK specifically in CRH neurons of the PVH was sufficient to increase selection of an HCD and reduce that of an HFD. In contrast, expression of shRNA specific for AMPK or for CPT1c in these neurons attenuated the fasting-induced increase in HCD selection. Expression of an shRNA specific for AMPK in CRH neurons also inhibited the increase in HCD selection induced by expression of CA-AMPK in the PVH. Furthermore, expression of an AMPK shRNA in these neurons also resulted in downregulation of the amount of CPT1c mRNA but not that of CPT1a mRNA in the PVH. AMPK had been shown to regulate the abundance of CPT1c mRNA [75]. These findings suggested that the AMPK-CPT1c axis in CRH neurons of the PVH is necessary for the fasting-induced increase in the selection of an HCD over an HFD (**Figure 8**).

CPT1c is localized to both the endoplasmic reticulum (ER) [76] and mitochondria [77], both of which contribute to intracellular Ca^{2+} signaling in a cooperative manner [78]. We found that the AMPK activator AICAR (5-aminoimidazole-4-carboxamide-1-β-D-ribofuranoside) increased the intracellular Ca^{2+} concentration in CRH neurons isolated from the PVH [10], and this effect was attenuated by the CPT1 inhibitor etomoxir. The shRNA-mediated depletion of AMPK or CPT1c in these neurons also blocked the Ca^{2+} response to AICAR, indicating that activation of the AMPK-CPT1c axis increases the intracellular Ca^{2+} concentration in CRH neurons of the PVH. These results suggested that activation of the AMPK-CPT1c system leads to increase synaptic activity in these neurons and in HCD selection by triggering an increase in intracellular Ca^{2+} concentration in CRH neurons. Activation of AMPK in these neurons inhibits ACC, decreases the abundance of malonyl-CoA and activates CPT1c. It also increases expression of the CPT1c gene (**Figure 8**).

AMPK activity is regulated by the glycolytic pathway as well as by cellular energy level (Section 3.1) [4, 5, 44]. Increased glucose levels in the brain inhibit AMPK activity in the PVH and ARC [7]. The i.c.v. injection of glucose in mice also inhibited the fasting-induced selection of an HCD in the two-diet choice approach [10]. The glucose-induced inhibition of AMPK may result in increased ACC activity, an increase in the amount of malonyl-CoA, and consequent inhibition of CPT1c activity in AMPK-regulated CRH neurons. The AMPK-CPT1c system may thus act as a glucose sensor in AMPK-regulated CRH neurons of the PVH.

4. Concluding remarks

Homeostatic regulation of feeding is essential for maintenance of total energy balance and whole-body metabolism. NPY/AgRP neurons and POMC neurons in the ARC are the most important neurons in the homeostatic regulation of feeding. New technologies have revealed that the activity of NPY/AgRP neurons changes in response to feeding and fasting. Of note, the activity of these neurons declines rapidly after the onset and before the completion of feeding behavior. Their activity also changes in response to the smell or anticipation of food. The neuronal activity thus appears to be correlated with food values. The evidence suggests that NPY/AgRP neurons are regulated by anticipatory stimuli related to food reward as well as by energy and nutrient levels in the body.

In addition to the regulation of total calorie intake, that of macronutrient intake appears to be important for maintenance of whole-body metabolism. We found that carbohydrate selection is increased in mice during refeeding after fasting and that this increase is associated with a rapid decrease in plasma ketone body levels. AMPK-regulated CRH neurons in the PVH are necessary and sufficient for this fasting-induced carbohydrate selection. CRH neurons are necessary for stress responses, and social stress can result in carbohydrate craving in humans. AMPK-regulated CRH neurons in the PVH may thus contribute to stress-induced carbohydrate craving. Identification of the neural circuits in which AMPK-regulated CRH neurons in the PVH of mice are embedded should shed new light on the physiological and molecular mechanisms responsible for macronutrient selection.

Acknowledgements

I thank all members of my lab who have contributed to the studies described in this review. The work was supported by a Grant-in-Aid for Scientific Research (B) (20H03736) from the Ministry of Education, Culture, Sports, Science, and Technology of Japan as well as by a grant from the Japan Agency for Medical Research and Development (JP19gm0610011h9906).

Author details

Yasuhiko Minokoshi[1,2]

1 Department of Homeostatic Regulation, Division of Endocrinology and Metabolism, National Institute for Physiological Sciences, Okazaki, Japan

2 Department of Physiological Sciences, School of Life Science, The Graduate University for Advanced Studies SOKENDAI, Okazaki, Japan

*Address all correspondence to: minokosh@nips.ac.jp

References

[1] Rossi MA, Stuber GD. Overlapping brain circuits for homeostatic and hedonic feeding. Cell Metabolism. 2018;**27**:42-56. DOI: 10.1016/j.cmet.2017.09.021

[2] Duerrschmid C, He Y, Wang C, Li C, Bournat JC, Romere C, et al. Asprosin is a centrally acting orexigenic hormone. Nature Medicine. 2017;**23**:1444-1453. DOI: 10.1038/nm.4432

[3] Mullican SE, Rangwala SM. Uniting GDF15 and GFRAL: Therapeutic opportunities in obesity and beyond. Trends in Endocrinology and Metabolism. 2018;**29**:560-570. DOI: 10.1016/j.tem.2018.05.002

[4] Hardie DG. AMPK--sensing energy while talking to other signaling pathways. Cell Metabolism. 2014;**20**:939-952. DOI: 10.1016/j.cmet.2014.09.013

[5] Lin SC, Hardie DG. AMPK: Sensing glucose as well as cellular energy status. Cell Metabolism. 2018;**27**:299-313. DOI: 10.1016/j.cmet.2017.10.009

[6] Minokoshi Y, Kim YB, Peroni OD, Fryer LGD, Müller C, Carling D, et al. Leptin stimulates fatty-acid oxidation by activating AMP-activated protein kinase. Nature. 2002;**415**:339-343. DOI: 10.1038/415339a

[7] Minokoshi Y, Alquier T, Furukawa N, Kim Y-B, Lee A, Xue B, et al. AMP-kinase regulates food intake by responding to hormonal and nutrient signals in the hypothalamus. Nature. 2004;**428**:569-574. DOI: 10.1038/nature02440

[8] Simpson SJ, Le Couteur DG, James DE, George J, Gunton JE, Solon-Biet SM, et al. The geometric framework for nutrition as a tool in precision medicine. The Journal of Nutrition, Health & Aging. 2017;**4**:217-226. DOI: 10.3233/NHA-170027

[9] Simpson SJ, Le Couteur DG, Raubenheimer D. Putting the balance in diet. Cell. 2015;**161**:18-23. DOI: 10.1016/j.cell.2015.02.033

[10] Okamoto S, Sato T, Tateyama M, Kageyama H, Maejima Y, Nakata M, et al. Activation of AMPK-regulated CRH neurons in the PVH is sufficient and necessary to induce dietary preference for carbohydrate over fat. Cell Reports. 2018;**22**:706-721. DOI: 10.1016/j.celrep.2017.11.102

[11] Andermann ML, Lowell BB. Toward a wiring diagram understanding of appetite control. Neuron. 2017;**95**:757-778. DOI: 10.1016/j.neuron.2017.06.014

[12] Balland E, Dam J, Langlet F, Caron E, Steculorum S, Messina A, et al. Hypothalamic tanycytes are an ERK-gated conduit for leptin into the brain. Cell Metabolism. 2014;**19**:293-301. DOI: 10.1016/j.cmet.2013.12.015

[13] Farooqi S, O'Rahilly S. Genetics of obesity in humans. Endocrine Reviews. 2006;**27**:710-718. DOI: 10.1210/er.2006-0040

[14] Luquet S, Perez FA, Hnasko TS, Palmiter RD. NPY/AgRP neurons are essential for feeding in adult mice but can be ablated in neonates. Science. 2005;**10**:683-685. DOI: 10.1126/science.1115524

[15] Luo SX, Huang J, Li Q, Mohammad H, Lee C-Y, Krishna K, et al. Regulation of feeding by somatostatin neurons in the tuberal nucleus. Science. 2018;**361**:76-81. DOI: 10.1126/science.aar4983

[16] Zhang X, van den Pol AN. Rapid binge-like eating and body weight gain

driven by zona incerta GABA neuron activation. Science. 2017;**356**:853-859. DOI: 10.1126/science.aam7100

[17] Chen Y, Lin YC, Kuo TW, Knight ZA. Sensory detection of food rapidly modulates arcuate feeding circuits. Cell. 2015;**160**:829-841. DOI: 10.1016/j.cell.2015.01.033

[18] Beutler LR, Chen Y, Ahn JS, Lin Y-C, Essner RA, Knight ZA. Dynamics of gut-brain communication underlying hunger. Neuron. 2017;**96**:461-475. DOI: 10.1016/j.neuron.2017.09.043

[19] Chen Y, Lin Y-C, Zimmerman CA, Essner RA, Knight ZA. Hunger neurons drive feeding through a sustained, positive reinforcement signal. eLife. 2016;**5**:e18640. DOI: 10.7554/eLife.18640

[20] Betley JN, Xu S, Cao ZFH, Rong Gong R, Magnus CJ, Yu Y, et al. Neurons for hunger and thirst transmit a negative-valence teaching signal. Nature. 2015;**521**:180-185. DOI: 10.1038/nature14416

[21] Kim KS, Seeley RJ, Sandoval DA. Signalling from the periphery to the brain that regulates energy homeostasis. Nature Reviews. Neuroscience. 2018;**19**:185-196. DOI: 10.1038/nrn.2018.8

[22] Yanagi S, Sato T, Kangawa K, Nakazato M. The homeostatic force of ghrelin. Cell Metabolism. 2018;**27**:786-804. DOI: 10.1016/j.cmet.2018.02.008

[23] Schwartz MW, Woods SC, Porte D Jr, Seeley RJ, Baskin DG. Central nervous system control of food intake. Nature. 2000;**404**:661-671. DOI: 10.1038/35007534

[24] Xu J, Bartolome CL, Low CS, Xinchi Yi X, Chien C-H, Wang P, et al. Genetic identification of leptin neural circuits in energy and glucose homeostases. Nature. 2018;**556**:505-509. DOI: 10.1038/s41586-018-0049-7

[25] Fiorenza CG, Chou SH, Mantzoros CS. Lipodystrophy: Pathophysiology and advances in treatment. Nature Reviews. Endocrinology. 2011;**7**:137-150. DOI: 10.1038/nrendo.2010.199

[26] Aotani D, Ebihara K, Sawamoto N, Kusakabe T, Aizawa-Abe M, Kataoka S, et al. Functional magnetic resonance imaging analysis of food-related brain activity in patients with lipodystrophy undergoing leptin replacement therapy. The Journal of Clinical Endocrinology and Metabolism. 2012;**97**:3663-3671. DOI: 10.1210/jc.2012-1872

[27] Romere C, Duerrschmid C, Bournat J, Constable P, Jain M, Xia F, et al. Asprosin, a fasting-induced glucogenic protein hormone. Cell. 2016;**165**:566-579. DOI: 10.1016/j. cell.2016.02.063

[28] Betley JN, Cao ZF, Ritola KD, Sternson SM. Parallel, redundant circuit organization for homeostatic control of feeding behavior. Cell. 2013;**155**:1337-1350. DOI: 10.1016/j.cell.2013.11.002

[29] Wu Q , Clark MS, Palmiter RD. Deciphering a neuronal circuit that mediates appetite. Nature. 2012;**483**:594-597. DOI: 10.1038/nature10899

[30] Garfield AS, Li C, Madara JC, Shah BP, Webber E, Steger JS, et al. A neural basis for melanocortin-4 receptor-regulated appetite. Nature Neuroscience. 2015;**18**:863-781. DOI: 10.1038/nn.4011

[31] Atasoy D, Betley JN, Su HH, Sternson SM. Deconstruction of a neural circuit for hunger. Nature. 2012;**488**:172-177. DOI: 10.1038/nature11270

[32] Chia Li C, Navarrete J, Liang-Guallpa J, Lu C, Funderburk SC, Chang RB, et al. Defined Paraventricular hypothalamic populations exhibit differential responses to food contingent

on caloric state. Cell Metabolism. 2019;**29**:681-694. DOI: 10.1016/j.cmet.2018.10.016

[33] Coutinho EA, Okamoto S, Ishikawa AW, Shigefumi Yokota S, Wada N, Hirabayashi T, et al. Activation of SF1 neurons in the ventromedial hypothalamus by DREADD technology increases insulin sensitivity in peripheral tissues. Diabetes. 2017;**66**:2372-2386. DOI: 10.2337/db16-1344

[34] Minokoshi Y, Haque MS, Shimazu T. Microinjection of leptin into the ventromedial hypothalamus increases glucose uptake in peripheral tissues in rats. Diabetes. 1999;**48**:287- 291. DOI: 10.2337/diabetes.48.2.287

[35] Toda C, Shiuchi T, Lee S, Yamato-Esaki M, Fujino Y, Suzuki A, et al. Distinct effects of leptin and a melanocortin receptor agonist injected into medial hypothalamic nuclei on glucose uptake in peripheral tissues. Diabetes. 2009;**58**:2757-2765. DOI: 10.2337/db09-0638

[36] Shiuchi T, Haque MS, Okamoto S, Inoue T, Kageyama H, Lee S, et al. Hypothalamic orexin stimulates feeding-associated glucose utilization in skeletal muscle via sympathetic nervous system. Cell Metabolism. 2009;**10**:466-480. DOI: 10.1016/j.cmet.2009.09.013

[37] Suber GD, Wise RA. Lateral hypothalamic circuits for feeding and reward. Nature Neuroscience. 2016;**19**:198-205. DOI: 10.1038/nn.4220

[38] Sakurai T. The role of orexin in motivated behaviours. Nature Reviews. Neuroscience. 2014;**15**:719-731. DOI: 10.1038/nrn3837

[39] Fu O, Iwai Y, Narukawa M, Ishikawa AW, Ishii KK, Murata K, et al. Hypothalamic neuronal circuits regulating hunger-induced taste modification. Nature Communications. 2019;**10**:4560. DOI: 10.1038/s41467-019-12478-x

[40] Campos CA, Bowen AJ, Roman CW, Palmiter RD. Encoding of danger by parabrachial CGRP neurons. Nature. 2018;**555**:617-622. DOI: 10.1038/nature25511

[41] Palmiter RD. The Parabrachial nucleus: CGRP neurons function as a general alarm. Trends in Neurosciences. 2018;**41**:280-293. DOI: 10.1016/j.tins.2018.03.007

[42] Cheng W, Gonzalez I, Pan W, Tsang AH, Adams J, Ndoka E, et al. Calcitonin receptor neurons in the mouse nucleus tractus solitarius control energy balance via the non-aversive suppression of feeding. Cell Metabolism. 2020;**31**:301-312. DOI: 10.1016/j.cmet.2019.12.012

[43] Sternson SM, Shepherd GM, Friedman JM. Topographic mapping of VMH --> arcuate nucleus microcircuits and their reorganization by fasting. Nature Neuroscience. 2005;**8**:1356-1363. DOI: 10.1038/nn1550

[44] Zhang CS, Hawley SA, Zong Y, Li M, Wang Z, Gray A, et al. Fructose-1,6-bisphosphate and aldolase mediate glucose sensing by AMPK. Nature. 2017;**548**:112-116. DOI: 10.1038/nature23275

[45] Xue B, Kahn BB. AMPK integrates nutrient and hormonal signals to regulate food intake and energy balance through effects in the hypothalamus and peripheral tissues. The Journal of Physiology. 2006;**574**:73-83. DOI: 10.1113/jphysiol.2006.113217

[46] Dagon Y, Hur E, Zheng B, Wellenstein K, Cantley LC, Kahn BB. p70S6 kinase phosphorylates AMPK on serine 491 to mediate leptin's effect on food intake. Cell Metabolism. 2012;**16**:104-112. DOI: 10.1016/j.cmet.2012.05.010

[47] Claret M, Smith MA, Batterham RL, Selman C, Choudhury AI, Fryer LGD, et al. AMPK is essential for energy homeostasis regulation and glucose sensing by POMC and AgRP neurons. The Journal of Clinical Investigation. 2007;**117**:2325-2336. DOI: 10.1172/JCI31516

[48] Andrews ZB, Liu ZW, Walllingford N, Erion DM, Borok E, Friedman JM, et al. UCP2 mediates ghrelin's action on NPY/AgRP neurons by lowering free radicals. Nature. 2008;**454**:846-851. DOI: 10.1038/nature07181

[49] Kong D, Dagon Y, Campbell JN, Guo Y, Yang Z, Yi X, et al. A postsynaptic AMPK→p21-activated kinase pathway drives fasting-induced synaptic plasticity in AgRP neurons. Neuron. 2016;**91**:25-33. DOI: 10.1016/j.neuron.2016.05.025

[50] Kohno D, Sone H, Minokoshi Y, Yada T. Ghrelin raises [Ca2+]i via AMPK in hypothalamic arcuate nucleus NPY neurons. Biochemical and Biophysical Research Communications. 2008;**366**:388-392. DOI: 10.1016/j.bbrc.2007.11.166

[51] Yang Y, Atasoy D, Su HH, Sternson SM. Hunger states switch a flip-flop memory circuit via a synaptic AMPK-dependent positive feedback loop. Cell. 2011;**146**:992-1003. DOI: 10.1016/j.cell.2011.07.039

[52] Mann JI. Diet and risk of coronary heart disease and type 2 diabetes. Lancet. 2002;**360**:783-789. DOI: 10.1016/s0140-6736(02)09901-4

[53] Roberts CJ, Campbell IC, Troop N. Increases in weight during chronic stress are partially associated with a switch in food choice towards increased carbohydrate and saturated fat intake. European Eating Disorders Review. 2014;**22**:77-82. DOI: 10.1002/erv.2264

[54] Rutters F, Nieuwenhuizen AG, Lemmens SG, Born JM, Westerterp-Plantenga MS. Acute stress-related changes in eating in the absence of hunger. Obesity. 2009;**17**:72-77. DOI: 10.1038/oby.2008.493

[55] Solon-Biet SM, McMahon AC, Ballard JW, Ruohonen K, Wu LE, Cogger VC, et al. The ratio of macronutrients, not caloric intake, dictates cardiometabolic health, aging, and longevity in ad libitum-fed mice. Cell Metabolism. 2014;**19**:418-430. DOI: 10.1016/j.cmet.2014.02.009

[56] Simpson SJ, Raubenheimer D. Geometric models of macronutrient selection. In: Berthoud HR, Seeley RJ, editors. Neural and Metabolic Control of Macronutrient Intake. New York: CRC Press; 2000. pp. 29-42

[57] Leung PM, Rogers QR, Harper AE. Effect of amino acid imbalance in rats fed ad libitum, interval-fed or force-fed. The Journal of Nutrition. 1968;**95**:474-482. DOI: 10.1093/jn/95.3.474

[58] Hao S, Sharp JW, Ross-Inta CM, McDaniel BJ, Anthony TG, Wek RC, et al. Uncharged tRNA and sensing of amino acid deficiency in mammalian piriform cortex. Science. 2005;**307**:1776-1778. DOI: 10.1126/science.1104882

[59] Koehnle TJ, Russell MC, Gietzen DW. Rats rapidly reject diets deficient in essential amino acids. The Journal of Nutrition. 2003;**133**:2331- 2335. DOI: 10.1093/jn/133.7.2331

[60] Maurin AC, Jousse C, Averous J, Parry L, Bruhat A, Cherasse Y, et al. The GCN2 kinase biases feeding behavior to maintain amino acid homeostasis in omnivores. Cell Metabolism. 2005;**1**:273-277. DOI: 10.1016/j.cmet.2005.03.004

[61] Leung PM, Larson DM, Rogers QR. Food intake and preference of olfactory

bulbectomized rats fed amino acid imbalanced or deficient diets. Physiology & Behavior. 1972;**9**:553-557. DOI: 10.1016/0031-9384(72)90011-x

[62] Leib DE, Knight ZA. Re-examination of dietary amino acid sensing reveals a GCN2-independent mechanism. Cell Reports. 2015;**13**:1081-1089. DOI: 10.1016/j.celrep.2015.09.055

[63] Hunsicker KD, Mullen BJ, Martin RJ. Effect of starvation or restriction on self-selection of macronutrients in rats. Physiology & Behavior. 1992;**51**:325-330. DOI: 10.1016/0031-9384(92)90148-u

[64] Welch CC, Grace MK, Bilington CJ, Levine AS. Preference and diet type affect macronutrient selection after morphine, NPY, norepinephrine, and deprivation. American Journal of Physiology. Regulatory, Integrative and Comparative Physiology. 1994;**35**:R426-R433. DOI: 10.1152/ajpregu.1994.266.2.R426

[65] Leibowitz SF. Macronutrients and brain peptides: What they do and how they respond. In: Berthoud HR, Seeley RJ, editors. Neural and Metabolic Control of Macronutrient Intake. New York: CRC Press; 2000. pp. 389-406

[66] Ritter S, Koegler FH, Wiater M. Effects of metabolic blockade on macronutrient selection. In: Berthoud HR, Seeley RJ, editors. Neural and Metabolic Control of Macronutrient Intake. New York: CRC Press; 2000. pp. 189-202

[67] Seeley DJ, Berthoud HR. Neural and metabolic control of macronutrient selection: Consensus and controversy. In: Berthoud HR, Seeley RJ, editors. Neural and Metabolic Control of Macronutrient Intake. New York: CRC Press; 2000. pp. 489-496

[68] Minokoshi Y, Nakajima KI, Okamoto S. Homeostatic versus hedonic control of carbohydrate selection. Journal of Physiology; 2020. DOI: 10.1113/JP280066

[69] Woods A, Azzout-Marniche D, Foretz M, Stein S, Lemarchand P, Ferré P, et al. Characterization of the role of AMP-activated protein kinase in the regulation of glucose-activated gene expression using constitutively active and dominant negative forms of the kinase. Molecular and Cellular Biology. 2000;**20**:6704-6711. DOI: 10.1128/mcb.20.18.6704-6711.2000

[70] Ramot A, Jiang Z, Tian JB, Nahum T, Kuperman Y, Justice N, et al. Hypothalamic CRFR1 is essential for HPA axis regulation following chronic stress. Nature Neuroscience. 2017;**20**:385-388. DOI: 10.1038/nn.4491

[71] Jiang Z, Rajamanickam S, Justice NJ. Local corticotropin-releasing factor signaling in the hypothalamic paraventricular nucleus. The Journal of Neuroscience. 2018;**38**:1874-1890. DOI: 10.1523/JNEUROSCI.1492-17.2017

[72] Fu O, Iwai Y, Kondoh K, Misaka T, Minokoshi Y, Nakajima KI. SatB2-expressing neurons in the parabrachial nucleus encode sweet taste. Cell Reports. 2019;**27**:1650-1656.e4. DOI: 10.1016/j.celrep.2019.04.040

[73] Tempel DL, Leibowitz SF. Adrenal steroid receptors: Interactions with brain neuropeptide systems in relation to nutrient intake and metabolism. Journal of Neuroendocrinology. 1994;**6**:479-501. DOI: 10.1111/j.1365-2826.1994.tb00611.x

[74] Dus M, Lai JS, Gunapala KM, Min S, Tayler TD, Hergarden AC, et al. Nutrient sensor in the brain directs the action of the brain-gut axis in drosophila. Neuron. 2015;**87**:139-151. DOI: 10.1016/j.neuron.2015.05.032

[75] Zaugg K, Yao Y, Reilly PT, Kannan K, Kiarash R, Mason J, et al.

Carnitine palmitoyltransferase 1C promotes cell survival and tumor growth under conditions of metabolic stress. Genes & Development. 2011;**25**:1041-1051. DOI: 10.1101/gad.1987211

[76] Sierra AY, Gratacés E, Carrasco P, Clotet J, Ureña J, Serra D, et al. CPT1c is localized in endoplasmic reticulum of neurons and has carnitine palmitoyltransferase activity. The Journal of Biological Chemistry. 2008;**283**:6878-6885. DOI: 10.1074/jbc. M707965200

[77] Dai Y, Wolfgang MJ, Cha SH, Lane MD. Localization and effect of ectopic expression of CPT1c in CNS feeding centers. Biochemical and Biophysical Research Communications. 2007;**359**:469-474. DOI: 10.1016/j.bbrc.2007.05.161

[78] Pizzo P, Pozzan T. Mitochondria-endoplasmic reticulum choreography: Structure and signaling dynamics. Trends in Cell Biology. 2007;**17**:511-517. DOI: 10.1016/j.tcb.2007.07.011

4

Significance of Trans Fatty Acids and Omega-3 Fatty Acids in Japanese Men with Coronary Heart Disease

Shinji Koba, Tetsuya Takao, Fumiko Shimizu, Mutsumi Ogawa, Yuuya Yokota, Fumiyoshi Tsunoda, Ken Arai, Toshiro Shinke and Akikazu Takada

Abstract

Trans fatty acids (TFA) are found naturally in ruminant foods (R-TFA) by biohydrogenation in ruminant animals or industrially produced oils (IP-TFA) by partial hydrogenation of vegetable or fish oils. The intake of TFA mainly IP-TFA is associated with an elevated risk of coronary heart disease (CHD), while some prospective cohort studies showed that R-TFA were associated with a lower risk for sudden cardiac death (SCD). Our case-control study showed that *trans*-C18:2 isomers (IP-TFA) were significantly higher, and palmitelaidic acid (R-TFA) levels were lower in patients with acute coronary syndrome (ACS) compared with healthy men. Eicosapentaenoic acid (EPA) and docosahexaenoic acid (DHA) have different effects on cardiometabolic risk factors. Delta-5 desaturase (D5D) is a key enzyme in the conversion of linoleic acid and alpha-linoleneic acid to arachidonic acid (AA) and EPA, respectively. Previous studies reported that low D5D estimated from the ratio of AA to dihomo-gamma linolenic acid predicts the incident cardiovascular disease. In our cross-sectional study with 436 men with ACS, various atherogenic lipid markers such as small dense LDL cholesterol and malondialdehyde-modified LDL were significantly inversely associated with D5D activity. We found that the EPA/AA may be a superior risk marker than DHA/AA in terms of correlation with atherogenic lipid profiles.

Keywords: trans fatty acid, omega-3 fatty acids, delta-5 desaturase, coronary heart disease

1. Introduction

Fatty acids (FA) are biologically -active molecules with a wide array of effects [1]. FA are classified as saturated or unsaturated on the basis of the absence or presence of double bonds. Monounsaturated FA (MUFA) have one double bond; polyunsaturated FA (PUFA) have more than one double bond. UFA usually occur in the *cis* configuration, and *trans* FA (TFA) are UFA containing at least one double bond in the*trans* configuration. FA status can be expressed as composition (each as a percent of total) or as concentration (mass/volume or cell count). PUFA with double bonds starting from the sixth position from the methyl end of FA are termed as omega-6 series and those from the third position as omega-3 series. Both omega-3 and omega-6 long-chain PUFA are particularly important in humans in order to maintain the function of brain and central nervous system. These PUFA are incorporated into the cell membrane. Numerous studies have demonstrated that, eicosapentaenoic acid (EPA) and docosahexaenoic acid (DHA), omega-3 PUFA which are present in fish oils, protect against coronary heart disease (CHD) [2]. Harris and von Schacky proposed a metric called the "Omega-3 index," which is the content of EPA + DHA in red blood cell (RBC) membranes (expressed as a weight percent of total FA) as a risk factor for death from CHD and especially sudden cardiac death (SCD) [3]. The Omega-3 index is highly responsive to changes in EPA + DHA intake and the levels in RBCs reflect those of other tissues [4]. The Omega-3 index has been used in multiple observational cohort and interventional studies around the world. It has been associated with the lower risk for CHD, SCD, acute coronary syndromes (ACS), all-cause mortality, and other health conditions such as impaired cognitive function, depression, aggressive behaviors, and bipolar disease [4]. EPA and DHA are usually considered as good friends for cardiovascular health, whereas arachidonic acid (AA), omega-6 PUFA, is the most important substrate for the synthesis of the strongest pro-inflammatory eicosanoids. However, in recent years, the complex biochemistry of the eicosanoids, docosanoids, and octadecanoids has become clearer, with some omega-6 PUFA metabolites being pro- and others anti-inflammatory [5, 6]. According to a meta-analysis of prospective cohort studies investigating plasma FA (palmitic, oleic, EPA, DHA, and AA) and CHD outcome, relative risk and 95% of confidence interval (CI) for CHD for these five FAs was, respectively, 1.15 (CI 0.96–1.37), 1.09 (CI 0.97–1.23), 0.78 (CI 0.65–0.94), 0.79 (CI 0.67–0.93), and 0.83 (CI 0.74–0.92), which suggest the statistically significant protective associations with EPA, DHA, and AA [7].

TFA can be found naturally in ruminant foods (R-TFA) by biohydrogenation in ruminant animals or industrially produced oils (IP-TFA) by partial hydrogenation of vegetable or fish oils. TFA were, initially, considered as safe, and partially hydrogenated oils (PHO) were responsible for high intakes in the 1970s to 1980s, when margarines were advocated over butter to reduce SFA intakes [8]. PHO are contained in hard margarine, fatty spreads, and vegetable shortening, deep-fried food, refined vegetable oils such as salad oil, and confectionery made using these products [9]. Since the early 1990s, however, numerous studies have suggested that high TFA intakes may be associated with CHD [10]. Cohort studies and their meta-analyses provide concordant evidence that the intake of TFA mainly IP-TFA is associated with the elevated risk of CHD [9]. In this chapter, we would like to focus on the role of TFA and omega-3 PUFA with special relation on their effects on blood lipids and CHD.

2. IP-TFA and RP-TFA on human health

There is a considerable overlap of TFA in IP-TFA and R-TFA (**Figure 1**) [11]. For fatty acids with 18 carbon atoms, a peak concentration of trans double bonds in IP-TFA is found in position 9, as elaidic acid, while a distinct preference for the double bond in R-TFA is in position 11.

Numerous studies have suggested that IP-TFA increase LDL cholesterol (LDL-C) and lipoprotein (a) [Lp(a)], which is a lipoprotein that promotes atherosclerosis and decrease HDL cholesterol (HDL-C), compared with other FA, whereas the effect on triglyceride is inconsistent [9, 12]. However, the threshold of effects of

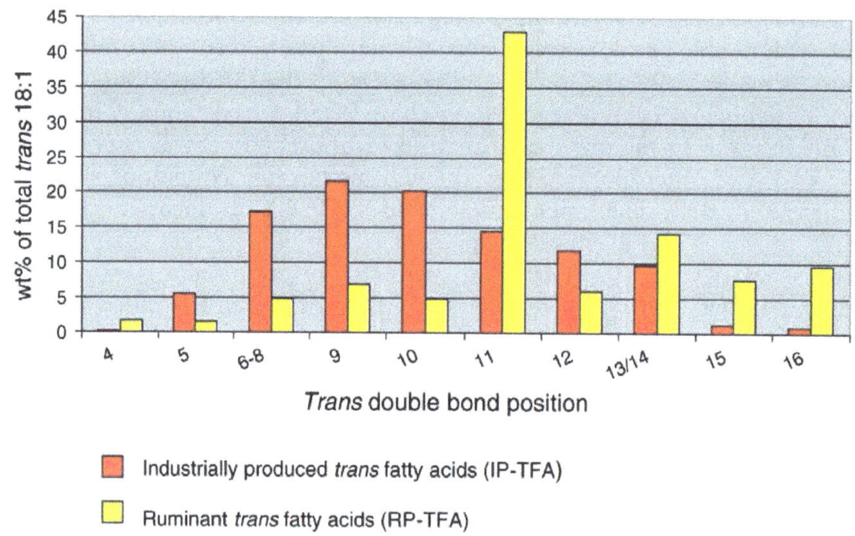

Figure 1.
Isomeric distribution of trans-octadecenoic acids in industrially produced and ruminant trans fatty acids (mean wt% of trans-18:1 fatty acids) adapted from [11].

TFA may exist in the relationship between TFA and lipid levels, and direct evidence of the dose-response relations were not observed from clinical trials when the dietary intake of TFAs was as low as <3%E [9, 10]. The consumption of TFA is cur-rently decreasing in many countries. The average daily TFA intake of the Japanese is 0.92–0.96 g, or 0.44–0.47%E, which is lower than the <1% target recommended by the World Health Organization [9].

The Seven Countries Study (United States (US), Finland, the Netherlands, Italy, Yugoslavia, Greece, and Japan) that was initiated in 1958 was the first to show true differences in prevalence, incidence, and mortality for CHD among populations with different geographical, ethnic, and cultural characteristics. The study reported that the intake of elaidic acids, the major IP-TFA, was strongly associated with the intake of SFA, serum levels of total cholesterol, and 25-year CHD mortality rates [13]. The cross-sectional study of Japanese patients undergoing coronary angiog-raphy (CAG) that was conducted from 2008 to 2012 failed to show the differences in levels of elaidic acid and linoelaidic acids (the two major IP-TFA, although the latter can be formed by frying in nonhydrogenated vegetable oils [14]) between patients with and without CHD [15]. They showed significantly higher elaidic acid levels in younger patients with CHD (≤66 years) compared with elder CHD patients and/or patients with metabolic syndrome compared with patients without metabolic syndrome [15]. Their group also reported that serum levels of elaidic acids were significantly higher in CHD patients with vulnerable plaque evaluated by optical coherence tomography compared with those without it (12.9 ± 4.9 vs. 10.3 ± 4.3 μmol/L, respectively, p = 0.001) [16]. Our case-control study with 66 male patients with ACS and 49 healthy men, which was conducted from 2013 to 2014, has reported that total FA and TFA levels were similar between ACS and control subjects [17]. Palmitelaidic acid, R-TFA, levels were lower in ACS patients, especially in middle-aged ACS patients (0.17 ± 0.06 vs. 0.20 ± 0.06 of total FA, in ACS and control, respectively, $p < 0.01$) (**Figure 2**). Both proportional and absolute concentrations of palmitelaidic acid were significantly directly associated with HDL-C (rho = 0.269 and rho = 0.216, respectively), EPA + DHA (rho = 0.458 and rho = 0.620, respectively), and EPA + DHA/AA ratios (rho = 0.474 and rho = 0.475, respectively). Linoleic *trans* isomers (total C18:2 TFA), (IP- or frying-derived TFA)

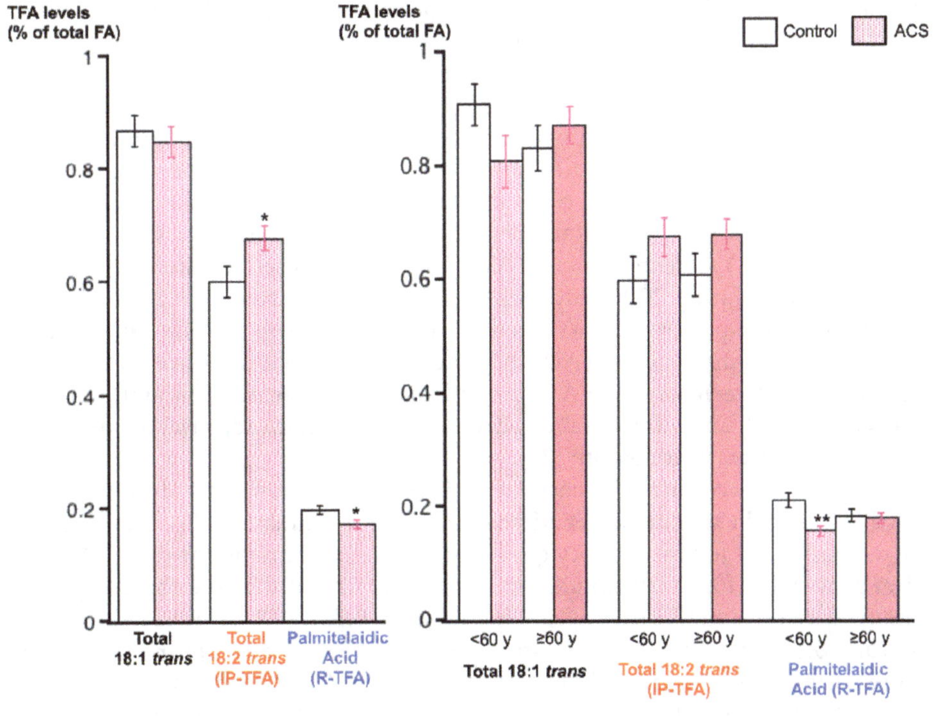

Figure 2.
*The comparison of trans fatty acids (TFA) between control and ACS patients. Left panel: comparison in whole subjects and Right panel: comparison separated by age. Data are expressed as mean ± standard error (SE), and the error bar represents SE. The number of subjects is 49 (<60 years 24; ≥60 years 25) in control and 67 (<60 years 25; ≥60 years 42) in ACS. *P < 0.05, **p < 0.01 vs. control. Figure was made by Ref. [17].*

were significantly higher in ACS patients (0.68 ± 0.17 vs. 0.60 ± 0.20 of total FA, in ACS and control, respectively) (**Figure 2**). Absolute concentration of *trans*-C18:2 isomers were significantly directly associated with LDL-C and non-HDL-C in ACS men. In conclusion of our case-control study, total *trans*-C18:1 isomers were comparable between ACS and control [17]. Differences between ACS and controls in C18:1 trans varied by specific C18:1 trans species [17]. Palmitelaidic acid (R-TFA) was lower in ACS patients, especially in middle-aged patients. Palmitelaidic acid was significantly directly associated with HDL-C, EPA + DHA, and EPA + DHA/AA ratios [17]. Linoleic trans isomers (IP-TFAs) were higher in ACS.

The Nurses' Health Study was initiated in 1976 and enrolled 121,799 female registered nurses aged 30–55 years in the United States. TFA content in RBC membrane was measured in 32,826 women from 1989 to 1990. During 6 years of follow-up, 166 incident cases of CHD were ascertained and matched with 327 controls. TFA in RBC membrane was significantly correlated with dietary intake of TFA (correla-tion coefficient = 0.44, p < 0.01). Increases in total TFA, *trans*-C18:1 isomers, and *trans*-C18:2 isomers in RBC membrane were significantly associated with CHD after adjustment of covariates [18]. In the Cardiovascular Health Study, a prospective cohort of older US adults (≥65 years), plasma phospholipid TFA was measured in 5888 men and women from 1992 to 1993. Plasma TFA was compared between 214 cases of fatal CHD and 214 matched controls. Neither plasma *trans*-C18:1 isomers nor palmitelaidic acids but linoelaidic acid (*trans*-C18:2 isomers) were significantly associated with fatal CHD [19]. During 31,494 person-years, 1735 total deaths and 639 fatal and nonfatal CHD events occurred. Neither plasma *trans*-C18:1 isomers nor palmitelaidic acids but linoelaidic acid (*trans*-C18:2 isomers) were significantly associated with total mortality mainly due to the cardiovascular disease (CVD) and increased risk of CHD [20]. Lemaitre et al. measured TFA in RBC membrane in 179 married cases of out-of-hospital primary cardiac arrest between the ages of 25 and 74 years, from 1998 to 1999, and 285 age- and sex-matched controls from the population-based study [21]. Not *trans*-C18:1 isomers but linoelaidic acid (*trans*-C18:2 isomers) were associated with three-fold increase in risk of primary cardiac arrest after adjustment for medical and lifestyle risk factors (odds ratio for inter-quintile range, 3.1; 95% CI: 1.7–5.4). In the Bergen Coronary Angiography Cohort (BECAC), serum TFA (palmitelaidic acid, an R-TFA; and *trans* C18:1 isomers; primarily IP-TFA) were measured in 1367 Norwegian patients underwent CAG for suspected CHD during 2000–2001 who were followed throughout 2006 [22]. The serum TFA was positively correlated with plasma levels of the NO inhibitor asymmetric dimethylarginine (ADMA). They reported that there are no significant associations between serum TFA and incident acute myocardial infarction (AMI), death from CVD, and all-cause mortality after multivariate adjustments during the median of 5.8 years of follow-up [22].

Lemaitre et al. confirmed a correlation between TFA content (C16:1, C18:1, and C18:2 isomers) in subcutaneous adipose tissue and estimated TFA intake using a self-administered food frequency questionnaire in 51 adult volunteers in 1996 [23]. After adjustment for energy intake, age, and body mass index, the correlation coefficients between total TFA and TFA intake were 0.76 (95% CI: 0.51–0.89) among men and 0.52 (95% CI: 0.17–0.75) among women [23]. A case-control study in the United Kingdom compared TFA (*trans*-C18:1 and C18:2 isomers) in abdominal adipose tissue obtained by necropsy from 66 cases of SCD due to the first episode of CHD ages of <65 years from 1990 to 1991 and by biopsy from 286 healthy age- and sex-matched controls [24]. Not linoelaidic acid (*trans*-C18:2 isomers) but *trans*-oleic acid (*trans*-C18:1 isomers) were unexpectedly inversely associated with SCD. In an international multicenter study in eight European countries and Israel (EURAMIC), adipose tissue aspiration samples were obtained from 671 men with AMI, aged of ≤70 years, and 717 men without a history of AMI as control from 1991 to 1992. The *trans*-oleic acid (*trans*-C18:1 isomers) were similar between AMI and controls [25]. A case-control study in Norway compared subcutaneous adipose tissue TFA between 100 patients with the first episode of AMI and 98 population controls, both men and postmenopausal women aged between 45 and 75 years [26]. TFA mainly *trans*-oleic acid (*trans*-C18:1 isomers) was significantly higher in AMI than those in control [26]. A case-control study in Costa Rican population com-pared adipose tissue TFA between 482 cases aged <75 years with the first episode of nonfatal AMI during 1994 and 482 population controls adjusted for sex, age, and area of residence [27]. Not *trans*-C18:1 isomers but high *trans*-C18:2 isomers were significantly associated with the increased risk of nonfatal AMI [27]. We found that not *trans*-C18:1 isomers but *trans*-C18:2 isomers (IP-TFA) were associated with the increased risk of ACS even in Japan [17] that was in good agreement with previous reports [18–21, 27].

A 2010 survey of the Hawaii-Los Angeles-Hiroshima Study reported that serum elaidic acid concentrations in the native Japanese living in Hiroshima were significantly lower than those in the Japanese-Americans living in Los Angeles [28]. The study reported a significant association between serum levels of elaidic acid and insulin resistance or diabetes among native Japanese [28]. Similarly, our study with Japanese and American older men (> age 50) showed that Japanese men had markedly lower levels of elaidic and linoelaidic acids (IP-TFA) while significantly higher levels of palmitelaidic acids (R-TFA), compared with American men [29].

The Ludwigshafen Risk and Cardiovascular Health (LURIC) study, a prospective cohort study of 3259 Caucasians hospitalized for CAG between 1997 and 2000 in southwestern Germany, was the first to show that higher levels of palmitelaidic acids (R-TFA) in RBC membranes were associated with the lower risk for SCD during a median of 10 years of follow-up (**Figure 3**) and that three *trans* isomers of C18:2n6 (IP-TFA) were not related to fatal cardiovascular outcomes [30]. Total TFA levels in LURIC patients (mean 0.96%) were much lower than those in US cohorts in the 1990s [31]. According to the TRANSFAIR study, a cross-sectional investiga-tion in eight countries in Europe, TFA intake is below 1%E and 79% of TFA intake was derived from milk and ruminant fat in Germany [32]. Some prospective cohort studies showed that R-TFA were associated with the lower risk for incident diabetes. In the Cardiovascular Health Study, a prospective cohort study comprising elder US adults from 1989 to 1990 from Medicare eligibility lists, plasma phospholipid FA were measured in 3736 adults in 1992 [33]. Higher *trans*-palmitoleate levels were associated with slightly lower adiposity and, independently, with higher HDL-C levels (1.9% across quintiles; $P = 0.040$), lower triglyceride levels (-19.0%; $P < 0.001$), a lower total cholesterol/HDL-C ratio (-4.7%; $P < 0.001$), lower C-reactive protein levels (-13.8%; $P < 0.05$), and lower insulin resistance (-16.7%, $P < 0.001$). *Trans*-palmitoleate was also associated with a substantially lower incidence of diabetes, with multivariate hazard ratios of 0.41 (95% CI, 0.27 to 0.64) and 0.38 (CI, 0.24 to 0.62) in quintiles 4 and 5 versus quintile 1 (P for trend <0.001) [33]. In the Multi-Ethnic Study of Atherosclerosis (MESA), a cohort of white, black, Hispanic, and Chinese Americans, plasma phospholipid FA and metabolic risk factors were measured in 2000–2002 in 2281 participants free of baseline diabetes [34]. They prospectively assessed the risk of new-onset diabetes (205 cases) from baseline to 2005–2007 [34]. Circulating *trans*-palmitoleate is associated with higher LDL-C but also with lower triglycerides, fasting insulin, blood pressure, and inci-dent diabetes [34]. Large genome-wide association studies have not identified any significant genetic determinants of circulating palmitelaidic acid (C16:1 n7t) levels

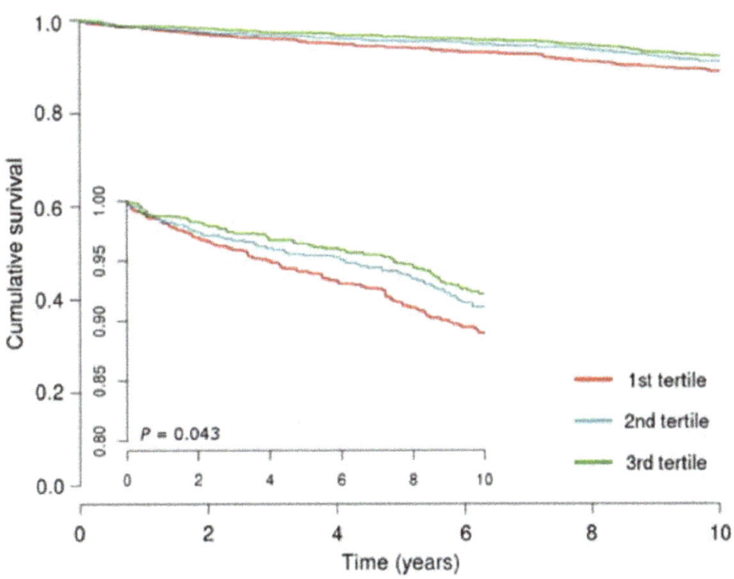

Figure 3.
Adjusted survival curves for sudden cardiac death. Tertiles of palmtelaidic acid (C16:1n7t) were balanced for body mass index, LDL-C, HDL-C. log-Triglyceride, log-fibrinogen, smoking, hypertension, diabetes, lipid-lowering therapy, and estimated glomerular filtration rate by inverse variance weighting. The inset shows the same data on a truncated y axis. Hazard ratios (95% confidence interval) for the second and third tertile compared with the first tertile were 0.82 (0.61–1.12) and 0.67 (0.48–0.93), respectively. The p-value of the robust score test was 0.043. Reproduced from [30].

in RBC or plasma phospholipids [35], suggesting that strong endogenous influences are not present [31].

According to these findings, dietary intake of R-TFA may be cardioprotective, contrary to IP-TFA. Further controlled studies are required to answer the questions how a high amount of R-TFA affects human health.

3. Omega-3 fatty acids and CHD

Numerous studies have demonstrated that omega-3 PUFA protect against CVD, and the ratios of serum levels of EPA and DHA to AA, omega-6 PUFA have been recognized as promising risk markers for CHD [2, 36]. Our case-control study showed that the ACS patients had significantly higher levels of saturated FA, mainly myristic and palmitic acids, and MUFA, mainly oleic acid, and lower levels of omega-3 PUFA, mainly EPA and DHA, and AA, omega-6 PUFA (**Figure 4**) [17]. The Japanese dietary style has markedly changed from the 1960s, and fish to meat ratios in food consumption are decreasing in the younger generation, while the ratios in the Western countries stayed the same or slightly increased [37]. The age profile of the fish/meat >1.0 was ≥40 years in 2000, ≥50 years in 2005 and 2010, and ≥ 60 years in 2015 in Japan. The EPA plus DHA to AA ratios were significantly lower in ACS patients and were further lower in ACS patients <60 years old (**Figure 4**) [17].

PUFA levels depend on dietary intake, bioavailability, and PUFA metabolism. In the biosynthesis of long chain PUFA from precursor PUFA, the crucial enzymes include elongase and desaturase (**Figure 5**) [38, 39]. Delta-5 desaturase (D5D) and

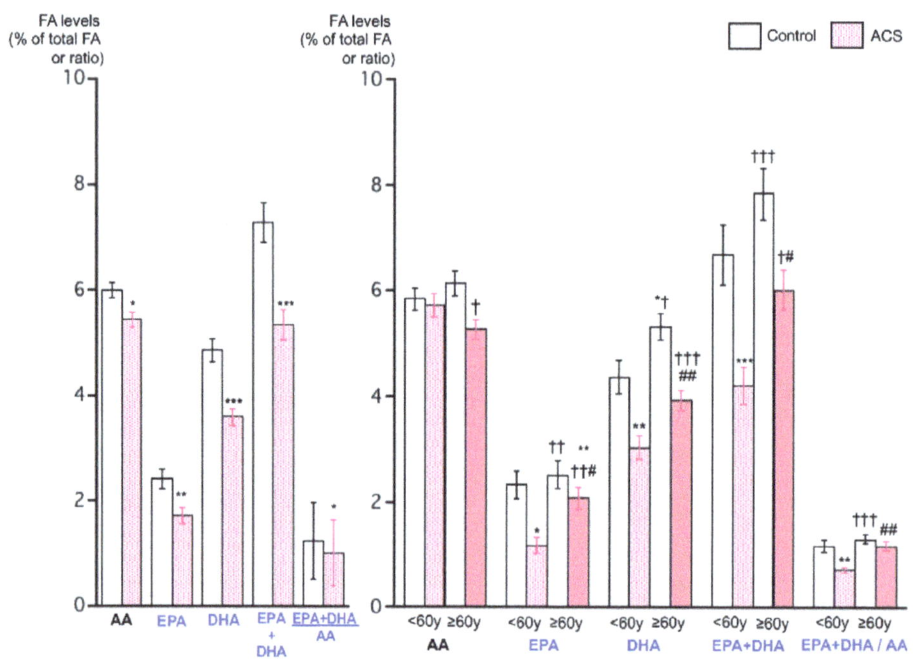

Figure 4.

*The comparison of trans fatty acids (TFA) between control and ACS patients. Left panel: comparison in whole subjects and Right panel: comparison separated by age. Data are expressed as mean ± standard error (SE), and the error bar represents SE. The number of subjects is 49 (<60 years 24; ≥60 years 25) in control and 67 (<60 years 25; ≥60 years 42) in ACS. (A) *p < 0.05, **p < 0.01 *p < 0.001 vs. control. (B) *p < 0.05, **p < 0.01 *p < 0.001 vs. control<60y; †P < 0.05, ††p < 0.01 †††p < 0.001 vs. ACS < 60y; #P < 0.05, ##p < 0.01 vs. control ≥60 years. Figure was made by Ref. [17].*

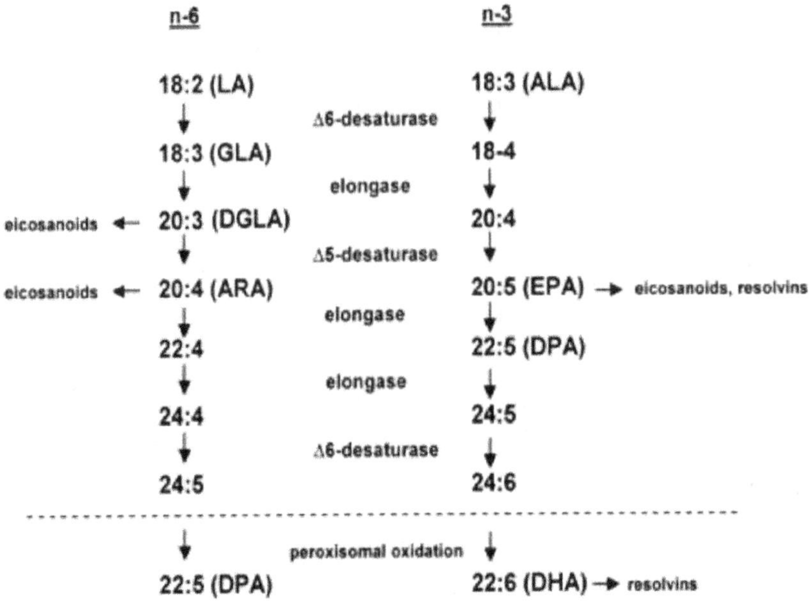

Figure 5.
The omega-3 and omega-6 FA metabolism. ALA, α-linolenic acid; ARA, arachidonic acid; DGLA, dihomo-γ-linolenic acid; DHA, docosahexaenoic acid; DPA, docosapentaenoic acid; EPA, eicosapentaenoic acid; GLA, γ-linolenic acid; LA, linoleic acid. Reproduced Ref. [38].

delta-6 desaturase (D6D) are two key enzymes in the synthesis of long-chain PUFA and are encoded by fatty acid desaturase 1 (FADS1) and FADS2 genes, respectively [39]. Previous studies have reported that the FADS1 gene polymorphism (less function) was associated with an increased CHD risk [40, 41]. D5D is involved in one step in the conversion of linoleic acid (LA, 18:2 *n*-6) and alpha-linoleneic acid (ALA, 18:3 *n*-3) to AA (20:4 *n*-6) and EPA (20:5 *n*-3), respectively, as the sole enzymatic source of endogenous AA and EPA. EPA and DHA are strongly influenced by the dietary intake of pre-formed PUFA, and, while human can readily retroconvert DHA to EPA, the elongation of ALA to EPA and DHA is minimal [38, 42]. However, contrary results have also been very recently reported [43]. The activities of D5D cannot be measured directly; generally, they are conventionally estimated from the ratio of AA to dihomo-gamma linolenic acid (DGLA, 20:3 *n*-6) [39, 44–46].

In our cross-sectional study with ACS patients alone, PUFA and various lipid markers such as small dense LDL cholesterol (sdLDL-C), malondialdehyde-modified LDL (MDA-LDL), and remnant lipoprotein cholesterol (RL-C) were assessed in 436 men with the first episode of ACS not take any lipid-lowering drugs [47]. Approximately 70% of ACS patients had low EPA/AA (<0.41) or DHA/AA (<0.93) according to the median levels in Japanese general population [48]. Serum levels of LDL-C, apolipoprotein B (apoB), and RL-C were significantly higher in the low EPA/AA or DHA/AA groups, while those of triglycerides and MDA-LDL were significantly higher in the low EPA/AA group alone. Thus, low EPA/AA is associ-ated with more atherogenic lipid biomarkers than low DHA/AA. Patients without any reperfusion at the culprit coronary artery on the initial CAG had significantly lower EPA levels and similar DHA and AA levels compared with the others. The levels of LDL-C, non-HDL-C, triglycerides, sdLDL-C, RL-C, MDA-LDL, and apoB decreased progressively and those of EPA, DHA, and HDL-C increased as D5D increased (**Figure 6**). While large buoyant LDL-C (lbLDL-C) estimated by subtracting the sdLDL-C concentration from the LDL-C concentration, and apoA-1 did not differ among quartiles of D5D. Previous prospective case-control studies

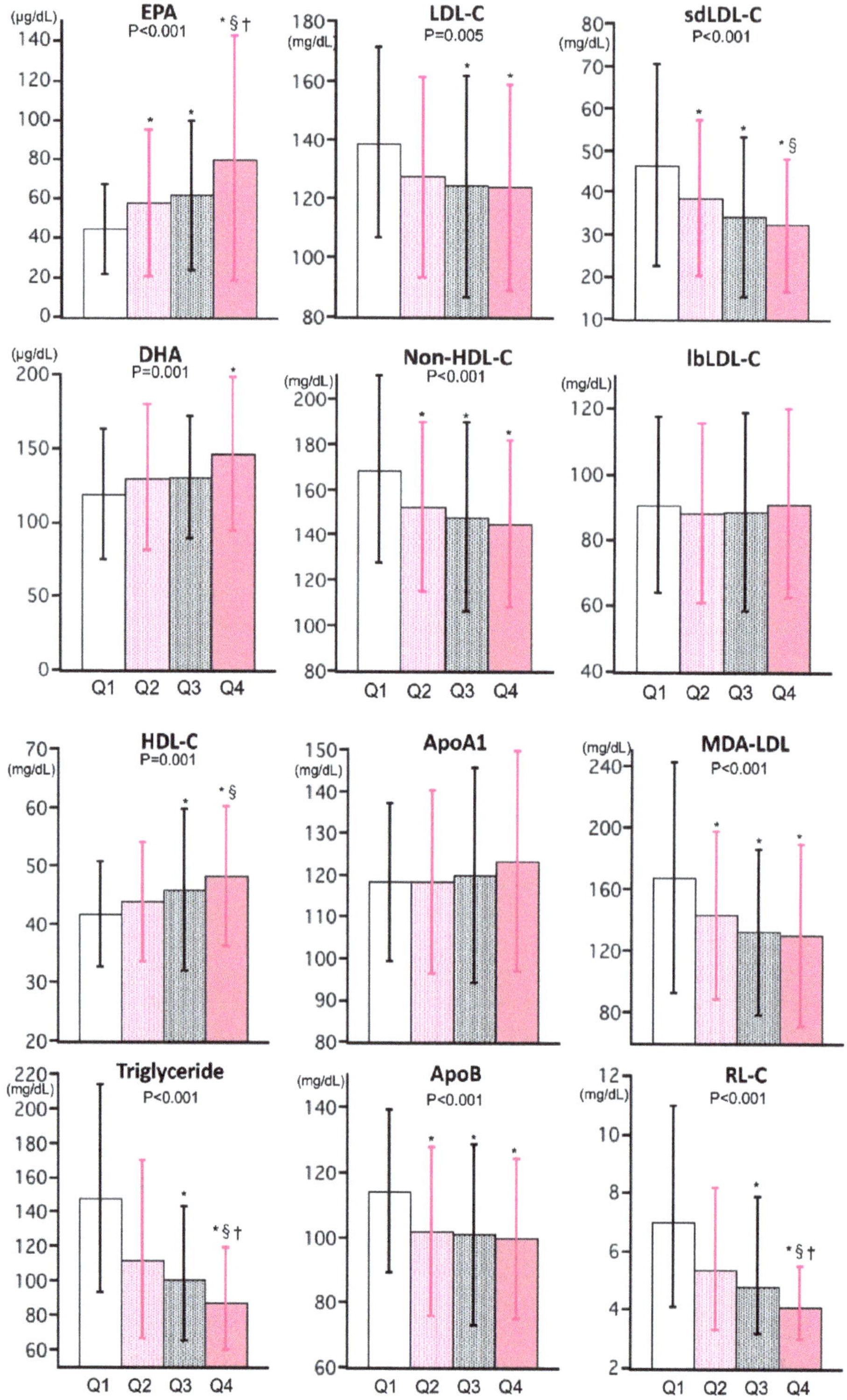

Figure 6.

*Comparisons of various lipid biomarkers between the quartiles of D5D estimated by AA/DGLA. Data are expressed as means ± standard deviation, or median (25% and 75% quartiles) (triglyceride and or RL-C). Abbreviations are presented in the main text. Kruskal-Wallis tests and analysis of variance (ANOVA) with Tukey's honest significant difference test was used to identify the differences between the groups. Q1: AA/ DGLA < 4.03; Q2: 4.04 ≤ AA/ DGLA < 5.07; Q3: 5.08 ≤AA/ DGLA < 6.29; Q4: AA/DGLA ≥ 6.29. *p < 0.05 vs. Q1, §p < 0.05 vs. Q2, †p < 0.05 vs. Q3 using Tukey--Kramer post-hoc test. Figure is made by Ref. [47].*

reported that low D5D predict the development of type 2 diabetes [49–51] and the risk of CVD [39]. In a Swedish population-based prospective cohort study of 2009 50-year old men, D5D was reported to have an inverse correlation with CVD mortality over a follow-up of 30 years [52]. The association of lower D5D with accu-mulation of atherogenic sdLDL, MDA-LDL, and RL-C in our study may provide the association between lower D5D and atherosclerotic CVD.

Previous studies reported that statins, 3-hydroxy-3-methylglutaryl coenzyme A (HMG-CoA) reductase inhibitor, have differential effects on the activities of D5D, D6D, and elongase, and any statins increased AA [53]. It is suggested that EPA/AA may better reflect the residual risk for CHD following statin treatment than DHA / AA. Some previous cross-sectional studies have demonstrated that EPA/AA but not DHA/AA was significantly associated with ACS [54, 55]. A cohort study of CHD patients underwent nonemergency percutaneous coronary intervention (PCI) found that lower EPA/AA (but not lower DHA/AA) was significantly associated with the incidence of major adverse cardiac events [56]. Our study showed that the EPA/AA is a superior risk marker than DHA/AA in terms of correlation with atherogenic lipid profiles in ACS patients.

Multiple studies have demonstrated that EPA and DHA have different effects on cardiometabolic risk factors [57, 58]. Innes and Calder reviewed 18 random-ized controlled trials that compare EPA or DHA (>2 g/day and purity ≥90%) and placebo on cardiometabolic risk factors [57]. The study durations were between 4 and 10 weeks. They reported the following results: (1) both EPA and DHA lowered triglycerides with DHA having a greater triglyceride-lowering effects than EPA; (2) while total cholesterol was largely unchanged by EPA and DHA, DHA increased HDL-C, particularly HDL_2 and increased LDL-C and LDL particle size; (3) both EPA and DHA inhibited platelet activity while DHA improved vascular function and lowered heart rate and blood pressure to a greater extent than EPA; and

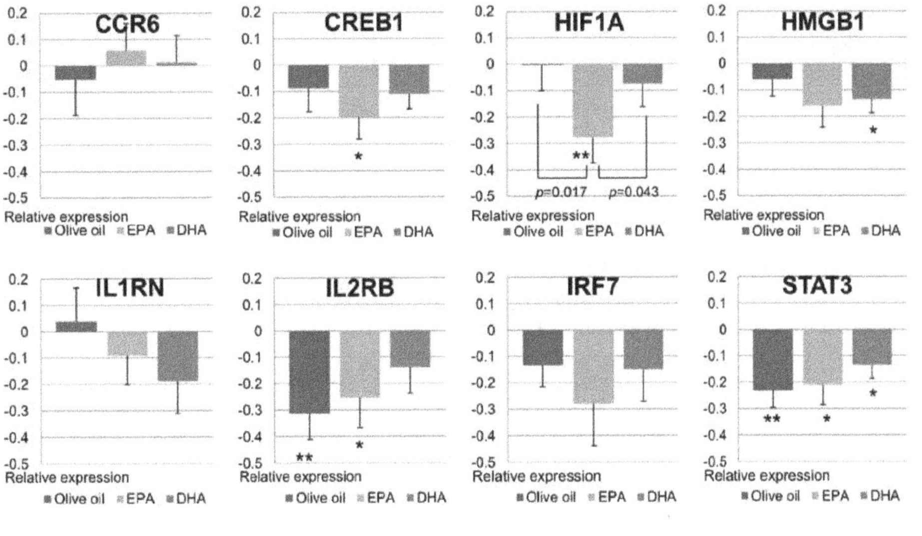

Figure 7.
*Relative changes in the expression of specific genes determined by quantitative real-time polymerase chain reaction (Q-PCR) in olive oil, EPA and DHA supplementation groups. Data are expressed as mean ± standard error. Differences within each group were determined by paired t test (**p < 0.01, *p < 0.05). Brackets indicate differences between two groups as determined with a 2-factor ANOVA with Tukey honestly significant difference correction. CCR6, chemokine (C-C motif) receptor 6; CREB1, cAMP responsive element binding protein 1; HIF1A, hypoxia-inducible factor 1-alpha; HMGB1, high mobility group box 1; IL1RN, interleukin 1 receptor antagonist; IL2RB, interleukin 2 receptor, beta; IRF7, interferon regulatory factor 7; STAT3, signal transducer and activator of transcription. Reproduced from [58].*

(4) the effects of EPA and DHA on inflammatory markers and glycemic control were inconclusive [57]. Tsunoda et al. assessed the effect of a six-week supplementation with either olive oil (6 g/day), EPA (1.8 g/day), or DHA (1.8 g/day) on gene expres-sion in peripheral blood mononuclear cells in healthy men and postmenopausal women [58]. EPA but not DHA or olive oil significantly affected the gene expression in the interferon signaling, receptor recognition of bacteria and viruses, G protein signaling, glycolysis, glycolytic shunting, S-adenosyl-L-methionine biosynthesis, cAMP-mediated signaling, as well as many other individual genes including hypoxia inducible factor 1 (**Figure** 7) [58]. They concluded that the effects of EPA and DHA were mediated by different pathways in human peripheral blood mononuclear cells and that EPA affected cellular immune responses including the interferon signaling pathway [58].

4. Conclusion

IP-TFA intake (estimated from plasma levels) is low in Japan, and accordingly, there is a little difference in IP-TFA levels between Japanese ACS patients and healthy controls. However, a certain IP-TFA is associated with the increased risk of CHD even in Japan. Although it is not clear whether R-TFA are cardioprotective or not, the ACS patients, especially middle-aged patients showed significantly lower levels of R-TFA and omega-3 FA. Although average EPA and DHA levels in Japan are much higher than in the United States [59], still higher levels of the marine omega-3 PUFA are associated with the lower cardiovascular disease risk. However, the Japanese dietary style has changed markedly in the younger generation since 1990 [37, 60]. The lack of fish intake and excessive oils and meat and poultry intakes have been recognized in subjects <60 years old in the present Japanese. Decreased biosynthesis of long-chain PUFA and imbalance of omega-3 and omega-6 FA are clearly associated with atherogenic lipid profiles in Japanese ACS patients. Multiple studies have demonstrated that EPA and DHA have different effects on cardio-metabolic risk factors. The EPA/AA may be a superior risk marker than DHA/AA in terms of correlation with atherogenic lipid profiles in clinical practice.

Abbreviations

AA	arachidonic acid
ACS	acute coronary syndromes
AMI	acute myocardial infarction
apoA1	apolipoprotein A1
apoB	apolipoprotein B
CAG	coronary angiography
CHD	coronary heart disease
CI	confidence interval
CVD	cardiovascular disease
DGLA	dihomo-gamma linolenic acid
DHA	docosahexaenoic acid
D5D	Delta-5 desaturase
D6D	delta-6 desaturase
EPA	eicosapentaenoic acid
FA	Fatty acids
FADS	fatty acid desaturase
HDL-C	HDL cholesterol

HMG-CoA	3-hydroxy-3-methylglutaryl coenzyme
lbLDL-C	large buoyant LDL-C
LDL-C	LDL cholesterol
Lp(a)	lipoprotein(a)
MDA-LDL	malondialdehyde-modified LDL
MUFA	Monounsaturated fatty acid
PCI	percutaneous coronary intervention
PHO	partially hydrogenated oils
PUFA	Polyunsaturated fatty acid
RBC	red blood cell
RL-C	remnant lipoprotein cholesterol
RTD	ruminant trans fatty acid
sdLDL-C	small dense LDL cholesterol
SCD	sudden cardiac death
TFA	*trans* fatty acid

Author details

Shinji Koba[1,2,3*], Tetsuya Takao[4], Fumiko Shimizu[4], Mutsumi Ogawa[4], Yuuya Yokota[1], Fumiyoshi Tsunoda[1], Ken Arai[1], Toshiro Shinke[1] and Akikazu Takada[5]

1 The Department of Medicine, Division of Cardiology, Showa University School of Medicine, Tokyo, Japan

2 The Department of Perioperative Medicine, Division of General Medicine, Showa University School of Dentistry, Tokyo, Japan

3 Showa University Research Institute for Sport and Exercise Sciences, Kanagawa, Japan

4 Faculty of Human Life and Environmental Sciences, Showa Women's University, Tokyo, Japan

5 The International Projects on Food and Health (NPO), Tokyo, Japan

*Address all correspondence to: skoba@med.showa-u.ac.jp

References

[1] Baum S, Kris Etherton P, Willett W, Lichtenstein A, Rudel L, Maki K, et al. Fatty acids in cardiovascular health and disease: A comprehensive update. Journal of Clinical Lipidology. 2012;**6**:216-234

[2] Superko HR, Superko SM, Nasir K, Agatston A, Garrett BC. Omega-3 fatty acid blood levels: Clinical significance and controversy. Circulation. 2013;**128**:2154-2161

[3] Harris WS, Von Schacky C. The Omega-3 index: A new risk factor for death from coronary heart disease? Preventive Medicine. 2004;**39**:212-220

[4] Harris WS. The Omega-6:Omega-3 ratio: A critical appraisal and possible successor. Prostaglandins, Leukotrienes, and Essential Fatty Acids. 2018;**132**:34-40

[5] Harris W, Shearer G. Omega-6 fatty acids and cardiovascular disease: Friend, not foe? Circulation. 2014;**130**:1562-1564

[6] Sala A, Proschak E, Steinhilber D, Rovati GE. Two-pronged approach to anti-inflammatory therapy through the modulation of the arachidonic acid cascade. Biochemical Pharmacology. 2018;**158**:161-173

[7] Chowdhury R, Warnakula S, Kunutsor S, et al. Association of dietary, circulating, and supplement fatty acids with coronary risk: A systematic review and meta-analysis. Annals of Internal Medicine. 2014;**160**:398-406

[8] Lichtenstein AH. Dietary trans fatty acids and cardiovascular disease risk: Past and present. Current Atherosclerosis Reports. 2014;**16**:433

[9] Kinoshita M, Yokote K, Arai H, Iida M, Ishigaki Y, et al. Japan atherosclerosis society (JAS) guidelines for prevention of atherosclerotic cardiovascular diseases 2017. Journal of Atherosclerosis and Thrombosis. 2018;**25**:846-984

[10] Liska DJ, Cook CM, Wang DD, Gaine PC, Baer DJ. Trans fatty acids and cholesterol levels: An evidence map of the available science. Food and Chemical Toxicology. 2016;**98**:269-281

[11] Stender S, Astrup A, Dyerberg J. Ruminant and industrially produced trans fatty acids: Health aspects. Food & Nutrition Research. 2008;**52**

[12] Mensink RP, Katan MB. Effect of dietary trans fatty acids on high-density and low-density lipoprotein cholesterol levels in healthy subjects. The New England Journal of Medicine. 1990;**323**:439-445

[13] Adachi H. Trans fatty acid and coronary artery disease- lessons from seven countries study. Circulation Journal. 2015;**79**:1902-1903

[14] Sebedio JL, Chardigny JM. Physiological effects of trans and cyclic fatty acids. In: Perkins EG, editor. Deep Frying. Chapter 9. 1996. pp. 183-209

[15] Mori K, Ishida T, Yasuda T, Hasokawa M, et al. Serum trans-fatty acid concentration is elevated in young patients with coronary artery disease in Japan. Circulation Journal. 2015;**79**:2017-2025

[16] Nagasawa Y, Shinke T, Toh R, Ishida T, et al. The impact of serum trans fatty acids concentration on plaque vulnerability in patients with coronary artery disease: Assessment via optical coherence tomography. Atherosclerosis. 2017;**265**:312-317

[17] Koba S, Takao T, Shimizu F, Ogawa M, et al. Comparison of plasma levels of different species of trans fatty

acids in Japanese male patients with acute coronary syndrome versus healthy men. Atherosclerosis. 2019;**284**:173-180

[18] Sun Q, Ma J, Campos H, Hankinson SE, Manson JE, Stampfer MJ, et al. A prospective study of trans fatty acids in erythrocytes and risk of coronary heart disease. Circulation. 2007;**115**:1858-1865

[19] Lemaitre RN, King IB, Mozaffarian D, Sotoodehnia N, Rea TD, Kuller LH, et al. Plasma phospholipid trans fatty acids, fatal ischemic heart disease, and sudden cardiac death in older adults: The cardiovascular health study. Circulation. 2006;**114**:209-215

[20] Wang Q, Imamura F, Lemaitre RN, Rimm EB, Wang M, King IB, et al. Plasma phospholipid trans-fatty acids levels, cardiovascular diseases, and total mortality: The cardiovascular health study. Journal of the American Heart Association. 2014;**3**

[21] Lemaitre RN, King IB, Raghunathan TE, et al. Cell membrane trans-fatty acids and the risk of primary cardiac arrest. Circulation. 2002;**105**:697-701

[22] Borgeraas H, Hertel JK, Seifert R, Berge RK, Bohov P, Ueland PM, et al. Serum trans fatty acids, asymmetric dimethylarginine and risk of acute myocardial infarction and mortality in patients with suspected coronary heart disease: A prospective cohort study. Lipids in Health and Disease. 2016;**15**:38

[23] Lemaitre RN, King IB, Patterson RE, Psaty BM, Kestin M, Heckbert SR. Assessment of trans-fatty acid intake with a food frequency questionnaire and validation with adipose tissue levels of trans-fatty acids. American Journal of Epidemiology. 1998;**148**:1085-1093

[24] Roberts TL, Wood DA, Riemersma RA, Gallagher PJ, Lampe FC. Trans isomers of oleic and linoleic acids in adipose tissue and sudden cardiac death. Lancet. 1995;**345**:278-282

[25] Aro A, Kardinaal AF, Salminen I, Kark JD, et al. Adipose tissue isomeric trans fatty acids and risk of myocardial infarction in nine countries: The EURAMIC study. Lancet. 1995;**345**:273-278

[26] Pedersen JI, Ringstad J, Almendingen K, Haugen TS, Stensvold I, Thelle DS. Adipose tissue fatty acids and risk of myocardial infarction—A case-control study. European Journal of Clinical Nutrition. 2000;**54**:618-625

[27] Baylin A, Kabagambe EK, Ascherio A, Spiegelman D, Campos H. High 18:2 trans-fatty acids in adipose tissue are associated with increased risk of nonfatal acute myocardial infarction in costa rican adults. The Journal of Nutrition. 2003;**133**:1186-1191

[28] Itcho K, Yoshii Y, Ohno H, Oki K, Shinohara M, et al. Association between serum elaidic acid concentration and insulin resistance in two Japanese cohorts with different lifestyles. Journal of Atherosclerosis and Thrombosis. 2017;**24**:1206-1214

[29] Takada A, Shimizu F, Ishii Y, Ogawa M, Takao T, Koba S, et al. Plasma fatty acid composition in men over 50 in the USA and Japan. Food and Nutrition Sciences. 2018;**9**:703-710

[30] Kleber ME, Delgado GE, Lorkowski S, Marz W, von Schacky C. Trans-fatty acids and mortality in patients referred for coronary angiography: The Ludwigshafen risk and cardiovascular health study. European Heart Journal. 2016;**37**:1072-1078

[31] Mozaffarian D. Natural trans fat, dairy fat, partially hydrogenated oils, and cardiometabolic health: The

Ludwigshafen risk and cardiovascular health study. European Heart Journal. 2016;**37**:1079-1081

[32] Hulshof KF, van Erp-Baart MA, Anttolainen M, et al. Intake of fatty acids in western Europe with emphasis on trans fatty acids: The TRANSFAIR study. European Journal of Clinical Nutrition. 1999;**53**:143-157

[33] Mozaffarian D, Cao H, King IB, Lemaitre RN, Song X, Siscovick DS, et al. Trans-palmitoleic acid, metabolic risk factors, and new-onset diabetes in U.S. adults: A cohort study. Annals of Internal Medicine. 2010;**153**:790-799

[34] Mozaffarian D, de Oliveira Otto MC, et al. Trans-Palmitoleic acid, other dairy fat biomarkers, and incident diabetes: The multi-ethnic study of atherosclerosis (MESA). The American Journal of Clinical Nutrition. 2013;**97**:854-861

[35] Mozaffarian D, Kabagambe EK, Johnson CO, Lemaitre RN, et al. Genetic loci associated with circulating phospholipid trans fatty acids: A meta-analysis of genome-wide association studies from the CHARGE Consortium. The American Journal of Clinical Nutrition. 2015;**101**:398-406

[36] Watanabe Y, Tatsuno I. Omega-3 polyunsaturated fatty acids for cardiovascular diseases: Present, past and future. Expert Review of Clinical Pharmacology. 2017;**10**:865-873

[37] Yokoyama S. Beneficial effect of retuning to "Japan diet" for the Japanese. Journal of Atherosclerosis and Thrombosis. 2019;**26**:1-2

[38] Arterburn LM, Hall EB, Oken H. Distribution, interconversion, and dose response of n-3 fatty acids in humans. The American Journal of Clinical Nutrition. 2006;**83**:1467S-1476S

[39] Tosi F, Sartori F, Guarini P, Olivieri O, Martinelli N. Delta-5 and delta-6 desaturases: Crucial enzymes in polyunsaturated fatty acid-related pathways with pleiotropic influences in health and disease. Advances in Experimental Medicine and Biology. 2014;**824**:61-81

[40] Lv X, Zhang Y, Rao S, Qiu J, Wang M, Luo X, et al. Joint effects of genetic variants in multiple loci on the risk of coronary artery disease in Chinese Han subjects. Circulation Journal. 2012;**76**:1987-1992

[41] Liu F, Li Z, Lv X, Ma J. Dietary n-3 polyunsaturated fatty acid intakes modify the effect of genetic variation in fatty acid desaturase 1 on coronary artery disease. PLoS One. 2015;**10**:e0121255

[42] Oscarsson J, Hurt Camejo E. Omega-3 fatty acids eicosapentaenoic acid and docosahexaenoic acid and their mechanisms of action on apolipoprotein B-containing lipoproteins in humans: A review. Lipids in Health and Disease. 2017;**16**:149-149

[43] Metherel A, Irfan M, Klingel S, Mutch D, Bazinet R. Compound-specific isotope analysis reveals no retroconversion of DHA to EPA but substantial conversion of EPA to DHA following supplementation: A randomized control trial. American Journal of Clinical Nutrition. 2019;**110**:823-831

[44] Ebbesson SOE, Voruganti V, Higgins P, et al. Fatty acids linked to cardiovascular mortality are associated with risk factors. International Journal of Circumpolar Health. 2015;**74**:28055

[45] Harris WS, Luo J, Pottala JV, Margolis KL, et al. Red blood cell fatty acids and incident diabetes mellitus in the women's health initiative memory study. PLoS One. 2016;**11**:e0147894

[46] Tsurutani Y, Inoue K, Sugisawa C, Saito J, Omura M, Nishikawa T. Increased serum Dihomo-gamma-linolenic acid levels are associated with obesity, body fat accumulation, and insulin resistance in Japanese patients with type 2 diabetes. Internal Medicine. 2018;**57**:2929-2935

[47] Arai K, Koba S, Yokota Y, Tsunoda F, Tsujita H, et al. Delta-5 desaturase activity, and lipid profiles in men with acute coronary syndrome. Journal of Atherosclerosis and Thrombosis. 2020. DOI: 10.5551/jat.55780. Online ahead of print

[48] Ninomiya T, Nagata M, Hata J, Hirakawa Y, et al. Association between ratio of serum eicosapentaenoic acid to arachidonic acid and risk of cardiovascular disease: The Hisayama study. Atherosclerosis (Amsterdam). 2013;**231**:261-267

[49] Hodge A, English D, O'Dea K, Sinclair A, et al. Plasma phospholipid and dietary fatty acids as predictors of type 2 diabetes: Interpreting the role of linoleic acid. American Journal of Clinical Nutrition. 2007;**86**:189-197

[50] Krachler B, Norberg M, Eriksson JW, et al. Fatty acid profile of the erythrocyte membrane preceding development of type 2 diabetes mellitus. Nutrition, Metabolism, and Cardiovascular Diseases. 2008;**18**:503-510

[51] Kröger J, Schulze M. Recent i nsights into the relation of Δ5 desaturase and Δ6 desaturase activity to the development of type 2 diabetes. Current Opinion in Lipidology. 2012;**23**:4-10

[52] Warensjö E, Sundström J, Vessby B, Cederholm T, Risérus U. Markers of dietary fat quality and fatty acid desaturation as predictors of total and cardiovascular mortality: A population-based prospective study. American Journal of Clinical Nutrition. 2008;**88**:203-209

[53] Bird JK, Calder PC, Eggersdorfer M. The role of n-3 long chain polyunsaturated fatty acids in cardiovascular disease prevention, and interactions with statins. Nutrients. 2018;**10**(6):775. DOI: 10.3390/nu10060775

[54] Nishizaki Y, Shimada K, Tani S, Ogawa T, et al. Significance of imbalance in the ratio of serum n-3 to n-6 polyunsaturated fatty acids in patients with acute coronary syndrome. The American Journal of Cardiology. 2014;**113**:441-445

[55] Iwamatsu K, Abe S, Nishida H, Kageyama M, Nasuno T, Sakuma M, et al. Which has the stronger impact on coronary artery disease, eicosapentaenoic acid or docosahexaenoic acid? Hypertension Research. 2016;**39**:272-275

[56] Domei T, Yokoi H, Kuramitsu S, Soga Y, et al. Ratio of serum n-3 to n-6 polyunsaturated fatty acids and the incidence of major adverse cardiac events in patients undergoing percutaneous coronary intervention. Circulation Journal. 2012;**76**:423-429

[57] Innes JK, Calder PC. The differential effects of eicosapentaenoic acid and docosahexaenoic acid on cardiometabolic risk factors: A systematic review. International Journal of Molecular Sciences. 2018;**19**

[58] Tsunoda F, Lamon-Fava S, Asztalos BF, et al. Effects of oral eicosapentaenoic acid versus docosahexaenoic acid on human peripheral blood mononuclear cell gene expression. Atherosclerosis. 2015;**241**:400-408

[59] Sekikawa A, Curb JD, Ueshima H, El-Saed A, Kadowaki T, et al. Marine-derived n-3 fatty acids and

atherosclerosis in Japanese, Japanese-American, and white men: A cross-sectional study. Journal of the American College of Cardiology. 2008;**52**:417-424

[60] Shijo Y, Maruyama C, Nakamura E, Nakano R, et al. Japan diet intake changes serum phospholipid fatty acid compositions in middle-aged men: A pilot study. Journal of Atherosclerosis and Thrombosis. 2019;**26**:3-13

5

Glucose or Sucrose Intakes and Plasma Levels of Essential and Nonessential Amino Acids

Akikazu Takada, Fumiko Shimizu, Yukie Ishii, Mutsumi Ogawa and Tetsuya Takao

Abstract

It is not known whether the administration of glucose or sucrose influences plasma levels of amino acids. We want to know whether plasma levels of amino acids and if the administration of glucose or sucrose are different in young and old men and are influenced by the administration of glucose or sucrose. We found that the levels of most amino acids in plasma are lower in old men than young men. When sucrose was administered to old men, levels of total amino acids decreased signifi-cantly in old men. In both old and young men plasma levels of total nonessential amino acids significantly decreased at 120 min. after the administration of glucose but not sucrose. On the other hand, total essential and branched amino acids levels decreased significantly after the administration of both glucose and sucrose in young and old men. From these results, responses to the administration of glucose were different from the response to sucrose between young and old men. Also glucose was more effective in decreasing plasma levels of various amino acids. These results seem to suggest that glucose was more effective in stimulating insulin release and young men were more responsive to sugar than old men in stimulating insulin release.

Keywords: amino acids, branched chain amino acids, tryptophan, serotonin, leucine, appetite, feeding

1. Introduction

Globally the prevalence of obesity nearly tripled between 1975 and 2016 (the World Health Organization) [1]. Foods such as fats, carbohydrates, or sugar are causes of such increase in alarming obesity pandemic. Carbohydrates were blamed for increase in obesity because consumption of carbohydrates results in increase in the release of insulin, and that insulin levels affect fat storage. Insulin secretion suppresses the release of fatty acids into circulation, thus storage of fat in fat cells.

According to the carbohydrate insulin model, decrease in the proportion of dietary carbohydrate to fat without changing protein or calories may reduce insulin secretion, mobilize fat from adipose tissue, and cause oxidation of circulating free fatty acids.

Recently, various data were presented to object to this theory. The intakes of isocaloric ketogenic diet were not shown to result in body fat loss and relatively small increases in energy expenditure [2].

The presence of signals about energetic value of food between gut and brain was proposed by experiments in which rodents were given isocaloric diets that varied in volume and rodents accurately took the volume of food consumed to maintain constant caloric intake across days [3].

The volumes and contents of foods we take will be conveyed to the brain by a gut-brain circuit [4], and it is proposed that intake of highly processed foods disturbs the circuitry resulting in the confusion of the processing of foods information in the brain. This may be the reason of overeating and obesity by the intakes of highly processed foods [1, 4].

We recently gave sucrose or glucose to healthy men and measured changes in plasma levels of various amino acids [5] and changes in body mass index [6]. We now review the results and discuss roles of sugar in maintaining plasma levels of amino acids. We also report that sugar intake did not result in increase in body mass index unless overtaken.

Many researchers paid attention to the central control of appetite and gut motor and hormonal functions [7–9]. Many studies have been performed on roles of tryptophan and leucine in the regulation of food intake and appetite [7–9]. Since serotonin is derived from tryptophan roles of serotonin in the regulation of appetite have been studied well (Review [10]).

Since intakes of carbohydrates considered to increase the release of insulin, which increase fat deposition, thus obesity, low carbohydrate diet has been popular in Japan lately. According to Noto et al. [11], high mortality rate was shown among people using low-carbohydrate-high protein diet.

Robert Atkins first proposed that intakes of meat may result decrease of fat, thus prevent obesity. He died by a serious head injury when he toppled down [12], the impaired muscle functions has been suspected for the results of low carbohydrate diet.

The ability of insulin to stimulate glucose uptake and to suppress protein degradation in skeletal muscle is increased after exercise. Decrease in amino acid availability may prevent the stimulatory effect of insulin on muscle protein synthesis after exercise.

Insulin is considered to regulate the metabolism of carbohydrate, lipid, protein, and amino acids [13]. Insulin inhibits protein degradation and the release of amino acids, and stimulates protein synthesis and amino acids uptake in skeletal muscles [14, 15]. When insulin levels were high, protein synthesis was stimulated in skeletal muscles [16]. In hyperglycemia plasma levels of alanine, phenylalanine, valine, leucine, isoleucine and tyrosine were shown to increase and the levels of histidine and glutamine decreased [17].

It is shown that when plasma levels of tryptophan were raised by taking tryptophan in foods or by injection of insulin, serotonin and tryptophan in the brain increased [18, 19]. It is also shown that intake of carbohydrate resulted in secretion of insulin, which increased plasma levels of tryptophan and lowered the plasma levels of competing amino acids such as branched neutral amino acids in rats [19]. Carbohydrate intake was shown to decrease plasma levels of free amino acids and glucose intake resulted in a decrease in large neutral amino acids such as methionine, phenylalanine, tyrosine, and tryptophan [20, 21]. Possibly plasma glucose and insulin may stimulate transporters of some amino acids of peripheral tissues, especially muscles, resulting in decrease in the concentration of such amino acids in plasma.

We administered glucose or sucrose solution to young and old men and examined plasma levels of various amino acids. In the present review we report the results [22, 23], and propose possible mechanisms with regard to the regulation of appetite.

2. Methods

We asked men older than 50 years old and men college students to participate in the experiments. We checked their health carefully and recruited them if there were no health problems such as diabetes, hypertension nor serious diseases experienced in the past. They did not smoke in the past. We also excluded people who took drugs for dyslipidemia, hyperglycemia, or hypertension.

Participants were randomly assigned to groups after fasting overnight. Depending on their group, each participant received a 550-mL solution containing 50 g of glucose or sucrose (or 500 mL water as a control). Either 50 g of glucose or sucrose was added and dissolved in each bottle containing 500 mL of water. Between 9:00 AM and 10:00 AM, blood was taken using a syringe, and participants were given either glucose or sucrose solution or water as a control. We measured blood glucose using a finger stick (TERUMO kit) before and 120 min after the administration of glucose or sucrose. Furthermore, other plasma factors were measured after plasma was separated from blood. Ethylenediaminetetraacetic acid (EDTA) was used as an anticoagulant.

Blood was centrifuged to obtain plasma. The amino acid and insulin levels were measured for backgrounds of these participants.

To know energy intakes of various foods we used BDHQ (brief-type self-administered diet history questionnaires). From these questionnaires, we calculated the intake of energy, carbohydrate, fat and protein.

The samples were analyzed by SRL, Inc. (Tokyo Japan) using the UF-Amino Station®, which is a liquid chromatography-mass spectrometry system with an automated pre-column derivatization for simultaneous determination of amino acids (Shimadzu Corporation, Kyoto, Japan). The original concept of this system was developed by Ajinomoto Co., Inc. (Tokyo Japan) as an automated method of analyzing major free amino acids in human plasma in the field of clinical chemistry.

The human plasma samples were cryopreserved with EDTANa2 before the analysis. The thawed samples were deproteinized with acetonitrile followed by the amino acid analysis. Pre-column derivatization in the UF-Amino Station was automatically performed using an automated sample injector with the regent APDSTAG® (Wako Pure Chemical Industries, Ltd., Osaka, Japan). Target free amino acids as derivatized compounds were separated under a reversed phase ultrahigh-performance liquid chromatography condition and determined by the liquid chromatograph mass spectrometer.

Insulin was measured by the CLEIA (chemiluminescent immunoassay) method.

3. Ethics

This work was approved by the ethical committees of Showa Women's University and the NPO "International projects on food and health" and was conducted in accordance with The Code of Ethics of the World Medical Association (Declaration of Helsinki) for experiments.

4. Statistics

The results are presented as means ± SD. Statistical significance of the differences between groups was calculated according by one-way ANOVA. When ANOVA indicated a significant difference ($P < 0.05$), the mean values of the treatment were compared using Tukey's least significant difference test at $P < 0.05$.

5. Results

5.1 Measurements of plasma levels of amino acids in old and young men

Table 1 shows the background of participants. There was no difference on energy intake between young and old men. Young men take more lipids and old men take more carbohydrate.

Table 2 shows plasma levels of amino acids of young and old men. Plasma levels of nonessential amino acids were higher in old men than young men. No differences were shown in plasma levels of total amino acids, and total essential and branched amino acids between young and old men.

Levels of phenylalanine, tyrosine, alanine, A-aminobutyric acid, citrulline, cysteine, glutamic acid, ornithine, and taurine were higher in old men, and serine were higher in young men.

5.2 The administration of glucose or sucrose in young and old men

Blood was taken before the experiments from old men and amino acids levels were measured at 0 min and 120 min after the administration of glucose (15 men) or sucrose (16 men) or water as a control (13 men). Amino acids levels of all blood samples were measured. Compared with the control group, essential amino acids (EAAs) such as histidine, lysine, methionine, phenylalanine, threonine, tryptophan, leucine, isoleucine, and valine and branched amino acids (BAAs) such as leucine, isoleucine, and valine decreased significantly 120 min after the administration or glucose or sucrose in old men. Nonessential amino acid (NEAA) levels decreased at 120 min after the administration of glucose only compared with the control group.

In 36 young men, amino acids levels in plasma were measured at 0 min and 120 min after the administration of glucose (12 men) or sucrose (13 men), with 11 men of a control group taking water only. Similarly, the EAA and BCAA levels decreased in comparison with the control group (11 men) after the administration of glucose or sucrose to young men. EAAs such as histidine, lysine, methionine, phenylalanine, threonine, tryptophan, leucine, isoleucine, and valine and BCAAs such as leucine, isoleucine, and valine decreased significantly after the

Subjects	Young (n = 36)	Old (n = 44)	ss
Age (years)	20.8±1.6	62.4±9.6	**
Height (m)	1.72±0.06	1.68±0.07	*
BMI	22.2±3.3	24.3±3.2	*
Energy intake(kcal/day)	1988±591.8	2115.1±460.2	
Protein intake (g/day)	69.3±25.1	66.6±28.8	
Lipid intake (g/day)	60.4±24.8	49.1±22.6	*
Carbohydrate intake (g/day)	78.9±13.1	198.6±89.4	**
Insulin (μU/ml)	6.87±4.19	6.19±3.79	

*$P<0.05$.
**$P<0.01$.

Table 1.
Background of participants.

Amino acids	Young men (n = 36)	Old men (n = 44)	ss
Histidine	78.5±7.7	78.7±7.5	
Lysine	185.9±28.6	190.9±28.7	
Methionine	27.3±3.6	27.6±4.9	
Phenylalanine	56.9±7.0	65.4±8.8	**
Threonine	131.4±21.5	136.5±27.4	
Tryptophan	65.8±9.1	58.7±9.2	
Isoleucine	67.9±11.2	67.5±8.5	
Leucine	129.8±16.8	133.8±17.5	
Valine	221.9±16.3	228.1±30.6	
Tyrosine	58.2±8.7	70.3±12.0	**
Alanine	356.0±68.8	415.9±75.7	**
A-Aminobutyric acid	20.9±5.3	21.7±6.5	**
Arginine	77.6±15.0	79.3±17.6	
Asparagine	45.0±6.1	47.3±5.7	
Aspartic acid	3.4±1.4	3.4±0.7	
Citrulline	22.2±3.6	27.0±6.2	**
Cysteine	14.1±4.1	23.6±6.7	**
Glutamic acid	37.0±11.6	45.0±16.	**
Glutamine	548.5±64.0	575.6±53.0	
Glycine	213.5±25.9	198.5±28.6	
Monoethanolamine	8.5±1.2	8.8±1.3	
Ornithine	59.4±12.5	72.5±13.9	**
Proline	172.8±58.4	169.2±56.9	
Serine	124.6±17.2	105.5±18.2	**
Taurine	49.9±1.5	67.7±3.1	**
Total amino acids	2751.7±215	2891.4±201.6	
Total essential AAs	695.3±89.0	985.4±94.9	
Total nonessential AAs	1786.4±153.3	1960.4±166.0	**
Total branched chain AAs	419.5±48.3	427.5±52.3	
Fisher ratio	3.7±0.4	3.2±0.4	

AAs: amino acids, ss: statistical significance.
**$P < 0.01$.

Table 2.
Plasma levels of amino acids in young and old men in Japan (nM).

administration of glucose or sucrose in young groups too. NEAA levels decreased after the administration of glucose in old and young men.

In **Figure 1**, changes in the levels of total amino acids at 120 min in old and young men after the administration of glucose or sucrose were compared to those levels in the control group. When glucose was taken the amounts of total amino acids significantly decreased in young and aged people. Sucrose administration resulted in a significant decrease in the total amino acids only in old men (**Figure 1**).

Decrease in plasma levels of total essential amino acids at 120 min after the administration of solutions containing 50 g of glucose or sucrose in young and old men were calculated.

Figure 2 shows changes in the decrease of total EAA levels at 120 min compared with the control group after glucose or sucrose administration in aged and young men. After the administration of both glucose and sucrose administration total EAAs significantly decreased in young and aged men at 120 min after the administration compared with the control group.

Figure 3 shows decrease in total NEAA levels at 120 min compared with the control group after glucose or sucrose administration in aged men. Glucose intake resulted in a significant decrease in the amounts of total NEAA levels in aged men. There was practically no further decrease in the total NEAAs after the administration of sucrose compared with the control group in either old or young men.

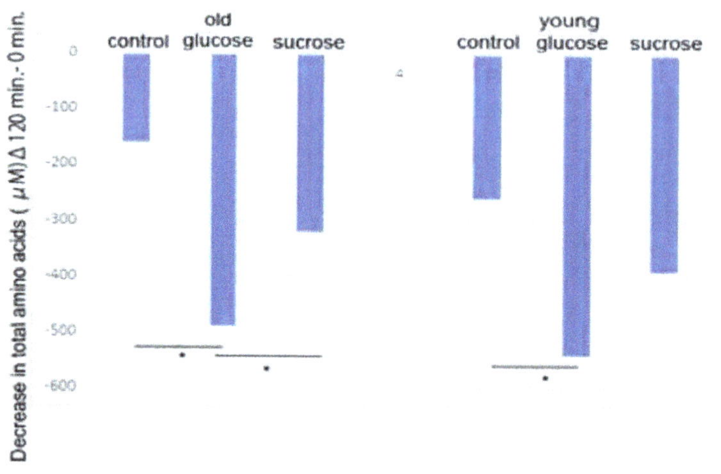

Figure 1.
Changes in total amino acids after the administration of glucose or sucrose in young and old men.

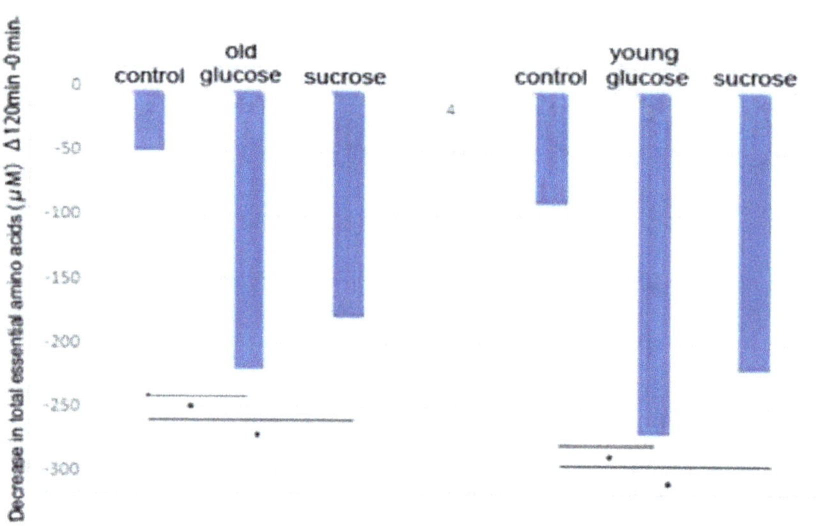

Figure 2.
Changes in total essential amino acids levels after the administration of glucose or sucrose in young and old men.

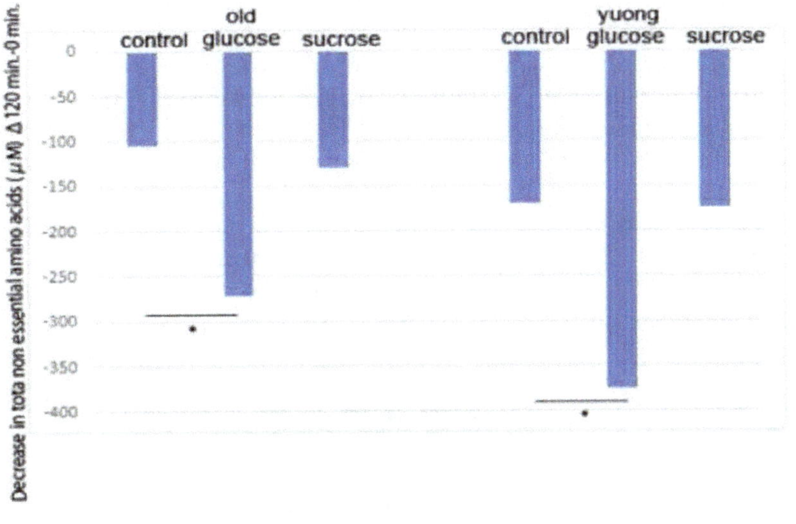

Figure 3.
Changes in total nonessential amino acids (NEAAs) after the administration of glucose or sucrose in young and old men.

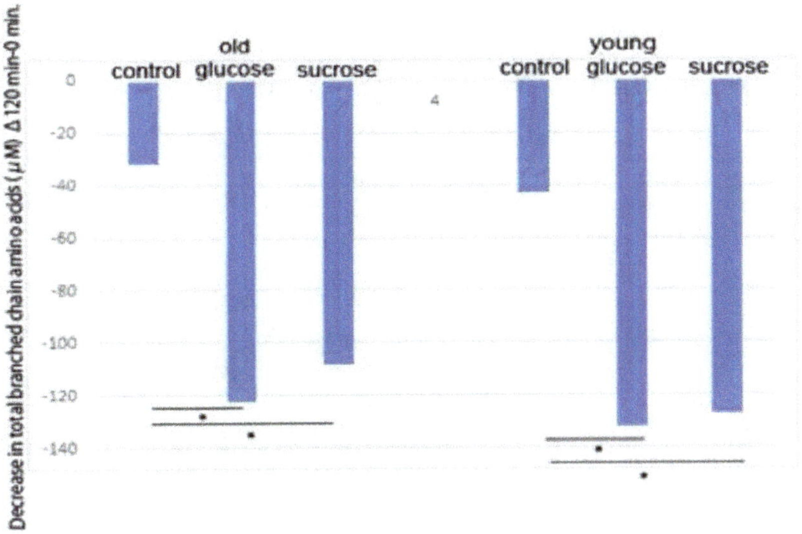

Figure 4.
Changes in total branched chain amino acids after the administration of glucose or sucrose in young and old men.

Figure 4 shows a decrease in the plasma levels of total BCAAs at 120 min after the administration of glucose or sucrose to old and young men. Both glucose and sucrose administrations significantly decreased total BCAA (leucine, isoleucine, and valine) levels in young and aged men at 120 min after the administration compared with the control group.

6. Discussion

Is carbohydrate needed for the transportation of amino acids from blood to the brain or peripheral organs.

As indicated by Burtman's group [18, 19], insulin is needed for the transportation of tryptophan to the brain.

Figure 5 illustrates the transportation of tryptophan from the blood to the brain. Insulin released upon intake of sugar facilitates the transportation of tryptophan. Burtman's group proposed that tryptophan competes with other long neutral amino acids for the transportation to the brain and that in the presence of insulin long neutral amino acids except for tryptophan are transported to the peripheral organ so that remaining tryptophan is now transported to the brain.

Figure 6 shows the hypothesis that in the presence of insulin long neutral amino acids are mainly transported to the peripheral organs and tryptophan is now transported to the brain.

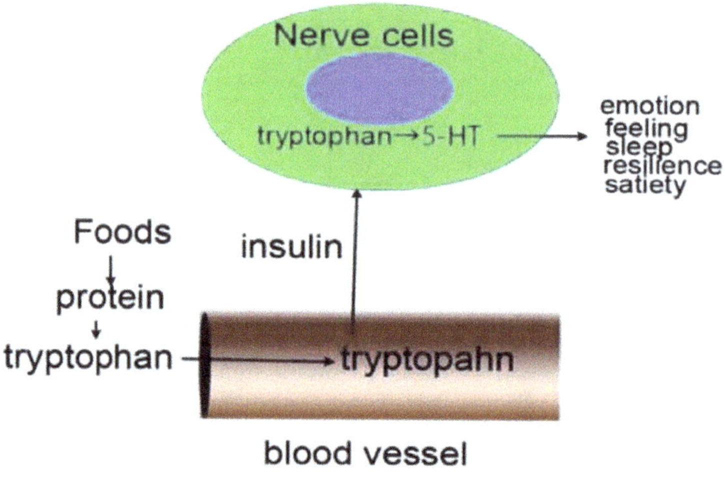

Figure 5.
The transportation of tryptophan from the blood to the brain.

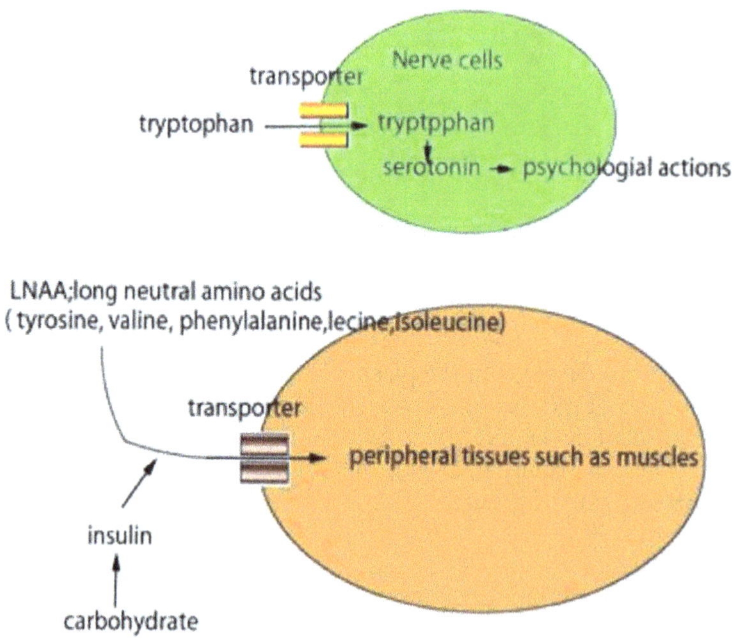

Figure 6.
Transportation of long neutral amino acids to the peripheral organs.

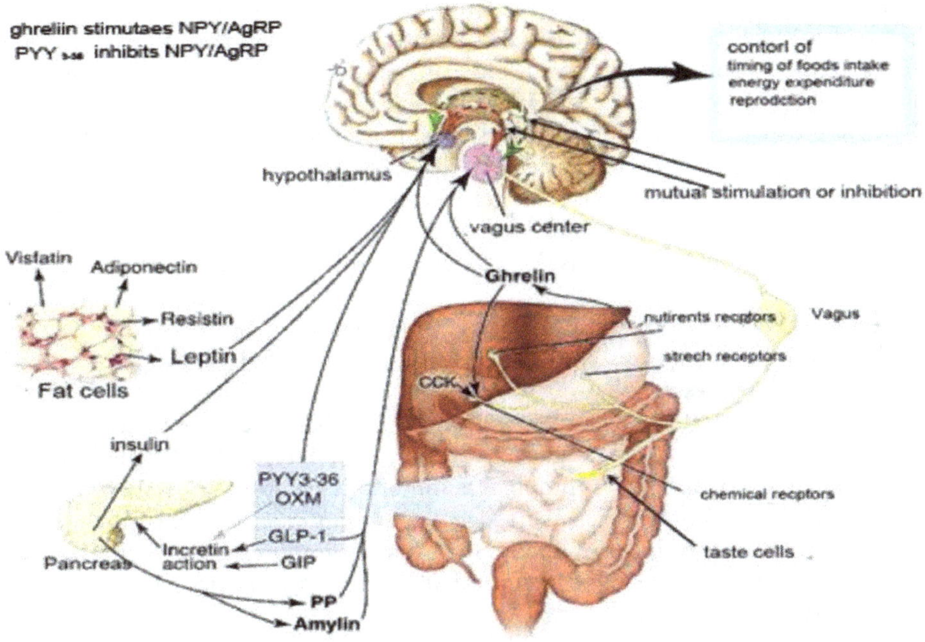

Figure 7.
Central and peripheral mechanisms of food intakes.

Intake of glucose or sucrose was shown to result in decrease in plasma levels of essential amino acids. Since insulin stimulate protein synthesis of the muscle [16] essential amino acids transported to the muscle are used muscular protein synthesis. This hypothesis explains why decrease in plasma levels of amino acids, especially essential amino acids after the administration of glucose or sucrose in men may be explained by this hypothesis.

Tryptophan is important for the stability of emotion, sleep and satiety.

There are many factors controlling hunger and satiety. As shown in **Figure 7**, ghrelin released from the stomach enhances foods intakes by stimulating NPY/AgRP NPY (neuropeptide Y)/AgRP (Agouti related peptide) in the arcuate nucleus. On the other hand PYY_{3-36} released from the colon inhibits NPY/AgRP. Leptin from fatty cells and insulin from the pancreas inhibit NPY/AgRP and stimulate melano-cortin-producing cells. Serotonin and leucine have been proposed to inhibit hunger.

In view of roles of tryptophan, thus serotonin in appetite controlling mechanisms, intakes of carbohydrates must be paid much attention.

Recently volumes and contents of intake amino acids are paid attention to.

7. Sensing of amino acids in the central nervous system

Ensuring sufficient consumption of proteins is needed for growth, reproduction, and species survival [24]. Evolutionally animals had mechanisms to keep adequate protein intake. Detection of decrease or increase of single amino acids can profoundly influence feeding behavior and food preference [24–27].

Hundred years ago, the marked reduction in energy intake and growth of animals maintained on diets containing very low protein amounts or imbalanced EAA ratios was first described. Harper and colleagues showed that the anorectic response to imbalanced amino acid diets is the cause rather than the consequence of growth failure. This suggestion supports the idea that dietary amino acids are important in the regulation of food intake [28–31].

Work by two independent groups demonstrated that mice could detect rapidly dietary EAA deficiency within the APC (anterior piriform cortex) occurs via a GCN2 (general control nonderepressible 2)-dependent mechanism; this pathway is also required for rejection of for EAA-imbalanced diets in drosophila [32]. The GCN2 pathway is an evolutionarily conserved pathway identified in yeast to mediate the detection of amino acid deficiency [33, 34].

From these observations, Hooley and Blouet [35] proposed a mechanism by which animals are able to detect lack or excess of protein. In these networks, leucine and tryptophan are considered a pivotal role in the regulation of feeding behaviors.

Figure 8 illustrates proposed protein sensing sites. APC is proposed to be a site to sense protein deficits and NTS (Nucleus tractus solitarius) is proposed to be a site to sense protein excess.

We here indicate that insulin, thus intake of carbohydrate is essential for the health of brain and peripheral organs. Especially insulin is needed for the transport of tryptophan to the brain. Tryptophan is important for feeding behavior and the production of serotonin, which is needed for emotion. Serotonin is further converted to melatonin in the pineal body. Melatonin is important for sleep. APC and NTS are sites to sense the excess and deficit of proteins. Tryptophan and leucine play important roles there.

In Section 1, we indicate that highly processed foods disturb the gut-brain circuitry so that the nutritional content in the processed foods is not accurately conveyed to the brain. It is possible that the way foods are processed and prepared

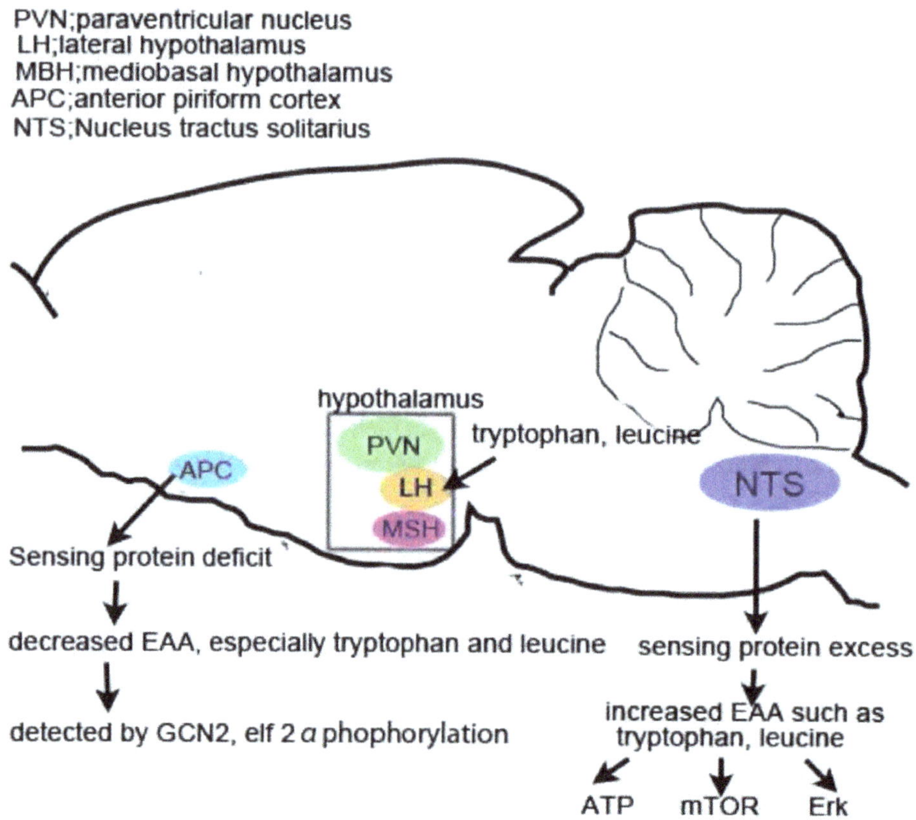

Figure 8.
Protein sensing sites.

affects physiology beyond the energy density or palatability of the foods, and that these disturbances promote overeating and metabolic dysfunction.

Small and DiFeliceantonio [4] proposed that information of carbohydrates after oxidation of glucose is conveyed to the midbrain and further to the cortex and that information of fat through PPAR γ is conveyed through vagus nerve and transmitted to the substantia nigra, further to the cortex, where unusual amounts of dopamine are released, leading to overeating.

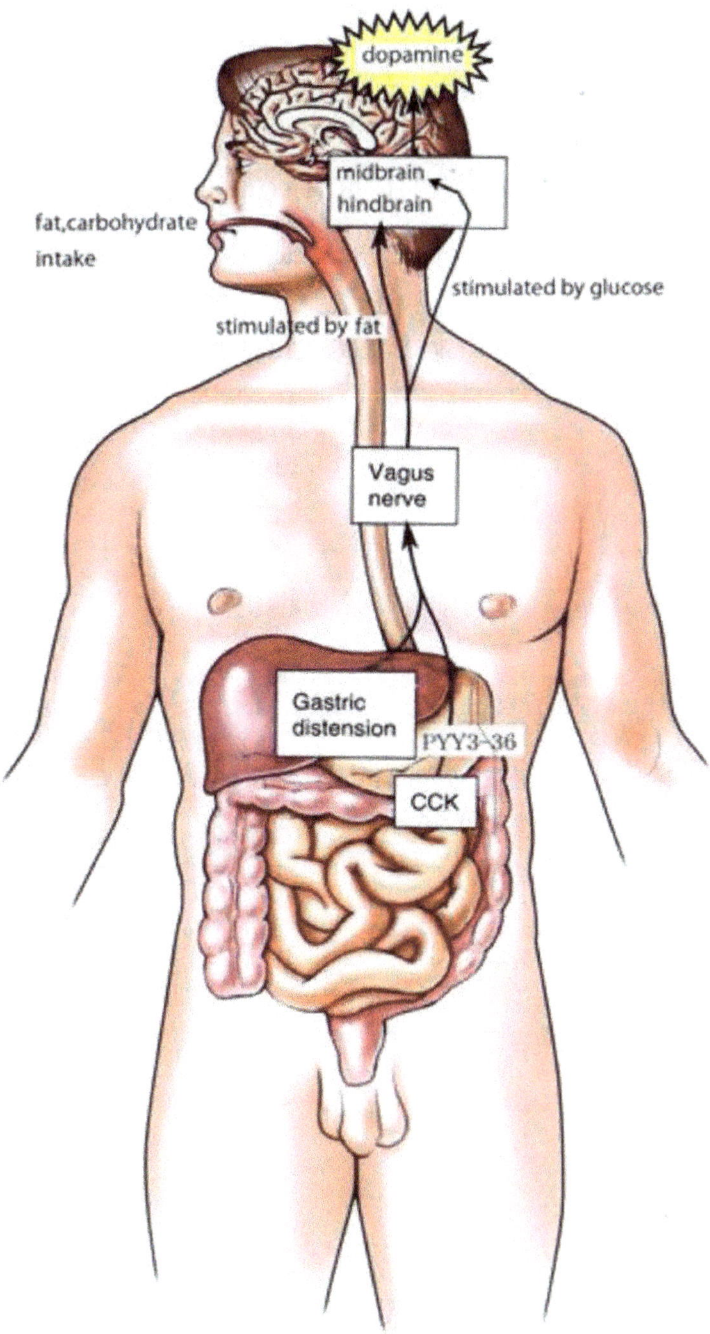

Figure 9.
Gut-brain circuitry of foods contents.

We propose that information of carbohydrates and fats in the processed foods is sent to the brain through vagus nerve, causing unexpected amounts of dopamine release. This may cause overeating.

Figure 9 shows our hypothesis. We propose that information of food intake is conveyed mainly through the vagus nerve to the brain. We report this hypothesis elsewhere.

Author details

Akikazu Takada[1*], Fumiko Shimizu[2], Yukie Ishii[2], Mutsumi Ogawa[2] and Tetsuya Takao[2]

1 International Projects on Food and Health (NPO), Tokyo, Japan

2 Faculty of Human Life and Environmental Sciences, Showa Women's University, Tokyo, Japan

*Address all correspondence to: takada-1a@kmd.biglobe.ne.jp

References

[1] Shell ER. New theory of obesity. Scientific American. 2019;**321**:31-37

[2] Hall KD, Chen KY, Guo J, Lam YY, Leibel RL, Mayer LE, et al. Energy expenditure and body composition changes after an isocaloric ketogenic diet in overweight and obese men. American Journal of Clinical Nutrition. 2016;**104**(2):324-333. DOI: 10.3945/ajcn.116.133561

[3] Adolph EF. Urges to eat and drink in rats. American Journal of Physiology. 1947;**151**(1):110-125

[4] Small DM, DiFeliceantonio AG. Processed foods and food reward. Science. 2019;**363**(6425):346-347. DOI: 10.1126/science.aav0556

[5] Takao T, Ogawa M, Ishii Y, Shimizu F, Takada A. Different glycemic responses to sucrose and glucose in old and young male adults. Journal of Nutrition and Food Sciences. 2016;**6**:460. DOI: 10.4172/2155-9600.1000460

[6] Shimizu F, Ogawa M, Takao T, Ishii Y, Takada A. Correlations among various foods uptakes and body mass index (BMI) or plasma parameters. Obesity Open Access. 2016;**2**(3):1-4. DOI: 10.16966/2380-5528.123

[7] Steinert RE, Luscombe-Marsh ND, Little TJ, Standfield S, Otto B, Horowitz M, et al. Effects of intra-duodenal infusion of L-tryptophan on ad libitum eating, antropyloroduodenal motility, glycemia, insulinemia, and gut peptide secretion in healthy men. Journal of Clinical Endocrinology and Metabolism. 2014;**99**:3275-3328

[8] Miller RL, Loewy AD. 5-HT neurons of the area postrema become c-Fos-activated after increases in plasma sodium levels and transmit interoceptive information to the nucleus accumbens. Amercian Journal of Physiology. 2014;**306**:R663-R673. DOI: 10.1152/ajpregu.00563.2013

[9] Meyer-Gerspach AC, Häfliger S, Meili J, Doody A, Rehfeld JF, Drewe J, et al. Effect of L-tryptophan and L-leucine on gut hormone secretion, appetite feelings and gastric emptying rates in lean and non-diabetic obese participants: A randomized, double-blind, parallel-group trial. PLoS ONE. 2016;**11**(11):e0166758. DOI: 10.1371/journal. pone.01667585

[10] Curzon G. Serotonergic aspects of feeding. In: Serotonin in the Central Nervous System and Periphery. Amsterdam, The Netherlands: Elsevier Science B.V.; 1995. pp. 43-51

[11] Noto H, Goto A, Tsujimoto T, Noda M. Low-carbohydrate diets and all-cause mortality: A systematic review and meta-analysis of observational studies. PLoS ONE. 2013;**8**(1):e55030

[12] Statements on Atkins' death. USA Today. February 2nd, 2004

[13] Felig P. Amino acid metabolism in man. Annual Review of Biochemistry. 1975;**44**:933-955

[14] Jefferson LS, Li JB, Rannels SR. Regulation by insulin of amino acid release and protein turnover in the perfused rat hemicorpus. Journal of Biological Chemistry. 1977;**252**:1476-1483

[15] Biolo G, Williams BD, Fleming RY, Wolfe RR. Insulin action on muscle protein kinetics and amino acid transport during recovery after resistance exercise. Diabetes. 1999;**48**:949-957

[16] Robinson MM, Soop M, Sohn TS, Morse DM, Schimke JM, et al. High insulin combined with essential amino acids stimulates skeletal muscle

mitochondrial protein synthesis while decreasing insulin sensitivity in healthy humans. Journal of Clinical Endocrinology and Metabolism. 2014;**99**:2574-2583

[17] Stancáková A, Civelek M, Saleem NK, Soininen P, et al. Hyperglycemia and a common variant of GCKR are associated with the levels of eight amino acids in 9,369 Finnish men. Diabetes. 2012;**61**:1895-1902

[18] Fernstrom JD, Wurtman RJ. Brain serotonin content: Increase following ingestion of carbohydrate diet. Science. 1971;**174**:1023-1025

[19] Fernstrom JD, Wurtman RJ. Brain serotonin content: Physiological regulation by plasma neutral amino acids. Science. 1972;**178**:414-416

[20] Lipsett D, Madras BK, Wurtman RJ, Munro HN. Serum tryptophan level after carbohydrate ingestion: Selective decline in non-albumin-bound tryptophan coincident with reduction in serum free fatty acids. Life Sciences II. 1873;**12**:57-64

[21] Pan RM, Mauron C, Glaeser B, Wurtman RJ. Effect of various oral glucose doses on plasma neutral amino acid levels. Metabolism. 1982;**31**:937-943

[22] Ogawa M, Takao T, Ishii Y, Takada A. Changes in plasma amino acid levels after the administration of glucose or sucrose to healthy young and aged males. Journal of Nutrition. 2016;**1**(2):008

[23] Shimizu F, Ishii Y, Ogawa M, Takao T, Matsuoka K, Kato K, et al. Plasma levels of various amino acids and their changes upon protein uptakes in Japanese young and old men and women. Integrative Food, Nutrition and Metabolism. 2017;**4**(6):1-5. DOI: 10.15761/IFNM.1000198

[24] Fontana L, Partridge L. Promoting health and longevity through diet: From model organisms to humans. Cell. 2015;**161**:106-118. DOI: 10.1016/ j.cell.2015.02.020

[25] Solon-Biet SM, Mitchell SJ, Coogan SCP, Cogger VC, Gokarn R, McMahon AC, et al. Dietary protein to carbohydrate ratio and caloric restriction: comparing metabolic outcomes in mice. Cell Reports. 2015;**11**:1529-1534. DOI: 10.1016/j. celrep.2015.05.007

[26] Gietzen DW, Hao S, Anthony TG. Mechanisms of food intake repression in indispensable amino acid deficiency. Annual Review of Nutrition. 2007;**27**:63-78. DOI: 10.1146/annurev. nutr.27.061406.093726

[27] Schwartz G. Central leucine sensing in the control of energy homeostasis. Endocrinology and Metabolism Clinics of North America. 2013;**42**:81-87. DOI: 10.1016/ j.ecl.2012.12.001 7

[28] Harper A, Benevenga N, Wohlhueter R. Effects of ingestion of disproportionate amounts of amino acids. Physiological Reviews. 1970;**50**:428-558

[29] Rogers QR, Morris JG, Freedland RA. Lack of hepatic adaptation to low and high levels of dietary protein in the adult rat. Enzyme. 1977;**55**:348-356

[30] Rogers QR, Egan AR. Amino acid imbalance in the liquid-fed lamb. Australian Journal of Biological Sciences. 1975;**26**:169-181

[31] Leung PM, Rogers QR. Effect of amino acid imbalance and deficiency on dietary choice patterns of rats. Physiology & Behavior. 1986;**37**:747-758

[32] Bjordal M, Arquier N, Kniazeff J, Pin JP, Leopold P. Sensing of amino acids in a dopaminergic circuitry promotes rejection of an incomplete diet

in drosophila. Cell. 2014;**156**:510-521. DOI: 10.1016/j.cell.2013.12.024

[33] Dong J, Qiu H, Garcia-Barrio M, Anderson J, Hinnebusch A. Uncharged tRNA activates GCN2 by displacing the protein kinase moiety from a bipartite tRNA-binding domain. Molecular Cell. 2000;**6**:269-679. DOI: 10.1016/ S1097-2765(00)00028-9

[34] Zhang P, McGrath BC, Reinert J, Olsen DS, Lei L, Gill S, et al. The GCN2 eIF2alpha kinase is required for adaptation to amino acid deprivation in mice. Molecular and Cellular Biology. 2002;**22**:6681-6688. DOI: 10.1128/MCB.22.19.6681

[35] Hooley N, Blouet C. Central amino acids sensing in the control of feeding behavior. Frontiers in Endocrinology. 2016;**7**:1-11. DOI: 10.3389/ fendo.2016.00148

6

Metabolic Programming and Nutrition

Poliana Guiomar de Almeida Brasiel
and Sheila Cristina Potente Dutra Luquetti

Abstract

Epidemiological and experimental studies have and continue to offer valuable insight into the Developmental Origins of Health and Disease (DOHaD) hypothesis, which emphasizes the importance of early-life nutritional and environmental changes on the increased risk of metabolic diseases in later life. It is now known that non-communicable chronic diseases that were previously associated with lifestyle and genetics have their origins early in life. It is well established that early life environmental signals, including nutrition, set the stage for long-term health and disease risk—effects that span multiple generations. This relationship began still in the intrauterine period and extends throughout the critical period of development. Many types of nutritional challenges including caloric restriction, macronutrient excess, and micronutrient insufficiencies have been shown to induce early life adaptations that produce long-term dysfunction. Several pathways have been suggested to underpin these associa-tions, including epigenetic reprogramming of germ cells. While the mechanisms still remain to be fully investigated, the relationship of nutrition factors in early life and metabolic diseases are clear. This chapter focuses on the role that the nutrition presents during critical periods of development and its repercussions into adulthood.

Keywords: metabolic programming, nutrition, epigenetics, developmental programming, obesity, microbiome

1. Introduction

In the development period, the fetus may be exposed to an altered risk of developing diseases in adulthood. In this regard, the hypothesis called Developmental Origins of Health and Disease (DOHaD) highlights the relationship between stimuli in the early stages of life and the subsequent development of the disease [1–3]. This model studies the adaptations that occur in the fetus in response to the intrauterine environment, leading to a permanent set of homeostatic systems to assist in immediate survival and improve success in an adverse postnatal environment. However, inappropriate interpretations or environmental changes can lead to an incompatibility between prenatal predictions and postnatal reality [4, 5].

Thus, these adaptations known as predictive adaptive responses can be disadvantageous in adulthood, resulting in an increased risk of diseases that can be transmitted to future generations. In this perspective, it was established that some nutritional changes early in life can lead to an increased risk for several diseases in adulthood [6, 7].

Various studies have shown an association between maternal malnutrition and exposure to hormones during critical periods of development, with metabolic changes, with an emphasis on chronic non-communicable diseases, thyroid disorders, among others [8, 9]. The mother's malnutrition characteristic is capable of interfering with the nutritional status of adult offspring. Maternal protein restriction during lactation led to low weight of the offspring at weaning. Caloric restriction resulted in greater weight gain and resistance to leptin in adult offspring [10].

Programming at a critical stage of development can lead to changes in tissues and organs, which extend throughout life; it may also present a latency period and manifest only in adult life. More studies are emerging to explain the possible mechanisms related to metabolic programming [11, 12].

The mechanisms involved are not entirely clear, but it is believed that there is a relationship between changes in the structural development of the organs and with persistent changes at the cellular level [13]:

- performance in epigenetic memory, with changes in the transcription process;
- alteration of the organ structure in vascularization, innervation, and juxtaposition, such as the position of hepatocytes, endothelial cells, and Kupffer cells, which during organogenesis can permanently modify metabolism;
- hyperplasia or hypertrophy;
- abnormal cell growth under specific metabolic conditions; and
- Metabolic differentiation process.

Molecular mechanisms suggested include acute or chronic changes in gene expression, through various avenues, where there is an epigenetic interrelation between certain genes, exposure to environmental factors, and biological events [5].

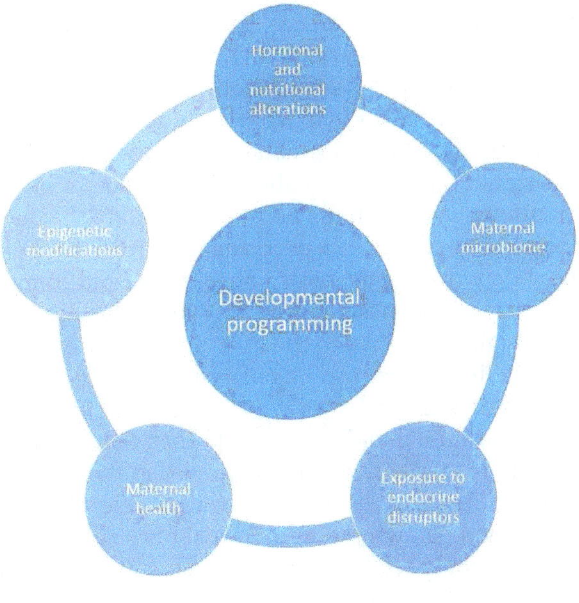

Figure 1.
A complex network that affects adult health and disease, including hormonal and nutrition alterations, epigenetic modifications, microbiota, and the exposure to endocrine disruptors.

As the epigenetic regulation during development changes, the dynamic epigenome has an unstable nature, providing a response and adaptation to environmental pressures, including nutritional changes [2]. **Figure 1** presents the principal mechanisms linked to developmental programming.

There is still a lot to be understood, although epigenetics helps to reveal how exposure to environmental factors, in critical periods of development, leads to changes in adult life, it is necessary to understand the post-epigenetic changes involved in the various processes that lead to the emergence of diseases [13].

2. The early-life origins of obesity

Obesity is defined by an excess of adipose tissue and occurs when an imbalance in the balance of energy exists [14]. The origin of obesity is a complex process that involves genetic and environmental factors and is often associated with the development of chronic complications, such as hyperglycemia, hypertriglyceridemia, low HDL levels, and hypertension. Individuals who have at least three of these criteria are clinically diagnosed as having metabolic syndrome, which increases the risk of developing metabolic diseases, such as type 2 diabetes and cardiovascular diseases [15, 16].

In 2016, more than 1.9 billion adults, 18 years and older, were overweight. Of these, over 650 million were obese; 41 million children under the age of 5 were over-weight or obese, as well as over 340 million children and adolescents aged 5–19 [14]. Recognizing its etiology is essential to face the global epidemic. This creates a challenge since the pathway to obesity in many individuals begins before birth; a predisposition to obesity can occur through epigenetic and other forms of early programming, and obesity and its metabolic consequences result from physiological changes set during fetal and early postnatal development [17–19].

It is known that a number of factors, including epigenetic signals, mitochondrial inheritance, milk composition, gut microbiota, and features of the maternal metabolic environment, such as insulin resistance, fatty acids, and inflammation, may cause developmental programming. In many cases, the effects of the prenatal perturbations are exacerbated by postnatal exposure to a high-calorie diet, accelerated postnatal growth, stress, or other factors [20–22].

The early-life origins of obesity are supported by a number of studies, which have shown that being exposed to inappropriately nutrition levels during critical periods of development (fetal and postnatal) is associated with increased risk of obesity, insulin resistance, and type 2 diabetes in child and adult life [23, 24]. The excessive or deficient nutritional status before birth alters the development of the fat cell, the adipocyte, and results in a permanent increase in the capacity to form new cells in adipose depots (adipogenesis) or to store lipid in existing adipocytes (lipogenesis) since the adipogenesis occurs primarily during late fetal and early postnatal life, and is highly sensitive to the nutritional environment at this time, in particular to the prevailing concentrations of insulin-like growth factors, glucose, insulin, and glucocorticoids [17, 25].

In addition, there are animal and human data that show that obese mothers are more likely to generate to an overweight baby and that these infants are at greater risk of obesity in later life. This "intergenerational cycle of obesity" already is a well-defined phenomenon, showing that maternal obesity, maternal diabetes, and an increase in nutrient supply to the developing fetus constitute major risk factors for obesity in postnatal life [26–28].

There is a greater propensity to develop altered energy metabolism in adult life, in particular, overweight and/or hyperphagia, after malnutrition during fetal development. This predisposition to develop obesity is particularly clear in the offspring of calorie-restricted dams and is also exacerbated when animals are exposed to an obesogenic environment in adulthood. Mechanisms contained in the deregula-tion of food intake and energy balance, due to perinatal nutrition, could be related to hypothalamic alterations and a lower capacity to respond to insulin and leptin signaling [29]. One potential mechanism of developmental programming is through permanent structural alterations of different organs. Different stress exposures (oxidative, immune, and inflammatory stresses, as well as maternal-placental-fetal endocrine disturbances) during the prenatal development could reprogram the telomere biology system [30, 31].

3. Metabolic pathways and epigenetics

During their lifetime, cells receive several external signals, like hormones, growth factors, cytokines, and other extracellular factors. This flow of metabolites, through complex metabolic networks, acts optimizing diverse epigenetic cofactors, thus relating nutrition and diet changes into cytoplasmic signaling and chromatin remodeling. Histone modifications—as DNA methylation, RNA interfer-ence, and non-coding RNA—inserted by the term epigenetics represent diverted ways by which cells control the expression of genes without any alteration in the underlying genetic material [32].

The produced metabolites remain the same for a given cell, but tissue function and nutrient availability will determine the metabolite requirements. In addition, metabolic challenges, such as calorie or oxygen restriction or even a high-fat diet, drive decisions about cell fate. Consistently, dramatic epigenetic changes have been associated with metabolic disorders, such as obesity, insulin resistance, type 2 diabetes, and cancer [32, 33].

The changes on the cellular and tissue level are followed by alterations in epigenetic regulation of gene expression. Epigenetic modifications refer to heritable changes in gene expression occurring without changes in DNA sequence. The epigenetic code is changed dramatically in the course of embryonic development to initiate varying patterns of gene expression in different developing tissues. This code consists of modifications of chromatin histones and DNA playing a central role in packing DNA by forming nucleosomes. Mechanisms of epigenetic regulation are DNA methylation at cytosine residues in promoter or enhancer gene regions, intragenic DNA methylation usually leading to transcriptional silencing, and posttranslational modifications of core histone proteins, such as acetylation usually resulting in transcriptional activation. Non-coding microRNAs which can govern gene activity at both transcriptional and posttranscriptional levels are one more recently discovered key component of epigenetic control. Another important factor is the microRNA expression that may be modulated by histone modifications or DNA methylation and vice versa, thereby causing feedback loops in epigenetic regulation [30, 34, 35].

The ability of the genotype to produce different phenotypes in response to different environments is termed "plasticity." The time of maximal plasticity appears to be during development. Nonetheless, heritable phenotypic variation at a later stage is also possible because of the individual's capability to respond to environmental conditions. Plasticity in developmental programming has evolved to provide the best chances of survival and reproductive success to the organism. When reflecting this theory to developmental data, adaptive growth and metabolic-related strategies for transition from one life history phase to the next and the timing of such transitions (inherent adaptive plasticity) have evolved [36, 37].

Adaptive plasticity enables a species to respond to an environmental change to survive and reproduce and may manifest itself as polyphenism or as a continuous variation in traits. In evolutionary terms, plastic and developmental responses in early life enable an organism to adjust its phenotype so that it can survive in the environment in which it will grow and reproduce. However, the adaptation is not always positive, and the outcome may be harmful and may result in teratogenesis, diseases, or death [36].

There are two types of adaptive responses (plasticity). The first type is the anticipatory or predictive adaptive responses, where the developing organism forecasts the future environment and then adjusts its phenotypic trajectory accordingly. The second type is the immediate adaptive responses that promote short-term maternal or fetal survival with some advantages in later life (developmental plasticity). These adaptive responses have a significant cost, and a cost-benefit analysis is performed to determine the true value of the adaptive response. The links between epigenetics, developmental programming, and plasticity in early growth and nutrition provide subsidies to understand aspects involved in child growth and development and their long-term impact [7, 36].

The nutrition is one of the most studied environmental epigenetic factors, and already associations have been observed between adverse prenatal nutritional conditions, postnatal health, and increased risk of disease. It is known that maternal and paternal diets influence metabolic phenotypes in offspring through epigenetic information transmission. Over molecular mechanisms with respect to the fetal origins of adult disease have been suggested including mitochondrial dysfunction and oxidative stress as among the earliest events described in offspring exposed to nutrient restriction. This in turn modifies the expression of critical genes and can affect health and longevity [38].

The foods contain nutrients and bioactive components that can modify epigenetic marks and alter the expression of genes. These compounds, including folate, vitamin B12, methionine, among others, can affect DNA methylation and histone, altering 1-carbon metabolism. The S-adenosylmethionine (AdoMet) and S-adenosylhomocysteine (AdoHcy), metabolites of 1-carbon metabolism, can alter the methylation of DNA and histones. Thus, nutrients and bioactive components, as well as conditions that may affect the levels of AdoMet or AdoHcy in the tissue, have the ability to modify the methylation of DNA and histones [11, 39].

In a study developed by our research group, we identified that the maternal intake of soybeans in lactation changed the lipid content of breast milk and programmed offspring for a phenotype of the lower metabolic risk. The difference in fat content of breast milk and the higher isoflavones content of soy diet are possible imprinting factors that could program the offspring [18]. This is particularly important because it highlights the dual role of nutritional alterations, whether as reprogramming strategies to prevent disease or leading to adult disease [40].

The metabolic mechanism linked to the programming induced by the adverse intrauterine environment is not completely clear, but fetal metabolic programming has already been indicated to contribute to changes in tissue development, number of cells, neural circuits, and so on. Epigenetic programming plays an important role in the differentiation and development of embryonic, tissue, and stem cells. The changes induced by epigenetic modification in cell or tissue function can be transmitted from fetuses to adults and induce the development of the metabolic syndrome in adult offspring. There is a vulnerable "window" for epigenetic programming when germ cells, embryos, and fetuses are in development [11, 41].

Figure 2 presents a scheme of developmental origins of health and disease. Epigenetic marks can be modulated by environmental factors, are heritable, perpetuate gene-expression changes that underlie programming, and may contribute to the onset of disease/health in later life.

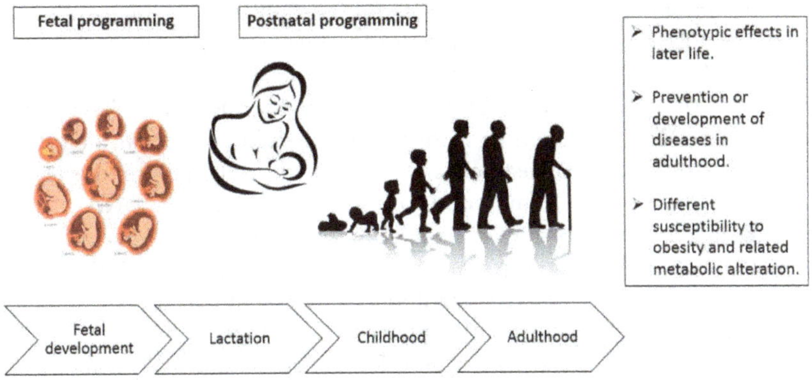

Figure 2.
Scheme demonstrative of developmental origins of health and disease, during prenatal and early postnatal life, involved in the susceptibility to obesity and metabolic changes.

4. Microbiome and metabolic health

The genetic set of the microbiome provides extensive metabolic and immunological potential. Genetic and environmental factors influence microbiota composition and function, and these complex host-microbe interactions contribute to health and disease state. The gut microorganisms have a significant role in epithelial barrier function, fermentation of dietary fiber, synthesis of vitamins, regulation of the immune system, and defense against pathogens. This community has also been found to play some important roles in angiogenesis, brain development, and behavior [15, 42].

Given the various functions of microbiota, alterations in this community (dysbiosis) have been associated with a range of non-communicable diseases, including obesity, diabetes, inflammatory bowel disease, metabolic syndrome, cancer, asthma, allergy, non-alcoholic fatty liver disease (NAFLD), and even certain neuropsychiatric disorders [43–46].

The early-life microbiota presents a unique microbial communities consisting of numerous bacteria and viruses. A part of this microbiota already has identified by using different kinds of technologies including 16S rRNA sequencing. Over the last decades, the paradigm of a sterile condition *in utero* is shifting to the possibility of the prenatal maternal-fetal coexist with commensal and symbiotic microbes. Recent studies also support a prenatal microbial milieu through bacterial presentation in placenta, amniotic fluid, umbilical cord, and meconium. In addition, there are emerging reports of the prenatal microbial composition on fetal and postnatal development [47–49].

A maternal condition during pregnancy and postnatal period can provide a critical window for susceptibility to microbiome development through environmental factors such as mode of delivery and maternal diet. The delivery mode has a crucial function in the early gut microbiota composition. Infants by vaginally delivery have higher levels of intestinal *Bacteroides, Lactobacilli*, and *Bifidobacterium*, which are commonly present in vaginal route, whereas infants by cesarean section (C-section) have higher level of *Enterococcus*, and *Clostridium* from skin, oral, or hospital environment [47, 50].

The gestational age is another important influencer for gut microbiome development. It is reported that the gut microbiota of preterm infants has shown delayed colonization by limited microbial diversity and this risk of gut dysbiosis.

The gut microbiota composition of preterm infants has *Enterobacter, Enterococcus, Escherichia*, and *Klebsiella* predominantly and relatively low level of gammaproteobacteria than those in full-term infants [51, 52].

It is known that breastfeeding influences the infant microbiota. The microbiome may affect the DNA methylation through breast milk, which influences the gut microbiome composition. Breastfeeding is associated with greater *Bacteroides* and *Bifidobacterium*, which are folate producers, thereby affecting DNA methylation. Breast milk oligosaccharides alter core microbiome community that secretes short-chain fatty acid (SCFA). Therefore, the strain of *Bifidobacterium* and *Lactobacillus* by breastfeeding could make intestinal contents more acidic with SCFA, which modulate a defense mechanism against pathogens and have epigenetic effects [53–55].

The microbial metabolites such as B vitamins, short-chain fatty acids, polyphenols, and omega 3 polyunsaturated fatty acids are reported to influence epigenetic mechanisms. Maternal gut microbe metabolites can change the host cellular levels of important epigenetic modifiers like histone acetyl transferases (HATs), histone deacetylases (HDACs), DNA methyltransferases (DNMTs), and DNA demethylases. The microbial SCFAs from the fermentation of dietary fiber were shown to maintain the nervous and immune systems through epigenetic modification. These, acetate and butyrate are the most abundant in the intestinal tract and can be produced with acetyl-CoA which is universal acetyl group donor for histone acetylation [45, 47].

Different essential functions for human health develop correspondingly with gut microorganism increase, including vitamin biosynthesis, energy extraction from the diet, gut barrier function, and immune system maturation. The immune system of neonates is immature and requires the exposure of gut bacteria to develop properly. Depending on the health of the mother, maternal bacterial communities may already be imbalanced when passed on to the infant. In children, metabolic diseases, including obesity, insulin resistance, and NAFLD, along with other related immune-based diseases, are associated with modifications in infant gut bacterial composition; however, the mechanisms involved are not entirely clear [43, 56].

5. Conclusions

It is known that there is a close relationship between maternal obesity, diet consumption during pregnancy and lactation, and their impact on the microbiota of both mother and infant, including their links to early gut colonization and innate immunity in the infants that drive an increased risk for metabolic diseases.

For the most effective confrontation of metabolic diseases, which represent a great burden of global health, it is important to consider the issues involving early nutrition, metabolic programming, and epigenetics. Thus, the adoption of health policies during critical stages of development, including pregnancy, lactation, and puberty, is essential to achieve long-term consistent results.

Author details

Poliana Guiomar de Almeida Brasiel* and Sheila Cristina Potente Dutra Luquetti
Department of Nutrition, Federal University of Juiz de Fora, MG, Brazil

*Address all correspondence to: brasiel.poliana@gmail.com

References

[1] Barker D, Bull A, Osmond C, Simmonds S. Fetal and placental size and risk of hypertension in adult life. BMJ. 1990;**301**:259-262

[2] Vickers MH. Early life nutrition, epigenetics and programming of later life disease. Nutrients. 2014;**6**:2165-2178

[3] Barker D. Fetal origins of coronary heart disease. BMJ. 1995;**311**:171-174

[4] Gluckman PD, Hanson MA, Cooper C, Thornburg KL. Effect of In utero and early-life conditions on adult health and disease. The New England Journal of Medicine. 2008;**359**(1):61-73

[5] Laker RC, Wlodek ME, Connelly JJ, Yan Z. Epigenetic origins of metabolic disease: The impact of the maternal condition to the offspring epigenome and later health consequences. Food Science and Human Wellness [Internet]. Beijing Academy of Food Sciences. 2013;**2**(1): 1-11. DOI: 10.1016/j.fshw.2013.03.002

[6] Fernandez-Twinn DS, Ozanne SE. Early life nutrition and metabolic programming. Annals of the New York Academy of Sciences. 2010;**1212**:78-96

[7] Gluckman P, Hanson M, Spencer H. Predictive adaptive responses and human evolution. Trends in Ecology & Evolution. 2005;**20**(10):527-533

[8] Passos M, da Fonte Ramos C, Dutra SP, de Moura EG. Transfer of iodine through the milk in protein-restricted lactating rats. The Journal of Nutritional Biochemistry. 2001;**12**(5):300-303

[9] Lisboa P, Fagundes A, Denolato A, Oliveira E, Bonomo I, Alves S, et al. Neonatal low-protein diet changes deiodinase activities and pituitary TSH response to TRH in adult rats. Experimental Biology and Medicine. 2008;**233**(1):57-63

[10] Passos M, Vicente L, Lisboa P, de Moura E. Absence of anorectic effect to acute peripheral leptin treatment in adult rats whose mothers were malnourished during lactation. Hormone and Metabolic Research. 2004;**36**(9):625-629

[11] Zhu Z, Cao F, Li X. Epigenetic programming and fetal metabolic programming. Front Endocrinol (Lausanne). 2019;**10**(764):1-15

[12] Vieira AM, Brasiel PGA, Ferreira MS, Aguiar AS, Luquetti SCPD. Relationship between the consumption of soy and its derivatives during critical periods of development and in adulthood and endocrine-metabolic disorders. Journal of Endocrinology and Metabolism. 2017;**7**(5):135-140

[13] Koletzko B, Symonds M, Olsen S, Programming PEN, Nutrition AE. Programming research: Where are we and where do we go from here? The American Journal of Clinical Nutrition. 2011;**94**:2036S-2043S

[14] WHO. Obesity and Overweight. World Health Organization (WHO). 2020. Available from: https://www.who.int/news-room/fact-sheets/detail/o

[15] Boulangé CL, Neves AL, Chilloux J, Nicholson JK, Dumas M. Impact of the gut microbiota on inflammation, obesity, and metabolic disease. Genome Medicine [Internet]. 2016;**8**:1-12. DOI: 10.1186/s13073-016-0303-2

[16] Alberti K, Zimmet P, Shaw J, Group ETFC. The metabolic syndrome —A new worldwide definition. Lancet. 2005;**366**:1059-1062

[17] Muhlhausler B, Smith SR. Early-life origins of metabolic dysfunction: Role of the adipocyte. Trends in Endocrinology and Metabolism. 2008;**20**:51-57

[18] Vieira AM, de Almeida Brasiel PG, Ferreira MS, Mateus K, Figueiredo MS, Lisboa PC, et al. Maternal soybean diet during lactation alters breast milk composition and programs the lipid profile in adult male rat offspring. Endocrine [Internet]. 2018;**60**:272-281. DOI: 10.1007/s12020-018-1572-x

[19] Rito AI, Buoncristiano M, Spinelli A, Salanave B, Kunešová M, Hejgaard T, et al. Association between characteristics at birth, breastfeeding and obesity in 22 countries: The WHO European Childhood Obesity Surveillance Initiative—COSI 2015/2017. Obesity Facts. 2019;**12**:226-243

[20] Isganaitis E. Developmental programming of body composition: Update on evidence and mechanisms. Current Diabetes Reports. 2019;**19**(8):60

[21] Jazwiec PA, Sloboda DM. Nutritional adversity, sex and reproduction: 30 years of DOHaD and what have we learned? The Journal of Endocrinology. 2019;**242**(1):T51-T68

[22] Neri C, Edlow AG. Effects of maternal obesity on fetal programming: Molecular approaches. Cold Spring Harbor Perspectives in Medicine. 2016;**6**:1-21

[23] Lukaszewski M, Eberlé D, Vieau D, Breton C. Nutritional manipulations in the perinatal period program adipose tissue in offspring. American Journal of Physiology. Endocrinology and Metabolism. 2013;**305**(10):E1195-E1207

[24] Rolland-Cachera MF, Deheeger M, Maillot M, Bellisle F. Early adiposity rebound: Causes and consequences for obesity in children and adults. International Journal of Obesity. 2006;**30**:S11-S17

[25] Patel M, Srinivasan M. Metabolic programming in the immediate postnatal life. Annals of Nutrition & Metabolism. 2011;**58**:18-28

[26] Morris MJ. Early life influences on obesity risk: Maternal overnutrition and programming of obesity. Expert Review of Endocrinology and Metabolism. 2009;**4**(6):625-637

[27] Millership SJ, Van De Pette M, Withers DJ. Genomic imprinting and its effects on postnatal growth and adult metabolism. Cellular and Molecular Life Sciences [Internet]. 2019;**76**(20):4009-4021. DOI: 10.1007/s00018-019-03197-z

[28] Montalvo-Martínez L, Maldonado-Ruiz R, Cárdenas-Tueme M, Reséndez-Pérez D, Camacho A. Maternal overnutrition programs central inflammation and addiction-like behavior in offspring. BioMed Research International. 2018;**2018**:8061389

[29] Sominsky L, Jasoni CL, Twigg HR, Spencer SJ. Hormonal and nutritional regulation of postnatal hypothalamic development. The Journal of Endocrinology. 2018;**237**(2):R47-R64

[30] Vaiserman AM. Birth weight predicts aging trajectory: A hypothesis. Mechanisms of Ageing and Development [Internet]. 2018;**173**:61-70. DOI: 10.1016/j.mad.2018.04.003

[31] Thompson LP, Al-hasan Y. Impact of oxidative stress in fetal programming. Journal of Pregnancy. 2012;**2012**:1-8

[32] Rabhi N, Hannou SA, Froguel P, Annicotte J-S. Cofactors as metabolic sensors driving cell adaptation in physiology and disease. Front Endocrinol (Lausanne). 2017;**8**:1-8

[33] Moody L, Wang H, Jung PM, Chen H, Pan Y. Maternal and post-weaning high-fat diets produce distinct DNA methylation patterns in hepatic metabolic pathways within specific genomic contexts. International Journal of Molecular Sciences. 2019;**20**(13):E3229

[34] Bannister AJ, Kouzarides T. Regulation of chromatin by histone

modifications. Cell Research [Internet]. 2011;**21**:381-395. DOI: 10.1038/cr.2011.22

[35] Wei J, Huang K, Yang C, Kang C. Non-coding RNAs as regulators in epigenetics (review). Oncology Reports. 2017;**37**(1):3-9

[36] Hochberg Z, Feil R, Constancia M, Fraga M, Junien C, Carel J, et al. Child health, developmental plasticity, and epigenetic programming. Endocrine Reviews. 2011;**32**:159-224

[37] Chui C, Li Y, Maloney CA, Cropley JE, Suter CM. Epigenetic programming by maternal nutrition: Shaping future generations. Epigenomics. 2010;**2**(4):539-549

[38] Tiffon C. The impact of nutrition and environmental epigenetics on human health and disease. International Journal of Medical Sciences. 2018;**19**(11):E3425

[39] Choi S, Friso S. Epigenetics: A new bridge between nutrition. Advances in Nutrition. 2010;**1**:8-16

[40] Hsu C-N, Tain Y-L. The good, the bad, and the ugly of pregnancy nutrients and developmental programming of adult disease. Nutrients. 2019;**11**(4):1-21

[41] Marousez L, Lesage J, Eberl D. Epigenetics: Linking early postnatal nutrition to obesity programming? Nutrición Hospitalaria. 2019;**11**(12):2966

[42] Stinson LF. Establishment of the early-life microbiome: A DOHaD perspective. Journal of Developmental Origins of Health and Disease. 2019:1-10

[43] Mulligan CM, Friedman JE. Maternal modifiers of the infant gut microbiota—Metabolic consequences. The Journal of Endocrinology. 2017;**235**(1):R1-R12

[44] Giorgetti G, Brandimarte G, Fabiocchi F, Ricci S, Flamini P, Sandri G, et al. Interactions between innate immunity, microbiota, and probiotics. Journal of Immunology Research. 2015:1-7

[45] Li Y. Epigenetic mechanisms link maternal diets and gut microbiome to obesity in the offspring. Frontiers in Genetics. 2018;**9**:1-13

[46] Stols-Gonçalves D, Tristão LS, Henneman P, Nieuwdorp M. Epigenetic markers and microbiota/metabolite-induced epigenetic modifications in the pathogenesis of obesity, metabolic syndrome, type 2 diabetes, and non-alcoholic fatty liver disease. Current Diabetes Reports. 2019;**19**(6):31

[47] Lee H. The interaction between gut microbiome and nutrients on development of human disease through epigenetic mechanisms. Genomics & Informatics. 2019;**17**(3):e24

[48] Smith-Brown P, Morrison M, Krause L, Davies PSW. Mothers secretor status affects development of childrens microbiota composition and function: A pilot study. PLOS One. 2016;**11**(9):e0161211

[49] Calatayud M, Koren O, Collado MC. Maternal microbiome and metabolic health program microbiome development and health of the offspring. Trends in Endocrinology and Metabolism [Internet]. 2019;**30**(10):735-744. DOI: 10.1016/j.tem.2019.07.021

[50] Zhou X, Du L, Shi R, Chen Z, Zhou Y, Li Z. Early-life food nutrition, microbiota maturation and immune development shape life-long health. Critical Reviews in Food Science and Nutrition. 2019;**59**:S30-S38

[51] Milani C, Duranti S, Bottacini F, Casey E, Turroni F, Mahony J, et al. The first microbial colonizers of the

human gut: Composition, activities, and health implications of the infant gut microbiota. Microbiology and Molecular Biology Reviews. 2017;**81**(4):e00036-e00017

[52] Montoya-Williams D, Lemas DJ, Spiryda L, Patel K, Carney OO, Neu J, et al. The neonatal microbiome and its partial role in mediating the association between birth by cesarean section and adverse pediatric outcomes. Neonatology. 2018;**114**(2):103-111

[53] Ramos-Roman MA. Breast milk: A postnatal link between maternal life choices and the prevention of childhood obesity. Clinical Therapeutics. 2018;**40**(10):1655-1658

[54] Pannaraj PS, Li F, Cerini C, Bender JM, Yang S, Rollie A, et al. Association between breast Milk bacterial communities and establishment and development of the infant gut microbiome. JAMA Pediatrics. 2017;**171**(7):647-654

[55] Pauwels S, Symons L, Vanautgaerden E, Ghosh M, Duca RC, Bekaert B, et al. The influence of the duration of breastfeeding on the infant's metabolic epigenome. Nutrients. 2019;**11**(6):E1408

[56] Jasarevic E, Bale TL. Prenatal and postnatal contributions of the maternal microbiome on offspring programming. Frontiers in Neuroendocrinology [Internet]. 2019;**55**:100797. DOI: 10.1016/j.yfrne.2019.100797

7

Mechanism of Thrombus Formation in Regard to Diet

Shinya Goto

Abstract

The majority of diseases causing sudden death or sudden onset of serious restriction of quality of life are thrombotic disease. Myocardial infarction is often caused by thrombotic occlusion of coronary arterial branches. Ischemic stroke is also caused by occlusion of cerebral arteries with thrombi. In patients admitted to the hospital and immobility, venous thromboembolism causing pulmonary embolism is a major cause of death. The risk of cardiovascular events is influenced by food intake. Yet, the mechanism between specific food intake and the risk of throm-botic disease is still to be elucidated. Recent progress of computer and information technology allows us to describe complex biological phenomena such as thrombosis from basic principles of physics and chemistry. Coupling blood flow, platelet, coagulation, and fibrinolysis allows us to understand the contributing role of each factor for thrombus formation. Yet, the precise role of food intake to influence the risk of thrombosis is still to be elucidated. Coupling basic research and large-scale clinical research will further clarify the role of various types of food intake in the risk of thrombosis.

Keywords: myocardial infarction, stroke, arterial thrombosis, platelet, coagulation

1. Introduction

Thrombosis is the leading cause of death in the world. Indeed, atherothrombosis including coronary artery diseases and cerebrovascular diseases is the top cause of death in various regions of the world [1]. Venous thrombosis including deep venous thrombosis and pulmonary embolism is the third cause of death in hospitalized patients [2]. Thrombosis is a disease caused by thrombi formed at various ves-sels. The major symptom differs substantially depending upon the site where the thrombi developed. Typically, arterial thrombosis such as myocardial infarction and ischemic stroke is symptomatic even when the thrombi are small (e.g., less than 1 mm in diameter) [3]. On the other hand, venous thrombosis is asymptomatic until thrombi become substantially large such as the ones that occlude several pulmonary arteries to cause pulmonary embolism [4]. In both arterial and venous thromboses, platelets are cells that contribute to initial thrombus formation. Coagulation and fibrinolysis are systems necessary to regulate the size of fibrin thrombi.

It is noteworthy that there is homogeneity in risk factors for various arterial/venous thromboses despite wide variation of clinical manifestation [5]. Framingham study demonstrated that cigarette smoking, diabetes mellitus (DM), dyslipidemia, and hypertension are strong predictors for the future onset of arterial thrombosis represented by acute myocardial infarction [6]. Recent international registries also confirm that these risk factors are contributing factors for the recurrence of cardiovascular events [7]. Moreover, international registries also suggested these parameters as risk factors of venous thrombosis [8]. These clinical observations suggested the presence of common pathways for the onset of arterial and venous thrombosis [9].

The Framingham registry suggested the contributory role of obesity and less exercise as the predictors for future prevalence of risk factors. These abnormalities represented as visceral obesity-related syndrome is named as "metabolic syndrome." In metabolic syndrome patients, insulin resistance is one of the major contributors [10]. Increased body weight, high blood pressure, and dyslipidemia are common manifestations of metabolic syndrome. Long-term exposure to a high-calorie diet and lack of good exercise are supposed as underlining mechanisms for the onset of metabolic syndromes. The risk of thrombotic disease including arterial and venous thrombosis is speculated to be high in patients with metabolic syndrome.

2. Platelet adhesion at the site of endothelial injuries

Blood is flowing to maintain homeostasis inside the human body. Blood cells have specific functions: erythrocytes bring oxygen to tissues, leukocytes protect from infection, and platelets stop bleeding promptly. As shown in **Figure 1**, large and heavy erythrocytes tend to be located in the center of blood flow. Small cells of platelets circulate interacting with endothelial cells [11]. In the case where endothelial cells have a physiological function, platelets do not interact with them [12]. Platelets collide with the vessel wall and promptly go back to the blood flow without platelet activation. On the other hand, when endothelial cell function was disturbed by physical or chemical stimuli, endothelial cells lose their ability to keep antithrombotic function. Then, platelets immediately start the interaction with endothelial cells [12]. At the time, von Willebrand factor (VWF) is expressed on the cell surface of stimulated endothelial cells. Platelets capture VWF through glycoprotein (GP)Ibα. GPIbα is expressed on the surface

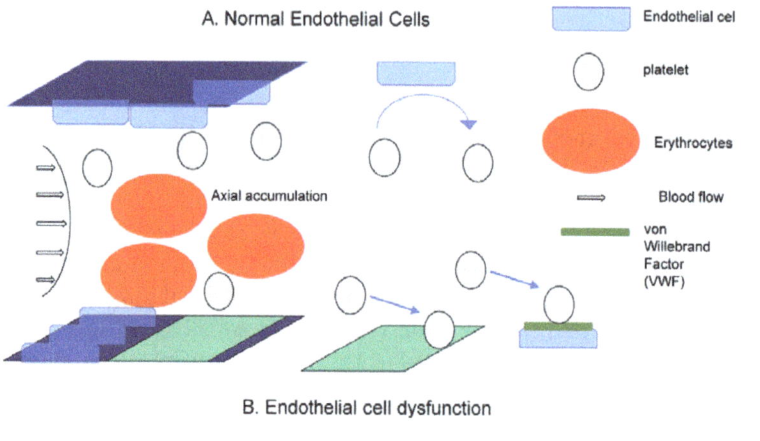

Figure 1.
Role of erythrocytes and blood flow in platelet adhesion at the site of endothelial injury. This figure demonstrates the three-dimensional distribution of erythrocytes, platelets, and endothelial cells. Erythrocytes accumulate in the center of blood flow by biorheological effects. Accordingly, platelets circulate close to endothelial cells. In the presence of normally functioning endothelial cells, platelets do not adhere nor are activated, but just return to blood flow (panel A). If the endothelial cell function was disturbed by various stimulations, platelets are adhered and activated through their interaction with von Willebrand factor (VWF).

of platelet regardless if they are activated or not [13]. Thus, initial adhesion of platelets at the site of endothelial cell damage occurs predominantly as a physical phenomenon, which occurs immediately without time-consuming biological process. Historically, the vast majority of vessel damage is caused by trauma. Rapid accumulation of platelets at the site of endothelial injury plays an important role to keep our blood in our vessel system for surviving.

The potential impact of erythrocytes for the onset and growth of thrombosis has first caught the interest of researchers in the 1960s [14]. Biorheological axial accumulation of flowing platelets was also recognized at the same time [15]. Clinical studies also support the notion that higher hematocrit values are related to higher risk of thrombotic diseases such as myocardial infarction [16]. These results strongly suggest the biophysical role of erythrocytes for thrombus formation. These rheological effects could hardly be controlled by food intake. In another aspect, erythrocytes also influence the function of platelet with biochemical modulation [17–19]. Indeed, erythrocytes are a huge source of ADP [20], which is one of the most potent platelet-stimulating agents [21, 22]. There is potential effects of food intake for influencing erythrocytes components which can influence thrombogenic-ity of platelet [23, 24].

Recent advances in computer technology allowed us to predict the structure and function of VWF bound with GPIbα from the physical movement of atoms and water molecules [25, 26]. By the method, physical force generated by VWF binding with GPIbα could be predicted. Platelet adhesion at injured vessel wall is summarized in **Figure 2**. Platelets are cells with a diameter of approximately 5 μm. But, when platelet adhered at the site of vessel damage, only part of platelet bound with VWF. Molecular dynamic prediction revealed that single bond of VWF and GPIbα could generate binding force approximately 70 pN [25]. Fluid dynamic force applied to platelets reaches to a couple hundred pN when the cell receives detach-ing force from arterial blood flow. Theoretically, several bonds between VWF and GPIbα are enough to stop platelets from adhering to the vessel wall. The mechanism of thrombus formation is a complicated process, but platelet adhesion under blood flow condition could now be constructed from physical movement of atoms and water molecules.

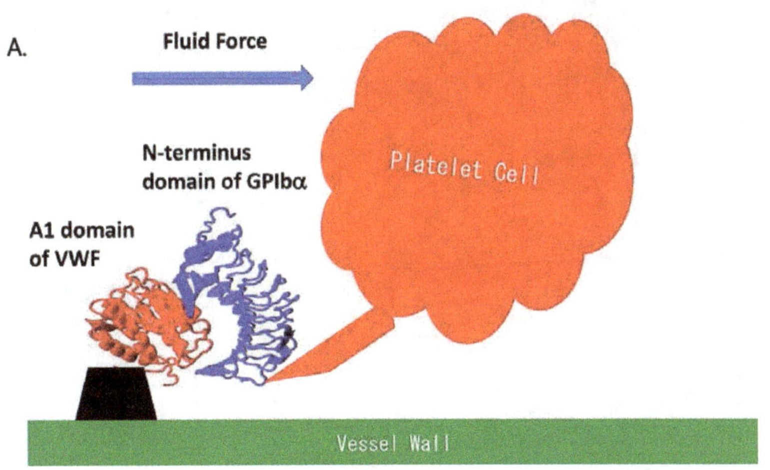

Figure 2.
Platelet adhesion at the site of endothelial damage under blood flow conditions. Platelet adhesion is mediated exclusively by its glycoprotein (GP)Ibα binding with von Willebrand factor (VWF). Adhered platelets receive fluid dynamic force, but platelets continue to adhere until the detaching force becomes larger than the binding force generated between VWF and GPIbα.

It is of particular importance that endothelial damage is not caused only by acute physical or chemical stimulation. In the recent era, human beings enjoy longer life than those who lived hundreds of years ago. Just like carrying human being, vessel system become old when people become old. Longer time exposure of vessel wall to atherogenic lipids such as LDL cholesterol and its related local biological reac-tion causes atherosclerosis [27, 28]. Antithrombotic potential of endothelial cell in patients with atherosclerosis is reduced when compared to younger normal ones. Moreover, plaque rupture exposes subendothelial thrombotic materials to vessel lumen. Thus, atherothrombotic events occur frequently [29] in the era of aging society. The initial event resulting in symptomatic atherothrombosis is always platelet adhesion at the site of endothelial injury.

By understanding the mechanism of atherosclerosis and atherothrombosis, it is rather easy to understand that various types of food intake influence the risk of thrombosis. As regards nutritional factor, there is a hot discussion concerning cholesterol. Some suggested potential benefit of cholesterol restriction for prevention of atherothrombosis. The other suggest there are no relationship between daily cholesterol intake and the risk of atherothrombotic event risk.

3. Activation of coagulation cascade and fibrinolysis

Symptomatic atherothrombotic events such as acute myocardial infarction occur when organ perfusing arterial branch was occluded by thrombi. The diameter of organ perfusing vessels is substantially larger than a single cell of platelet. Indeed, the diameter of platelets is just 2–5 μm, while the diameter of myocardial perfusing coronary arterial branches is 2–3 mm. The size of vessel diameter is typically 1000 more than the size of platelet diameter. It is nonrealistic to imagine that coronary arterial branches were occluded by platelet thrombi. Indeed, when coronary arte-rial thrombi causing myocardial infarction are aspirated by thrombo-aspiration therapy, the main component of occlusive thrombi was fibrin (**Figure 3**). It is

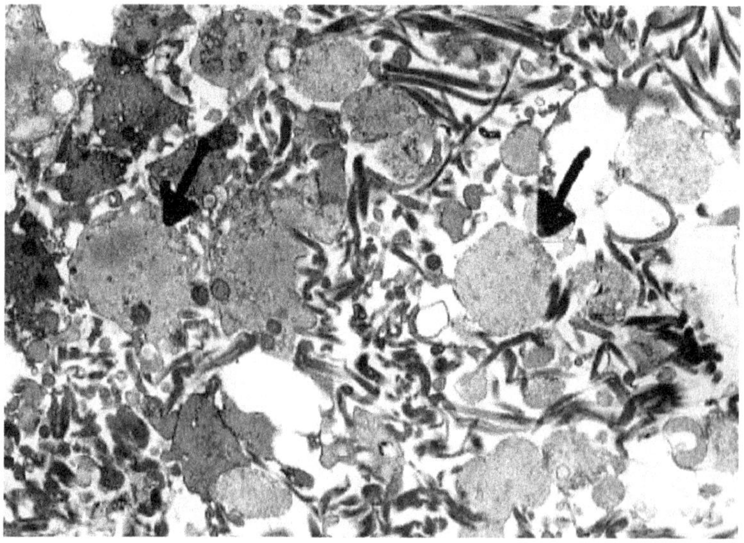

Figure 3.
Major components of thrombi causing acute myocardial infarction. Sample thrombi were aspirated from patients with acute myocardial infarction. The main results and study protocols were published elsewhere [53]. Here, electron microscopy results are shown. Fibrin fibrils could be seen around activated platelets (arrow).

noteworthy that fibrin fibrils are detected around activated platelets (**Figure 3** is the product in collaboration with Prof. Yujiro Asada at Miyazaki University).

The lipid components of activated platelet changed from the ones at the quiescent state. Negatively charged phospholipids appeared on the surface of activated platelets [22]. Then, various coagulation factors accumulated around the lipid to form pro-thrombin complex. On the activated platelet, thrombin generation occurs extremely efficiently. Indeed, thrombin generation rate in the absence of activated platelet and tissue factor is almost 0 as compared to that in its presence. At the site of atheroma rupture, large enough fibrin thrombi were formed as a result of the accumulation of activated platelet and exposure of tissue factor from the ruptured atheroma. Tissue factor accumulated in the atheroma is generated from inflammatory cells, which migrated into the atheroma. In the animal study, dietary lipid restriction reduces the amount of tissue factor accumulated in the atheroma [30]. The clinical factor of the reduction of the onset of myocardial infarction by the use of lipid-lowering therapy [31] may be related to reduction of lipid accumulation and subsequent reduction in tissue factor accumulated in the atheroma. Moreover, there are several publications indicating the impact of food intake for the lipid component of blood cells [23, 24]. The rate of fibrin formation at the site of endothelial damage and platelet accumulation should be modified by food from both activated platelet-derived procoagulant activity and the amount of tissue factors accumulated in the atheroma.

The process of thrombus formation at the site of endothelial injury is com-plex. We have attempted to develop the process model of thrombus formation as shown in **Figure 4** [32]. The model is still simple but includes various physically and chemically different events. First, the model implemented the effect of blood flow, which is a purely physical phenomenon. Second, the model includes platelet

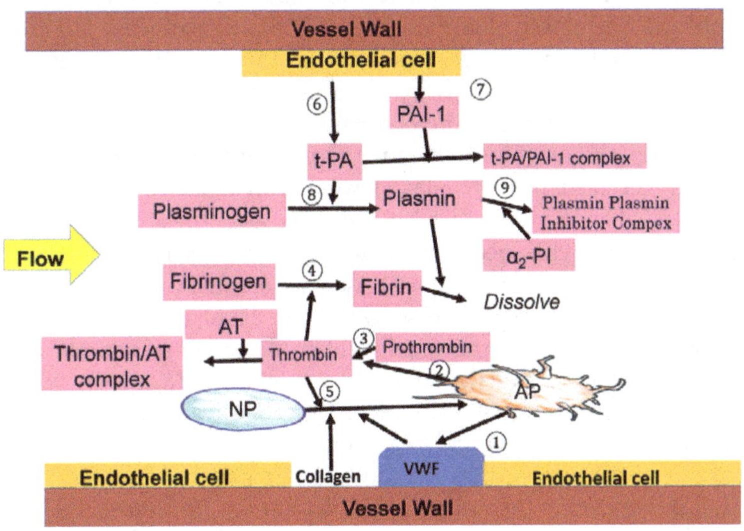

Figure 4.

Coupling model of blood flow, platelet, coagulation, and fibrinolysis. Thrombus formation at the site of endothelial injury is modeled. Nonactivated platelets (NP) adhered at the site of endothelial injury through von Willebrand factor (VWF) and collagen are exposed there. NP become activated platelets (AP) by their interaction with VWF/collagen (①). AP has a potential to convert prothrombin to thrombin on their membrane surface (②). After production of thrombin from prothrombin (③), thrombin converts soluble fibrinogen to fibrin thrombi. (④) thrombin also has a function to further activate platelets through thrombin receptor stimulation. (⑤) Fibrinolytic system is also incorporated in this model. Functional endothelial cells constitutively release both tissue-type plasminogen activator (t-PA: ⑥) and plasminogen activator inhibitor (PAI)-1 (⑦). T-PA converts plasminogen to plasmin, which has fibrinolytic activity (⑧) unless inactivated by binding with PAI-1. Plasmin is a strong enzyme able to degrade fibrin. Its function is immediately neutralized by its binding with a2-plasmin inhibitor to form plasmin a2-plasmin inhibitor complex (PIC: ⑨).

adhesion and activation. Platelet adhesion is implemented to be medicated by its GPIbα binding with von Willebrand factor (VWF) (① in **Figure 4**). GPIbα bind-ing with VWF is a chemical phenomenon, but the binding force is a physical one. We have implemented both in the same model. Platelets were implemented to be activated to change their biological roles (② in **Figure 4**). This process is a biological process. The detailed process model of platelet activation was published elsewhere [33]. Briefly, platelets were settled to be captured by VWF under blood flow condi-tion. Collagen exposed at the site of endothelial injury also interacts with platelet and contributed to platelet activation through its receptor, namely, GPVI [34]. Then, activated platelet was settled to have stronger capacity to bind with injured vessel wall, cohesion each other, and possess the capacity to express coagulogenic phospholipids. Then, prothrombin conversion to thrombin was settled to occur only on the surface of activated platelets (③ in **Figure 4**). Thrombin function is neutral-ized promptly by its interaction with antithrombin III. Thrombin implemented to have function to convert fibrinogen to fibrin (④ in **Figure 4**) and further activated platelet through thrombin receptor stimulations [35].

There are several coagulation factors, the function of which is regulated strongly by food intake. Gla-domain of coagulation factors plays crucial roles in the accumu-lation of coagulation factors around exposed negatively charged phospholipids on activated platelets [36]. Gla-domain also plays crucial roles for enzymatic func-tion of coagulation factors. Carboxylation of Gla-domain is mediated by vitamin K. Thus, coagulation cascade does not work well in the absence of vitamin K or in patients taking vitamin K inhibitor. It is noteworthy that there are many foods including fermented food that are known to contain abundant vitamin K. Strict food restriction is necessary to keep the anticoagulant effects of vitamin K inhibi-tors. Recently, a larger load of vitamin K on health is cautioned [37].

The amount of fibrin formed at the site of endothelial injury was reduced by the effect of intrinsic fibrinolysis. Fibrinolysis is a complex pathway, but the details of which is simplified to be incorporated as shown in **Figure 4**. Vascular endothelial cells have balanced roles for fibrinolysis by releasing both fibrinolytic tissue-type plas-minogen activator (t-PA: ⑥) and the one has antifibrinolytic effects of plasminogen activator inhibitor (PAI)-1 (⑦). Both of them are constitutively released from endo-thelial cells. But the rates of their releases were individually controlled in individual endothelial cells. When the rate of t-PA release increases, the amount of fibrin formed around the endothelial cells becomes smaller. It becomes larger in the case when the rate of PAI-1 release increases. Free t-PA has a potential to convert plasminogen to plasmin. (⑧) Plasmin is a strong protease, which can dissolve many functional proteins including fibrinogen. To avoid too much protein degradation, activity of plasmin is promptly neutralized by the function of α_2-plasmin inhibitor (α_2-PI: ⑨).

Previous publication suggested increased PAI-1 release after acute myocardial infarction and its role for the increased recurrence of myocardial infarction [38]. Animal experiments revealed that the food coloring agent of crocin reduces activ-ity of PAI-1 and prevents thrombosis [39]. In human, increased PAI-1 activity is reported at the time of too much intake of fat [40]. Total fibrinolytic activity in humans is also reported to be low in obese patients [41]. Decreased fibrinolytic activity in patients taking too much lipid is one potential reason of increased risk of thrombosis in these patients.

4. Role of various types of food intake for the risk of thrombosis

There are many reports suggesting the increase/decrease in the risk of throm-bosis by various food and beverage intake. Framingham study suggested that coffee consumption is related to lower risk of myocardial infarction [42]. However, the influence of coffee intake for the onset and recurrence of myocardial infarction is still under discussion because other reports suggested higher rate of sudden cardiac death in coffee intake in patients after myocardial infarction [43]. People have consensus that food intake should influence the risk of arterial and venous thrombosis. The problem is that it is still hard to state which food reduces/increases the risk of thrombosis.

Old epidemiological studies suggested that the risk of myocardial infarction increased in Japanese people who immigrated to Hawaii or California than that of the ones staying in Japan. They have the same genetic background. Environmental factors including food should contribute to the change in the risk of population when moved to the US than staying in Japan. Lower cardiovascular death rate in Japan is still noted in the international registry of patients with atherothrombosis or non-valvular atrial fibrillation. Despite epidemiological data, it is still hard to identify what food specifically modulated the rate of thrombosis.

There are many specific diets that potentially influence thrombotic risk. Among them, sodium intake should be one of the most established factors to avoid cardiovascular diseases. Low sodium intake clearly decreases the risk of heart failure [44], but its direct effects for thrombosis is still to be elucidated. Mediterranean diet is also related to lower risk of cardiovascular diseases [45]. But it is still difficult to identify the specific content of Mediterranean diet related to the reduction in the risk of CV disease. A plant-based diet seems beneficial in reducing the risk of cardiovascular disease, but it has both good qualities and bad qualities [46]. The relationship between food and the risk of cardiovascular diseases (mostly arterial thrombosis) is complex.

A recent publication suggested the positive correlation between red and processed meat intake and risk of cardiovascular diseases. This study also suggested the negative relationship between the intake of yogurt, cheese, and eggs and CV disease risk [47]. The observation study is useful to find potential contributing factors but still includes many potential biases. Just like drug or medical intervention, randomized trials comparing a variety of food intake with hard endpoint of cardiovascular death, myocardial infarction, and ischemic stroke will give us more insight. However, in reality, it is hard to design such trials because people have the right to eat whatever they like. It is hard to make a restriction in food intake for a long period of time. The combination of observational study and the study to clarify the mechanism will give us the best available evidence now.

5. Metabolic syndrome and thrombosis: view from the mechanism

Metabolic syndrome is characterized as the presence of three apparent characteristics including visceral obesity manifested as increasing waist circumference, dyslipidemia, hypertension, and high blood glucose. Underlining pathophysiology is insulin resistance and lipid accumulation. It is noteworthy that various cytokines (adipocytokines) were identified from adipose tissue. Adiponectin is the one identified as factor reducing the risk of thrombosis by preventing endothelial dysfunction [48]. Indeed, decreased plasma concentration of adiponectin observed in obese patients may suggest the potential regulatory role of adiponectin for the onset of thrombotic diseases [49]. Despite difficulty in understanding the precise relationship among various cytokines and adiponectin [50], an apparent link between metabolic syndrome and decreased adiponectin is noteworthy. Various parameters for coagulation and fibrinolysis are also influenced in metabolic syndrome patients [51]. It is reasonable to recommend regular exercise to prevent metabolic syndrome and future onset of thrombosis [52].

6. Conclusion

Obviously, food intake influences deeply the risk of thrombotic disease such as arterial and venous thrombotic diseases. Deeply reliable population-based clinical trials or nicely designed registry studies are awaited. Precise understand the mechanism of thrombotic disease from hard science such as re-construction of biological phenomena from the physical movement of atoms.

Acknowledgements

Shinya Goto acknowledges financial support from MEXT/JSPS KAKENHI 17 K19669, 18H01726, and 19H03661. SG acknowledges independent research grant support from Bristol-Myers Squibb (33999603). SG also acknowledges grant sup-port from Vehicle Racing Commemorative Foundation and Nakatani Foundation for Advancement of Measuring Technologies in Biomedical Engineering. SG received research funding from Sanofi, Pfizer, and Ono.

Author details

Shinya Goto
Department of Medicine (Cardiology), Tokai University School of Medicine, Isehara, Japan

*Address all correspondence to: sgoto3@mac.com

References

[1] Leys D. Atherothrombosis: A major health burden. Cerebrovascular Diseases. 2001;**11**(Suppl 2):1-4

[2] Lindblad B, Sternby NH, Bergqvist D. Incidence of venous thromboembolism verified by necropsy over 30 years. British Medical Journal. 1991;**302**:709-711

[3] Goto S. Propagation of arterial thrombi: Local and remote contributory factors. Arteriosclerosis, Thrombosis, and Vascular Biology. 2004;**24**:2207-2208

[4] Moser KM, Fedullo PF, LitteJohn JK, Crawford R. Frequent asymptomatic pulmonary embolism in patients with deep venous thrombosis. Journal of the American Medical Association. 1994;**271**:223-225

[5] Lowe GDO. Common risk factors for both arterial and venous thrombosis. British Journal of Haematology. 2008;**140**:488-495

[6] Wilson PW. Established risk factors and coronary artery disease: The Framingham study. American Journal of Hypertension. 1994;7:7S-12S

[7] Bhatt DL, Eagle KA, Ohman EM, Hirsch AT, Goto S, Mahoney EM, et al. Comparative determinants of 4-year cardiovascular event rates in stable outpatients at risk of or with atherothrombosis. Journal of the American Medical Association. 2010;**304**:1350-1357

[8] Weitz JI, Haas S, Ageno W, Angchaisuksiri P, Bounameaux H, Nielsen JD, et al. Global anticoagulant registry in the field – venous thromboembolism (GARFIELD-VTE). Thrombosis and Haemostasis. 2016;**116**:1172-1179

[9] Mackman N. New insights into the mechanisms of venous thrombosis. The Journal of Clinical Investigation. 2012;**122**:2331-2336

[10] McKeown NM, Meigs JB, Liu S, Saltzman E, Wilson PW, Jacques PF. Carbohydrate nutrition, insulin resistance, and the prevalence of the metabolic syndrome in the Framingham offspring cohort. Diabetes Care. 2004;**27**:538-546

[11] Goto S, Hasebe T, Takagi S. Platelets: Small in size but essential in the regulation of vascular homeostasis - translation from basic science to clinical medicine. Circulation Journal. 2015;**79**:1871-1881

[12] Kawamura Y, Takahari Y, Tamura N, Eguchi Y, Urano T, Ishida H, et al. Imaging of structural changes in endothelial cells and thrombus formation at the site of FeCl(3)-induced injuries in mice cremasteric arteries. Journal of Atherosclerosis and Thrombosis. 2009;**16**:807-814

[13] Goto S, Ikeda Y, Saldivar E, Ruggeri ZM. Distinct mechanisms of platelet aggregation as a consequence of different shearing flow conditions. The Journal of Clinical Investigation. 1998;**101**:479-486

[14] Hellem AJ, Borchgrevink CF, Ames SB. The role of red cells in haemostasis: The relation between haematocrit, bleeding time and platelet adhesiveness. British Journal of Haematology. 1961;**7**:42-50

[15] Repetti RV, Leonard EF. Axial accumulation of red cells: Probable causes and effects of interest in artificial organs. Transactions - American Society for Artificial Internal Organs. 1964;**10**:311-315

[16] Sorlie PD, Garcia-Palmieri MR, Costas R Jr, Havlik RJ. Hematocrit and risk of coronary heart disease: The

Puerto Rico health program. American Heart Journal. 1981;**101**:456-461

[17] Santos MT, Valles J, Marcus AJ, Safier LB, Broekman MJ, Islam N, et al. Enhancement of platelet reactivity and modulation of eicosanoid production by intact erythrocytes. A new approach to platelet activation and recruitment. The Journal of Clinical Investigation. 1991;**87**:571-580

[18] Valles J, Santos MT, Aznar J, Marcus AJ, Martinez-Sales V, Portoles M, et al. Erythrocytes metabolically enhance collagen-induced platelet responsiveness via increased thromboxane production, adenosine diphosphate release, and recruitment. Blood. 1991;**78**:154-162

[19] Rocca B, FitzGerald GA. Simply read: Erythrocytes modulate platelet function. Should we rethink the way we give aspirin? Circulation. 1997;**95**:11-13

[20] Bakhtiari N, Hosseinkhani S, Larijani B, Mohajeri-Tehrani MR, Fallah A. Red blood cell ATP/ADP & nitric oxide: The best vasodilators in diabetic patients. Journal of Diabetes and Metabolic Disorders. 2012;**11**:9

[21] Cattaneo M, Gachet C. ADP receptors and clinical bleeding disorders. Arteriosclerosis, Thrombosis, and Vascular Biology. 1999;**19**:2281-2285

[22] Goto S, Tamura N, Eto K, Ikeda Y, Handa S. Functional significance of adenosine 5′-diphosphate receptor (P2Y(12)) in platelet activation initiated by binding of von Willebrand factor to platelet GP Ibalpha induced by conditions of high shear rate. Circulation. 2002;**105**:2531-2536

[23] Vidgren HM, Agren JJ, Schwab U, Rissanen T, Hanninen O, Uusitupa MI. Incorporation of n-3 fatty acids into plasma lipid fractions, and erythrocyte membranes and platelets during dietary supplementation with fish, fish oil, and docosahexaenoic acid-rich oil among healthy young men. Lipids. 1997;**32**:697-705

[24] Murphy KJ, Meyer BJ, Mori TA, Burke V, Mansour J, Patch CS, et al. Impact of foods enriched with n-3 long-chain polyunsaturated fatty acids on erythrocyte n-3 levels and cardiovascular risk factors. The British Journal of Nutrition. 2007;**97**:749-757

[25] Shiozaki S, Takagi S, Goto S. Prediction of molecular interaction between platelet glycoprotein Ibalpha and von Willebrand factor using molecular dynamics simulations. Journal of Atherosclerosis and Thrombosis. 2016;**23**:455-464

[26] Goto S, Oka H, Ayabe K, Yabushita H, Nakayama M, Hasebe T, et al. Prediction of binding characteristics between von Willebrand factor and platelet glycoprotein Ibalpha with various mutations by molecular dynamic simulation. Thrombosis Research. 2019;**184**:129-135

[27] Libby P. Atherosclerosis: The new view. Scientific American. 2002;**286**:46-55

[28] Hansson GK. Inflammation, atherosclerosis, and coronary artery disease. The New England Journal of Medicine. 2005;**352**:1685-1695

[29] Ruggeri ZM. Platelets in atherothrombosis. Nature Medicine. 2002;**8**:1227-1234

[30] Aikawa M, Voglic SJ, Sugiyama S, Rabkin E, Taubman MB, Fallon JT, et al. Dietary lipid lowering reduces tissue factor expression in rabbit atheroma. Circulation. 1999;**100**:1215-1222

[31] Brown WV. The benefit of aggressive lipid lowering. Atherosclerosis. Supplements. 2000;**1**:15-19

[32] Ayabe K, Goto S, Oka H, Yabushita H, Nakayama M, Tomita A, et al. Potential different impact of inhibition of thrombin function and thrombin generation rate for the growth of thrombi formed at site of endothelial injury under blood flow condition. Thrombosis Research. 2019;**179**:121-127

[33] Tomita A, Tamura N, Nanazawa Y, Shiozaki S, Goto S. Development of virtual platelets implementing the functions of three platelet membrane proteins with different adhesive characteristics. Journal of Atherosclerosis and Thrombosis. 2015;**22**:201-210

[34] Goto S, Tamura N, Handa S, Arai M, Kodama K, Takayama H. Involvement of glycoprotein VI in platelet thrombus formation on both collagen and von Willebrand factor surfaces under flow conditions. Circulation. 2002;**106**:266-272

[35] Angiolillo DJ, Capodanno D, Goto S. Platelet thrombin receptor antagonism and atherothrombosis. European Heart Journal. 2010;**31**:17-28

[36] Huang M, Rigby AC, Morelli X, Grant MA, Huang G, Furie B, et al. Structural basis of membrane binding by Gla domains of vitamin K-dependent proteins. Nature Structural Biology. 2003;**10**:751-756

[37] Vermeer C. Vitamin K: The effect on health beyond coagulation - an overview. Food & Nutrition Research. 2012;**56**:5329. DOI: 10.3402/fnr.v56i0.5329

[38] Collet JP, Montalescot G, Vicaut E, Ankri A, Walylo F, Lesty C, et al. Acute release of plasminogen activator inhibitor-1 in ST-segment elevation myocardial infarction predicts mortality. Circulation. 2003;**108**:391-394

[39] Tsantarliotou MP, Lavrentiadou SN, Psalla DA, Margaritis IE, Kritsepi MG, Zervos IA, et al. Suppression of plasminogen activator inhibitor-1 (PAI-1) activity by crocin ameliorates lipopolysaccharide-induced thrombosis in rats. Food and Chemical Toxicology. 2019;**125**:190-197

[40] Byrne CD, Wareham NJ, Martensz ND, Humphries SE, Metcalfe JC, Grainger DJ. Increased PAI activity and PAI-1 antigen occurring with an oral fat load: Associations with PAI-1 genotype and plasma active TGF-beta levels. Atherosclerosis. 1998;**140**:45-53

[41] Basurto L, Sanchez L, Diaz A, Valle M, Robledo A, Martinez- Murillo C. Differences between metabolically healthy and unhealthy obesity in PAI-1 level: Fibrinolysis, body size phenotypes and metabolism. Thrombosis Research. 2019;**180**:110-114

[42] Noh HM, Park YS, Kim JH. Coffee consumption and coronary heart disease risk using the Framingham risk score. Asia Pacific Journal of Clinical Nutrition. 2017;**26**:931-938

[43] de Vreede-Swagemakers JJ, Gorgels AP, Weijenberg MP, Dubois-Arbouw WI, Golombeck B, van Ree JW, et al. Risk indicators for out-of-hospital cardiac arrest in patients with coronary artery disease. Journal of Clinical Epidemiology. 1999;**52**:601-607

[44] Kalogeropoulos A, Papadimitriou L, Georgiopoulou VV, Dunbar SB, Skopicki H, Butler J. Low- versus moderate-sodium diet in patients with recent hospitalization for heart failure: The PROHIBIT (prevent adverse outcomes in heart failure by limiting sodium) pilot study. Circulation. Heart Failure. 2020;**13**:e006389

[45] Lim CC, Hayes RB, Ahn J, Shao Y, Silverman DT, Jones RR, et al. Mediterranean diet and the association between air pollution and cardiovascular disease mortality risk. Circulation. 2019;**139**:1766-1775

[46] Baden MY, Liu G, Satija A, Li Y, Sun Q , Fung TT, et al. Changes in plant-based diet quality and Total and cause-specific mortality. Circulation. 2019;**140**:979-991

[47] Key TJ, Appleby PN, Bradbury KE, Sweeting M, Wood A, Johansson I, et al. Consumption of meat, fish, dairy products, and eggs and risk of ischemic heart disease. Circulation. 2019;**139**:2835-2845

[48] Ekmekci H, Ekmekci OB. The role of adiponectin in atherosclerosis and thrombosis. Clinical and Applied Thrombosis/Hemostasis. 2006;**12**:163-168

[49] Matsuzawa Y, Funahashi T, Kihara S, Shimomura I. Adiponectin and metabolic syndrome. Arteriosclerosis, Thrombosis, and Vascular Biology. 2004;**24**:29-33

[50] Matsushita K, Yatsuya H, Tamakoshi K, Wada K, Otsuka R, Takefuji S, et al. Comparison of circulating adiponectin and proinflammatory markers regarding their association with metabolic syndrome in Japanese men. Arteriosclerosis, Thrombosis, and Vascular Biology. 2006;**26**:871-876

[51] Alessi M-C, Juhan-Vague I. Metabolic syndrome, haemostasis and thrombosis. Thrombosis and Haemostasis. 2008;**99**:995-1000

[52] Katzmarzyk PT, Leon AS, Wilmore JH, Skinner JS, Rao DC, Rankinen T, et al. Targeting the metabolic syndrome with exercise: Evidence from the HERITAGE family study. Medicine and Science in Sports and Exercise. 2003;**35**:1703-1709

[53] Hoshiba Y, Hatakeyama K, Tanabe T, Asada Y, Goto S. Co-localization of von Willebrand factor with platelet thrombi, tissue factor and platelets with fibrin, and consistent presence of inflammatory cells in coronary thrombi obtained by an aspiration device from patients with acute myocardial infarction. Journal of Thrombosis and Haemostasis. 2006;**4**:114-120

8

Acidosis and Anion Gap

Md. Masudul Hassan

Abstract

The journey of exploring acid and base starts long before, but much advancement was seen in the last century. In 1890, Wilhelm Ostwald electronically measured hydrogen. Svante Arrhenius won the Noble prize in 1903 for the theory of ionization. In 1908, Henderson and Black showed that bicarbonate and phosphate equilibrate with CO_2 at normal body temperature. In 1923, Bronsted first put forward the idea of acid that ionizes in solution and donate hydrogen and the base accepts the hydrogen from the solution. Handerson invented the important bicarbonate buffer system and Hasselbalch First measured the actual blood pH. In 1909, S. P. S. Sorensen developed the pH scale. Later Hasselbalch-Henderson developed an equation that helped in relating pH to the blood bicarbonate and PCO_2. Acidosis has fatal consequences like CNS damage and death. Acidosis is rapidly stabilized by the body buffer systems. There are equal amounts of cations and anions in blood, but some of them are unmeasured. These unmeasured ions are mostly anions that produce an anion gap. Increased anion gap usually represents metabolic acidosis. Albumin and many other confounding factors influence the anion gap derangements. Accuracy in measuring anion gap is critically important for the evaluation of acidosis.

Keywords: anion gap, acidosis

1. Introduction

The journey of exploring acid and base starts long before, but in the last century the advancement was remarkable. In 1890, Wilhelm Ostwald electronically measured hydrogen [1]. Svante Arrhenius won the Noble prize in 1903 for the theory of ionization [2]. In 1908, Henderson and Black showed that bicarbonate and phosphate equilibrated with CO_2 at normal body temperature in different solution [3]. In 1923, Bronsted first put forward the idea of acid as a substance that ionizes in solution and donate hydrogen and the base accepts the hydrogen from the solution [4]. Bronsted, Henderson and Van Slyke described acid-base balance in the early part of nineteenth century [5]. Handerson invented bicarbonate as the most important buffer system of the body, and Hasselbalch first measured the real blood pH in the early part of nineteenth century [6–8]. In 1909, S. P. S. Sorensen developed the pH scale [8]. Later Hasselbalch-Henderson developed an equation that helped in relating pH to the blood bicarbonate and PCO_2 [7, 9, 10]. In the early 1980s, scientists introduced electrodes specific for each ion. Thereafter, serum electrolyte and the anion gap measurement become routine tools for assessing acidosis.

Acidosis has fatal consequences like CNS damage. Even death is not uncommon. Acidosis is characterized by a decrease in pH, and this change is rapidly corrected by the body buffer systems. Many clinical conditions develop acidosis, as well as ionic derangements and the only correction of the underlying cause can resolve it. There are equal numbers of cations and anions in the blood and among them there are some unmeasured anions. These unmeasured anions can contribute in the clinically important anion gap. In a healthy individual, there is an acceptable range of normal anion gap. But some conditions can increase or decrease this gap. Increased anion gap usually represents metabolic acidosis. Albumin and many other confounding factors influence the anion gap derangements. Accuracy in measuring anion gap is critically important for the evaluation of acidosis.

2. Normal acid-base balance

The body maintains its normal physiology by the strict balance of acid and base. The body maintains its normal arterial pH close to 7.4 at a range between 7.36–7.44, and the intracellular pH of the human body is 7.2 [11]. Normal acid-base balance is the balance between each hydrogen increase by the intake or production, and that is decreased by elimination. Acid-base balance is measured by measuring pH, CO_2 and HCO_3. In general, consuming animal protein add acid in the body, and consuming cereals and vegetables add alkali in the body. In oxidative metabolism, CO_2 is produced in the tissue, and at a similar rate, that is eliminated by the lungs. So, pCO_2 persists at about 5.33 kPa (40 mm of Hg). Different buffer systems of the body play a crucial role in removing excess H^+. Metabolism of carbohydrate and fat uses O_2 and produce CO_2 and H_2O. Normal lungs efficiently remove most of the CO_2. In oxidation of amino acids, carbon dioxide and water are produced along with the liberation of nitrogen as ammonia, a toxic material in the body. In the liver, the urea cycle utilizes the ammonia, where this toxic NH_3 combines with CO_2, and produce urea. In the proximal tubule and other renal epithelial cells, ammonia and bicarbonate are also produced from glutamine metabolism. Some of it returns to the body fluid through the renal veins and is metabolized in the liver. And the rest of the NH_3 excreted in the lumen. So, NH3 does not exist in the body fluid. Most of the NH_3 is excreted in the urine, and it plays an important role in removing H^+ to maintain normal acid-base balance. In the urine, NH_3 binds hydrogen ion to pro-duce NH_4, and it prevents excessive acidification of urine.

3. Respiratory and renal regulation of acid and base

Excess acid is eliminated from the body by the lungs and the kidneys. In the lungs, acid is eliminated in the form of CO_2, and in the kidneys, acid is excreted as acid phosphatase and ammonium. CO_2 is lipid soluble, and it crosses the cell membranes in the lungs. Most of the CO_2 produced in the tissue is eliminated by alveolar ventilation. Arterial and brain chemoreceptors can sense the acid and base excess, and respira-tory system responds with hyper or hypo ventilation. As a result, pH is increased or decreased by increasing and decreasing pCO_2 level. The regulation between CO_2 and H_2CO_3 level is critically maintained when the blood travels through the lung capillaries. When strong acid is added, some HCO_3^- become H_2CO_3 and blood PCO_2 is increased. In acidosis, carbonic acid dissociate to CO_2 and H_2O. As a result, respira-tory center is stimulated and it leads to hyperventilation. Hyperventilation eliminates these CO_2 to maintain normal pH. In alkalosis, CO_2 is retained by hypoventilation. This CO_2 combines with H_2O to produce H_2CO_3, and pH is maintained.

The kidneys excrete acids, both respiratory and nonrespiratory origin and retain HCO_3^- to stabilize the pH of blood. HCO_3^- is predominantly regulated in the kidneys. The nephron reabsorbs all filtered bicarbonate in exchange for H^+. The kidneys also produce new bicarbonate to neutralize acids. Tubular cells contain carbonic anhydrase, that converts CO_2 and H_2O to HCO_3^- and H^+. Newly formed HCO_3^- is shunted to peritubular capillaries and H^+ is excreted in tubular lumen. Bicarbonate is also produced from glutamine metabolism along with ammonium. Some NH_4 diffuses to body fluid and converts to urea in the liver. The rest of the them excreted in urine. The tubules are impermeable to bicarbonate, and it cannot be converted back to CO_2 and H_2O. So, the blood HCO_3 level is increased.

In the apical membrane of the kidney tubules, sodium is reabsorbed in exchange for the hydrogen ion. Salts like sulfates, phosphates, ammonia combines the hydro-gen ions and excrete it. The kidneys titrate less than half of the excreted acids and the rest is excreted as ammonium [11]. For every ammonium excreted in urine, one HCO_{3+}^- is reabsorbed. HCl and H_2SO_4 are produced during dietary protein metabo-lism reacts with $NaHSO_4$, and produce NaCl and Na_2SO_4. These Na salts are excreted by the kidneys as NH_4Cl, and $(NH_4)_2SO_4$.

The kidneys are largely responsible for K^+ excretion and most of it is reabsorbed in the proximal tubule and in the loop of Henly. In acidosis, K^+ secretion is decreased and K^+ absorption is increased in the collecting duct. In alkalosis, hypokalemia develops from increased K^+ secretion and reduced K^+ absorption in the collecting duct. H^+ and K^+ exchange occur in the tubules. Serum potassium level also influences the renal acid-base balance. In hyperkalemia, potassium is available in an increased amount in the filtrate, and hydrogen will be scarce for exchange with HCO_3 and there will be an imbalance. In hypokalemia, less potassium will be available for H^+ and K^+ exchange and hydrogen will be available to exchange with bicarbonate.

Na^+, K^+ and NH_4^+ are the principle urinary cations, and the principal urinary anion is chloride. Urinary anion gap helps in estimating renal NH_4^+ excretion, as NH_4^+ is the urinary unmeasured ion. Chloride is an important anion in neutralizing positive ions, reabsorbed in the proximal convoluted tubule and secreted in urine by the collecting duct. Secreted H^+ is also buffered by urinary buffer HPO_4^- to H_2PO_4, and is excreted in urine.

4. Acidosis and buffer

Acidosis results from a reduction in serum bicarbonate and cause secondary reduction of $PaCO_2$ resulting in a low blood pH. It develops from the addition of hydrogen or removal of HCO_3 from the body. $PaCO_2$ in blood is 38 ± 2 mm of Hg and HCO_3 is24 ± 2mmol/L.Metabolic acidosis is characterized by the blood pH <7.38 and bicarbonate <22 mmol/L [12].

Acid and base disorders are: respiratory acidosis and respiratory alkalosis, and metabolic acidosis and metabolic alkalosis [13]. In respiratory acidosis, $PaCO_2$ is increased and it is compensated by renal H^+ excretion, HCO_3 retention and HCO_3 generation. In respiratory alkalosis, decreased $PaCO_2$ is compensated by renal HCO_3 excretion. In metabolic acidosis, HCO_3 is reduced and it is compensated by hyper-ventilation and $PaCO_2$ reduction. HCO3 is increased in metabolic alkalosis, and it is compensated by increasing $PaCO_2$ by hypoventilation [14]. Usually, respiratory disorders cause derangements of CO_2 level in the blood, and change in HCO_3 level is developed from metabolic disturbances.

In the blood, Alkali is present mainly in the form of sodium bicarbonate, and bicarbonate is bound to other bases. Increase in $BHCO_3$ and decrease in H_2CO_3

results in alkalosis, and decrease in $BHCO_3$ and increase in H_2CO_3 results in acidosis [13]. The body contains many acids. They are hydrochloric acid, carbonic acid, citric acid, lactic acid, phosphoric acid and carboxylic acid. Acute metabolic acidosis is developed by the overproduction of organic acids, like lactic acid and keto acid. Chronic acidosis is caused by bicarbonate wasting and impaired urinary acidification.

Blood cells are more acidic than serum, which influences the distribution of electrolyte and water between them. These transports took place with the oxygenation and reduction of hemoglobin and shift of bases (Na^+, K^+) due to changes in pH. Under normal environment Na^+ and K^+ do not diffuse through the cell wall. Shifting of water and electrolyte through membrane results from the change in anion (HCO_3^- and Cl^-) and H^+ concentration, and that changes in cell volume. CO_2, relative electrolyte concentration and weak acid concentrations are three indepen-dent variables that regulate blood pH [15].

The body has different buffer systems to maintain the normal pH of the body. Elkinton Jr. reported that multiple level of buffering linked different series of ionic exchanges which includes hydrogen, sodium, potassium, and other anions. The buffers absorb excess hydrogen and hydroxyl ions. They help in the maintenance of neutrality during redistribution of the hydrogen ion [16].

A buffer system consists of a weak acid with its conjugate base, or a weak base with its conjugate acid. Blood is a strong solution, and it has many important components that maintain the buffer systems. These include hemoglobin, bicarbonate, carbonic acid, plasma proteins, RBCs and plasma phosphate [17]. HCO_3/CO_2 buffer is the most important buffer system of the body, and plays a major role in regulating pH of the blood. But, the rest of the buffer systems have minimum contribution in pH regulation. In dissolved state, bicarbonate and carbon dioxide ion remains in equilibrium. Bicarbonate reduces strong acid to carbonic acid, whereas carbonic acid neutralizes strong base (Eq. (1)).

$$CO_2 + H_2O <--> H_2CO_3 <--> H^+ + HCO_3^-. \quad (1)$$

When CO_2 and water is converted to HCO_3 and hydrogen ions, this hydrogen ion is then buffered by hemoglobin [18].

Proteins have a buffering capacity, including hemoglobin. Protein can accept and donate H^+, if there is H^+ excess or it is reduced. Hemoglobin has a distinct types of buffer action. When blood passes through the capillaries, it loses oxygen and took CO_2 to raise the $PaCO_2$ and maintain the pH. Hemoglobin plays an important role in transporting both oxygen and carbon dioxide. In 1914, Douglas, Haldane and Christiansen tried to prove that the hemoglobin binds more CO_2 in the reduced form than the oxygenated form [19].

The phosphate buffer system works in the internal environment of all cells. But, in the blood $H_2PO_4^-$ and HPO_4^{2-} are found in a very low concentration. Sodium dihydrogen phosphate neutralizes strong bases and sodium monohydrogen phos-phate neutralizes strong acids. The Phosphate buffer system plays an important role in the kidneys.

5. Acid base physiology

Two types of variables, dependent and independent, are important in acid-base balance [20]. Bicarbonate, hydroxyl ion, hydrogen ion or pH, weak acid, anion and carbon trioxide are dependent variables and they are determined by three independent variables pCO_2, total weak acid and net strong ion charge [21]. Lungs, kidneys, liver and gut regulated this balance. Traditional bicarbonate/carbon-di-oxide approach, base excess approach and Stewert's physicochemical methods are widely discussed for measuring the acid base disorders as well as to explore the physiology of body fluid.

6. Traditional physiological approach

HCO_3/CO_2 buffer system is the basis of this approach. Carbonic acid freely moves in the body fluid and dissociates into bicarbonate automatically when needed. Bicarbonate in the body acts as alkaline reserve. CO_2, pH and HCO_3 can be calculated by Hasselbalch-Henderson Equation (2) [7, 9].

$$pH = pK + \log_{10}\left[HCO_3^-/s.PCo_2\right] \quad (2)$$

This equation states that not only HCO_3 and CO_2, but also their ratio determines the pH. In this equation, PCO_2 is the respiratory component and HCO_3^- is the metabolic component of the acid base imbalance. This buffer system is the largest and inde-pendent buffer system of the body and whole body acts as an open system for CO_2. In traditional approach balance is determined by the influx and efflux of H^+ and HCO_3.

7. Base excess approach

Astrup and Siggaard-Anderson introduced base excess approach, which is close to the traditional approach [22, 23]. Base excess can be calculated from bicarbonate concentration and pH of the body [4]. It can estimate the acid base status of non-respiratory origin. If base excess is too high, then it is metabolic alkalosis. If base excess is too low, then it is metabolic acidosis. When a deviation of normal blood pH is corrected by administrating base, then it is called base deficit. Which is a characteristic of metabolic acidosis. Base deficit with increase anion gap suggest the addition of acid in the body fluid. If there is a base deficit with normal anion gap, then there is bicarbonate loss from the body.

8. Stewart approach

Here H^+/proton is the preliminary determinant in acid base disturbances, not the CO_2 [21]. The dependent variables are H^+, OH^-, CO_3^{2-}, HA (weak acid), A^-(weak anions), $HCO3^-$ and pH. The independent variables are strong ion difference (SID), total non-volatile weak acids (A_{tot}) and $PaCO_2$ [24]. Among them the strong ion difference has maximum effect on the hydrogen ion concentration. With that, acid base disorder can be divided into three categories: 1. respiratory (increase or decrease $PaCO\ )_2$ 2. SID changes (excess or deficit of strong ions or water) and 3. inorganic phosphate or albumin deficit or excess (A_{tot} changes). In Stewart approach, a large number of variables are needed to calculate SID. Sodium, potassium, calcium and magnesium are strong positive ions, and chloride and lactate are the negative ions [25]. Bicarbonate and albumin are the balancing ion in strong ion difference. Strong ion difference (mEq/L) = [strong cations] – [strong anions]. Weak acid dissociates in body fluid (Eq. (3)).

$$HA \leftarrow\rightarrow H^+ + A^- \quad (3)$$

A^- Resembles weak anions, that vary with pH. Strong ion difference is filled with this weak A^-, and HCO_{3+}^-, H^+, OH^-, CO_3^{2-} are also present in minute amount, but are less important. There are many unmeasured anions accounts for ion difference. For electrical neutrality, strong ion difference and the total charge of weak ions must be equal [26]. Normal SID is dominated by sodium and chloride. But other negligible, but measurable ions are present there. Here narrowing of SID from an increase in $[Na^+]$ has alkalizing effect, whereas an increase in $[Cl^-]$ has acidifying effect. From the ionic basis metabolic acid base disturbances are about four major types [25]: (1) The water effect, and it is produced by dilutional effect on SID. Free water intake and intravenous infusion can produce it. (2) The chloride effect is caused by chloride change, and administration of normal saline is the common cause. (3) The protein effect is produced by a change in albumin concentration. (4) There are other factors, and those are influenced by unmeasured anions, that cause a wide anion gap.

9. Anion gap

In vivo, true ion gap cannot exist. There are many anions and cations in the blood. Blood cations and anions must be equal. Sodium, chloride and bicarbonate have the highest concentrations, and they are calculated for anion gap for their largest variability in different pathologic conditions. Anion gap is the difference between serum sodium ion and bicarbonate plus chloride. There are wide variations in the reported anion gap. Widely accepted anion gap is 8–12 mmol/L [15]. Anion gap is clinically important for assessing acidosis. Normal anion gap (hyperchlo-remic) acidosis and increased anion gap acidosis [27] are two important types of anion gap acidosis. Common serum cation levels are sodium 138.8 ± 4.56 mmol/L, potassium 4.05 ± 0.21 mmol/L, magnesium 0.98 ± 0.05 mmol/L [28] and calcium 2.2–2.7 mmol/L [29]. And normal serum anion levels are chloride 97.7 ± 3.42 mmol/L and acetate 0.23 ± 0.04 mmol/L [28]. The sum of cations and anions should be equal (Eq. (4)).

$$Na^+ + K^+ + Mg^+ + Ca^+ + Protein^+ = Cl^- + OA^- + HCO_3^- + SO_4^{-2} + HPO_4^{-2}/HPO_4^- + Protein^- \quad (4)$$

There are other ions which are not commonly measured, are unmeasured anions and cations [30]. Under normal conditions, albumin and phosphate accounts for this anion gap. There are many clinical conditions, where urate, lactate, ketone bodies, sulfate, salicylates, penicillin's, citrate, pyruvate, and acetates are also responsible for increased anion gap [5]. So, anion gap [31] is Eq. (5)

$$Na - \left(Cl^+ + HCO_3^-\right) = UA - UC \quad (5)$$

10. Unmeasured anion

Presence of unmeasured anion in blood is the anion gap and it represents metabolic acidosis [32]. When unmeasured anions like lactate and pyruvate donates proton then that proton is buffered by bicarbonate. And bicarbonate consumption increases the anion gap. The most common causes include lactic acidosis, diabetic ketoacidosis, uremia and acidosis due to drugs and toxins. Methanol, propylene glycol, ethylene glycol, salicylate, and some inborn error of metabolism are other causes of unmeasured anions [33]. Both lactate and β-hydroxybutyrate are increased in both Gram-positive septiceamia [34] and starvation [35]. Krebs cycle intermediate citrate, isocitrate, malate, α-ketogluterate, succinate and D-lactate are increased in different types of acidosis. Intestinal ischemia and short bowel syndrome cause increase in D-lactate [35]. Plasma proteins are mostly anionic compris-ing 75% of the unmeasured anion [36–38]. Treatment with Sodium thiosulfate that has no hydrogen can cause severe metabolic acidosis [39].

11. Increased anion gap

It usually indicates acidosis. Increase blood lactate, ketoacidosis, uremia (in advanced renal failure), drugs (salicylate and penicillin), ethylene glycol, methanol are contributor of high anion gap acidosis. But the increase anion gap can be due to laboratory error, hyperphosphatemia [30]. Massive rhabdomyelysis, hippurate, oxalate can also cause increased anion gap acidosis [31]. Diabetes, starvation and alcohol are the most common cause of ketoacidosis. In alcoholic ketoacidosis, primary keto acid is β-hydroxybutyrate. It can be missed in conventional assessment of ketonuria. High anion gap and normal lactate level are characteristics of alcoholic acidosis [40]. Starvation alone can cause high anion gap acidosis [41]. In the third trimester of pregnancy, short period of starvation can cause ketogenesis with a very high anion gap acidosis [42]. Septic shock, hypoxemia, hypovolemic shock, cyanide, mesenteric ischemia, CO poisoning, causes hypoxic type of L-lactic acidosis [43]. Non-hypoxic, L-lactic acidosis develops from seizure, thiamine deficiency, metformin, methanol, ethylene glycol, salicylate, propylene glycol, niacin, isoniazide, iron, propofol, toluene, paraldehyde, non-nucleoside reverse transcriptase inhibitor (NNRTI) drugs [12]. Recurrent 5-oxoprolinuria from inborn errors of metabolism is a rare cause if high anion gap metabolic acidosis [44]. Uremia results from not only reduced ammonia secretion but also reduced filtration of sulfate and phosphate anions, and increases the anion gap [45]. Polyclonal gammopathies are also contributor of increased anion gap [46]. Serum albumin is an important contributor to the anion gap and hypoalbu-minemia is a common comorbid condition. That is why, albumin correction is crucial for the anion gap calculation [36, 37]. To explore the cause of the metabolic acidosis anion gap must be corrected for albumin as well as lactate [43]. A high anion gap can be masked by a concomitant low anion gap results from hypoalbuminemia.

12. Reduced anion gap

In anion gap calculation, sodium is the only cation that is measured. But, hypercalcemia, hyperkalemia and hypermagnesemia can produce significant decrements in anion gap. So, clinical correlation and correction of such abnormality is important. Plasma proteins comprise two third of the unmeasured anion, and hypoalbuminemia is a common cause for the low anion gap [31, 36, 37]. The reduced anion gap is usually seen in delusional states, hypernatremia, hypoalbuminemia, hypermagnesemia, hypercalcemia, bromide intoxication, hyperviscosity associated diseases etc. [47]. Sometimes it can be due to laboratory error, paraproteinemia [48, 49], or iodide [30, 50], gastrointestinal bicarbonate loss and diarrhea [31]. It has been reported that Lithium carbonate intoxication can also produce low or absent anion gap [51]. Non-sodium containing paraprotein IgG in multiple myeloma increase the unmeasured cations and reduce the anion gap [48, 52, 53]. Hypercalcemia and hypoalbuminemia in paraproteinemia also contribute to low anion gap [52].

13. Normal anion gap

Measuring anion gap is a routine for evaluating acidosis, and normal anion gap is sometimes misleading. As we know, the increase in anion gap is usual in meta-bolic acidosis. And acidosis is due to acid retention or ingestion. Normal anion gap acidosis is due to loss of HCO_3^- from the body. Hyperchloremic normal anion gap acidosis is characterized by acidosis with excess chloride ions [54]. Here, the low HCO_3 level is a characteristic feature. Reduced negatively charged bicarbonate is compensated by the negatively charged chloride movement into the extracellular space, and normal anion gap is maintained. The causes of gastrointestinal and renal loss of bicarbonate are diarrhea, ureteral diversions, pancreatic and biliary fistulas, toluene ingestion, acetazolamide, ifosfamide, topiramite, tenofovir, renal tubular acidosis. These are the causes of normal anion gap acidosis. Rapid infu-sion of 0.9% normal saline can also cause hyperchloremic metabolic acidosis [55]. If the blood anion gap is normal, but there is acidosis, then the urinary anion gap Eq. (6) is calculated [12].

$$[Na^+] + [K^+] - [Cl^-] \tag{6}$$

The urinary anion gap is negative in diarrhea, sodium infusion and proximal renal tubular acidosis. Whereas, positive urinary anion gap is found in both type 1 and type 4 renal tubular acidosis. Renal tubular acidosis is sometimes the only presenting feature of many chronic diseases and conditions associated with poly-clonal gummopathies.

14. Metabolic acidosis and anion gap

Metabolic acidosis results from gain of anions and loss of cations. Potassium chloride, hydrogen chloride, sodium chloride, arginine hydrochloride, calcium chloride, ammonium chloride, lysine hydrochloride can cause hyperchloremia and increase anion gap. Hyperphosphatemia increases the anion gap. But renal tubular acidosis [33], amiloride and triamterene cause a non anion gap hyperchloraemic acidosis and hyperkalemia due to impaired bicarbonate production.

Anion gap should be measured for all types of metabolic acidosis. High anion gap metabolic acidosis is a subtype of non-respiratory acidosis. Mnemonics were used for remembering the causes of high gap metabolic acidosis such as KUSMALE (Ketoacidosis, Uraemia, Salicylate poisoning, Methanol, ParAldehyde, Lactate, Ethylene glycol) and MUD PILES (Methanol, Metformin uremia, Diabetic keto-acidosis, Paraldehydes, iron, isoniazid, Lactate, ethylene glycol, Salicylates and starvation). As paraldehyde induced acidosis is extremely rare and recently three anion gap generating organic acid has been recognized. They are Short bowel syndrome producing D-lactic acid, chronic paracetamol use induced 5-oxoproline (or pyroglutamic acid) especially in malnourished woman and high dose propyl-ene glycol (used in lorazepum, phenobarbital) infusions generate acidosis. Also, Iron and Isoniazid can cause lactic acidosis. So, GOLD MARK is a new acronym for metabolic acidosis [Glycols (ethylene and propylene), Oxyproline, L-lactate, D-lactate, Methanol, Aspirin, Renal failure, Ketoacidosis] [56]. Metabolic acidosis also caused by renal bicarbonate loss in type 2 renal tubular acidosis, renal dysfunc-tion in type 4 renal tubular acidosis, type 1 renal tubular acidosis and ingestion of ammonium chloride [31]. Acute rheumatism causes lactate induced acidosis also [57]. Symptomatic correction of acidosis will not eliminate the problem. If the clinical features suggest acidosis, then it should be assessed for anion gap as well.

Following anion gap measurement accordingly history of drug, toxins and diseases need to be evaluated for managing the exact pathology thus acidosis will be properly treated.

15. Albumin, phosphate, lactate and corrected anion gap

At normal blood pH 7.4 plasma proteins are mostly anionic. It has been estimated that anion gap decreases by 2.5 mEq/L for every 10 gm/L drop of serum albumin [36, 37]. Several studies had observed that 2–2.5 times changes in albumin influences in anion gap changes [58]. Albumin contributes a greater part of the normal anion gap [46]. Phosphate and lactate contribute some anion gap as well [59]. Consideration of all of these contributors are important in explaining changes in anion gap. Calculation of anion gap is crucial in critically ill patients. Anion gap should be adjusted for Eq. (7) albumin, phosphate and lactate with the following equation [59].

$$\text{Anion gap} = \{(\text{Na}) + (\text{K}) - (\text{Cl}) - (\text{HCO}_3)\} - \{2 \times \text{albumin g/dl} + 0.5 \times \text{phosphate mg/dl}\} - \{\text{lactate mmol/L}\} \quad (7)$$

Author details

Md. Masudul Hassan[1,2,3]

1 Bangladesh College of Physicians and Surgeons, Dhaka, Bangladesh

2 Department of Rheumatology, Bangabandhu Sheikh Mujib Medical University, Dhaka, Bangladesh

3 DHCRL and IB Hospital, Dhaka, Bangladesh

*Address all correspondence to: masud292@yahoo.com

References

[1] Severinghaus JW, Astrup PB. History of blood gas analysis. II. pH and acid base balance measurements. Journal of Clinical Monitoring and Computing. 1985;**1**:259. DOI: 10.1007/BF02832819

[2] Malkin HM. Historical review: Concept of acid-base balance in medicine. Annals of Clinical and Laboratory Science. 2003;**33**(3):337-344

[3] Henderson LJ, Black OF. A study of the equilibrium between carbonic acid, sodium bicarbonate, mono-sodium phosphate, and di-sodium phosphate at body temperature. American Journal of Physiology-Legacy Content. 1908;**21**(4):420-426

[4] Astrup P, Jorgensen K, Andersen OS, et al. Acid–base metabolism: New approach. Lancet. 1960;**i**:1035-1039

[5] Kimura S, Shabsigh M, Morimatsu H. Traditional approach versus Stewart approach for acid-base disorders: Inconsistent evidence. SAGE Open Medicine. 2018;**6**:2050312118801255. DOI: 10.1177/2050312118801255

[6] Henderson LJ. Concerning the relationship between the strength of acids and their capacity to preserve neutrality. The American Journal of Physiology. 1908;**21**:173-179

[7] Hasselbalch KA. Die Berechnung des Wasserstoffzahl des Blutes aus der freien und gebunden Kohlensäure desselben, und die Sauerstoffbindung des Blutes als Funktion der Wasserstoffzahl. Biochemische Zeitschrift. 1916;**78**:112-144

[8] Myers RJ. One-hundred years of PH. Journal of Chemical Education. 2010;**87**(1):30-32. DOI: 10.1021/ed800002c

[9] Henderson LJ. The theory of neutrality regulation in the animal organism. American Journal of Physiology-Legacy Content. 1908;**21**:427-448

[10] Warburg EJ. Studies on carbonic acid compounds and hydrogen ion activities in blood and salt solution—A contribution to the theory of the equation of L. J. Henderson and K. A. Hasselbalch. The Biochemical Journal. 1922;**16**:153-340

[11] Hamm LL, Nakhoul N, Hering-Smith KS. Acid-base homeostasis. Clinical Journal of the American Society of Nephrology. 2015;**10**(12):2232-2242. DOI: 10.2215/CJN.07400715

[12] Berend K, de Vries AP, Gans RO. Physiological approach to assessment of acid-base disturbances. The New England Journal of Medicine. 2014;**371**(15):1434-1445. DOI: 10.1056/NEJMra1003327

[13] Austin JH, Cullen GE. Hydrogen ion concentration of the blood in health and disease. Medicine. 1925;**4**(3):275-343

[14] Trulock EP III. Chapter 49: Arterial blood gases. In: Walker HK, Hall WD, Hurst JW, editors. Clinical Methods: The History, Physical, and Laboratory Examinations. 3rd ed. Boston: Butterworths; 1990. Available from: https://www.ncbi.nlm.nih.gov/books/NBK37

[15] Kellum JA. Determinants of blood pH in health and disease. Critical Care. 2000;**4**:6. DOI: 10.1186/cc644

[16] Elkinton JR. Whole body buffers in the regulation of acid-base equilibrium. The Yale Journal of Biology and Medicine. 1956;**29**(3):191-210

[17] Viikari SJ, Harjola P, Maamies T. Clinical studies on the buffer capacity of the blood. Scandinavian

Journal of Clinical and Laboratory Investigation. 1954;**6**(2):122-128. DOI: 10.3109/00365515409134852

[18] Ferry RM, Green AA. Studies in the chemistry of hemoglobin. The Journal of Biological Chemistry. 1929;**81**:175

[19] Doisy EA, Briggs AP, Eaton EP, Chambers WH. Evaluation of buffers of the blood. The Journal of Biological Chemistry. 1922;**54**:305

[20] Stewart PA. Independent and dependent variables of acid-base control. Respiration Physiology. 1978;**33**(1):9-26

[21] Stewart PA. Modern quantitative acidbase chemistry. Canadian Journal of Physiology and Pharmacology. 1983;**61**:1444-1461

[22] Astrup P. A simple electrometric technique for the determination of carbon dioxide tension in blood and plasma, total content of carbon dioxide in plasma, and bicarbonate content in separated plasma at a fixed carbon dioxide tension (40 mm Hg). Scandinavian Journal of Clinical and Laboratory Investigation. 1956;**8**(1):33-43

[23] Andersen OS. The pH-log pCO_2 blood acid-base nomogram revised. Scandinavian Journal of Clinical and Laboratory Investigation. 1962;**14**:598-604

[24] Jones NL. A quantitative physicochemical approach to acid-base physiology. Clinical Biochemistry. 1990;**23**(3):189-195

[25] Magder S, Emami A. Practical approach to physical-chemical acid-base management. Stewart at the bedside. Annals of the American Thoracic Society. 2015;**12**:111-117. DOI: 10.1016/j. pbiomolbio.2015.01.00

[26] Morgan TJ. The meaning of acid–base abnormalities in the intensive care unit – Effects of fluid administration. Critical Care. 2004;**9**:204. DOI: 10.1186/cc2946

[27] Kraut J, Madias N. Metabolic acidosis: Pathophysiology, diagnosis and management. Nature Reviews. Nephrology. 2010;**6**:274-285. DOI: 10.1038/nrneph.2010.33

[28] Chapp AD, Schum S, Behnke JE, et al. Measurement of cations, anions, and acetate in serum, urine, cerebrospinal fluid, and tissue by ion chromatography. Physiological Reports. 2018;**6**(7):e13666. DOI: 10.14814/phy2.13666

[29] Goldstein DA. Chapter 143: Serum Calcium. In: Walker HK, Hall WD, Hurst JW, editors. Clinical Methods: The History, Physical, and Laboratory Examinations. 3rd ed. Boston: Butterworths; 1990. Available from: https://www.ncbi.nlm.nih.gov/books/NBK250

[30] Kraut JA, Madias NE. Serum anion gap: Its uses and limitations in clinical medicine. Clinical Journal of the American Society of Nephrology. 2007;**2**:162-174

[31] Lee S, Kang KP, Kang SK. Clinical usefulness of the serum anion gap. Electrolyte Blood Press. 2006;**4**(1):44-46. DOI: 10.5049/EBP.2006.4.1.44

[32] Selk N, Rodby RA. Unexpectedly severe metabolic acidosis associated with sodium thiosulfate therapy in a patient with calcific uremic arteriolopathy. Seminars in Dialysis. 2011;**24**(1):85-88. DOI: 10.1111/j.1525-139X.2011.00848.x

[33] Seifter JL. Integration of acid–base and electrolyte disorders. The New England Journal of Medicine. 2014;**371**:1821-1831

[34] Barnardo DE, Cohen RD, Iles RA. "Idiopathic" lactic and

betahydroxybutyric acidosis. British Medical Journal. 1970;**4**(5731):348-349. DOI: 10.1136/bmj.4.5731.348-a

[35] Forni LG, McKinnon W, Hilton PJ. Unmeasured anions in metabolic acidosis: Unravelling the mystery. Critical Care. 2006;**10**(4):220. DOI: 10.1186/cc4954

[36] Figge J, Jabor A, Kazda A, Fencl V. Anion gap in hypoalbuminemia. Critical Care Medicine. 1998;**26**:1807-1810

[37] Durward A, Mayer A, Skellet S, Taylor D, Hanna S, Tibby SM, et al. Hypoalbuminemia in critically ill children : Incidence, prognosis, and influence on the anion gap. Archives of Disease in Childhood. 2003;**88**:419-422

[38] Rocktaeschel J, Morimatsu H, Uchino S, Bellomo R. Unmeasured anions in critically ill patients: Can they predict mortality? Critical Care Medicine. 2003;**31**(8):2131-2136

[39] Hunt GM, Ryder HF. Metabolic acidosis after sodium thiosulfate infusion and the role of hydrogen sulfide. Clinical case reports. 2018;**6**(8):1595-1599. DOI: 10.1002/ccr3.1673

[40] Noor NM, Basavaraju K, Sharpstone D. Alcoholic ketoacidosis: A case report and review of the literature. Oxford Medical Case Reports. 2016;**2016**(3):31-33. DOI: 10.1093/omcr/omw006

[41] Mubarik A, Jupalli A, Iqbal AM, Muddassir S, Eddib A. Isolated starvation ketoacidosis: A rare cause of severe metabolic acidosis presenting with a pH less than 7. Cureus. 2019;**11**(2):e4086. DOI: 10.7759/cureus.4086

[42] Sinha N, Venkatram S, Diaz-Fuentes G. Starvation ketoacidosis: A cause of severe anion gap metabolic acidosis in pregnancy. Case Reports in Critical Care. 2014;**2014**. Article ID: 906283, 4 pages. DOI: 10.1155/2014/906283

[43] Moviat M, van Haren F, van der Hoeven H. Conventional or physicochemical approach in intensive care unit patients with metabolic acidosis. Critical Care. 2003;**7**(3):R41-R45

[44] Tailor P, Raman T, Garganta CL, Njalsson R, Carlsson K, Ristoff E, et al. Recurrent high anion gap metabolic acidosis secondary to 5-oxoproline (pyroglutamic acid). American Journal of Kidney Diseases. 2005;**46**(1):e4-e10

[45] Ishihara K, Szerlip HM. Anion gap acidosis. Seminars in Nephrology. 1998;**18**(1):83-97

[46] Kirschbaum B. Hyperglobulinemia with an increased anion gap. The American Journal of the Medical Sciences. 1998;**316**(6):393-397

[47] Emmett M, Narins RG. Clinical use of the anion gap. Medicine (Baltimore). 1977;**56**(1):38-54

[48] Keshgegian AA. Anion gap and immunoglobulin concentration. American Journal of Clinical Pathology. 1980;**74**(3):282-284

[49] Qujeq D, Mohiti J. Decreased anion gap in polyclonal hypergammaglobulinemia. Clinical Biochemistry. 2002;**35**(1):73-75

[50] Fischman RA, Fairclough GF, Cheigh JS. Iodide and negative anion gap. The New England Journal of Medicine. 1978;**298**:1035-1036

[51] Kelleher SP, Raciti A, Arbeit LA. Reduced or absent serum anion gap as a marker of severe lithium carbonate intoxication. Archives of Internal Medicine. 1986;**146**:1839-1840

[52] Murray T, Long W, Narins RG. Multiple myeloma and anion gap.

The New England Journal of Medicine. 1975;**292**:574-575

[53] De Troyer A, Stolarczyk A, De Beyl DZ, Stryckmans P. Value of anion-gap determination in multiple myeloma. The New England Journal of Medicine. 1977;**296**:858-860

[54] Sharma S, Hashmi MF, Aggarwal S. Hyperchloremic Acidosis. [Updated: 13 September 2019]. In: StatPearls [Internet]. Treasure Island (FL): StatPearls Publishing; 2019. Available from: https://www.ncbi.nlm.nih.gov/books/NBK4823

[55] Prough DS, Bidani A. Hyperchloremic metabolic acidosis is a predictable consequence of intraoperative infusion of 0.9% saline. Anesthesiology. 1999;**90**(5):1247-1249

[56] Mehta AN, Emmett JB, Emmett M. GOLD MARK: An anion gap mnemonic for the 21st century. Lancet. 2008;**372**(9642):892. DOI: 10.1016/S0140-6736(08)61398-7

[57] Parsons LG, Edgar SH. The Acid-Base equilibrium of the blood in acute rheumatism. Archives of Disease in Childhood. 1929;**4**(23):291

[58] Feldman M, Soni N, Dickson B. Influence of hypoalbuminemia or hyperalbuminemia on the serum anion gap. The Journal of Laboratory and Clinical Medicine. 2005;**146**(6):317-320

[59] Zampieri FG, Park M, Ranzani OT, et al. Anion gap corrected for albumin, phosphate and lactate is a good predictor of strong ion gap in critically ill patients: A nested cohort study. Revista Brasileira de Terapia Intensiva. 2013;**25**(3):205- 211. DOI: 10.5935/0103-507X.20130036

9

Effects and Issues of Diet Fat on Cardiovascular Metabolism

Yasuhiro Nishikawa

Abstract

Diet is a foundation of treatment for lifestyle-related diseases, such as high blood pressure, diabetes, and dyslipidemia. For these diseases, diet therapy has been disregarded in management of hyperlipidemia. Fat has more diversity of biological effects compared to those of protein and carbohydrate. New emerging evidences have resulted in a clear shift of recognition of fatty acids in diet therapy. The PREDIMED study has shown recently the amazing result that a calorie-unlimited, high-fat Mediterranean diet caused about 30% reduction in cardiovascular disease in obese subjects compared with a low-fat diet. Many authorities have removed restriction of intake of fat from their guidelines. The important, new message from recent medical and nutritional science is that people need to consume more "good fat" rather than limiting intake of fat to prevent cardiometabolic diseases. In this chapter, I would like to focus on the role of fatty acids with special relation on their effects on blood lipids and cardiovascular events.

Keywords: saturated fat, unsaturated fat, complex and refined carbohydrate, Mediterranean diet, olive oil, n-3 fish oil, primary and secondary prevention, LDL cholesterol, antioxidant, diet guidelines

1. Introduction

Diet therapy has been disregarded in management of hyperlipidemia. Statistical data for the US between 1990 and 2016 show that in addition to tobacco consumption, poor diet and subsequent obesity are one of the major reasons for mortality [1]. Generally, information about the benefits of nutritional interventions has not adequately been translated into action in medical training or practice [2]. In a 2017 online survey of 646 cardiologists in the US [3], 90% reported that they had not received adequate nutrition education to be able to counsel their patients, even though 95% believed it was their personal responsibility to do so.

Compared with pharmacological trials, high-level evidence about diet therapy is limited. Among the three macronutrients, data around fat have been especially controversial. This is partially due to the more diverse roles of fat compared to protein or carbohydrate. Fat is not only a source of energy production but also a major component of hormones, and cell and nuclear membranes, and a carrier for the fat-soluble vitamins. Furthermore, essential fatty acids are involved in many physiological processes such as inflammation, cell proliferation, wound healing, and blood coagulation. The data about diet therapy are frequently inconsistent even for apparently solid recommendations in authorized guidelines. In this chapter, I would like to focus on the role of fatty acids with special relation on their effects on blood lipids and cardiovascular events.

2. Incidence of formal diet consultation in Japan

In Japan, formal professional dietary intervention is not so common. Generally, registered dietitians provide recommendations for meals according to the patients' disease conditions from medical, nutritional, and hygienic aspects. Statistical data from the two university hospitals in Tokyo indicate that the number of dietary referrals from physicians for patients with dyslipidemia is less than 5% of total cases, which is in sharp contrast to those with diabetes at more than 50% [4, 5]. There are several reasons to explain the fewer consultations, including scanty data in diet intervention trials in Japanese population, weak recognition of effectiveness of diet therapy for dyslipidemia among physicians, and most importantly, patients find it easier to take statins than follow diet therapy. Compared with LDL cholesterol reduction by diet therapy, statins are more powerful, with up to 50% reduction in LDL cholesterol. Results in the PREDIMED study have clearly shown that a Mediterranean diet enriched with extra-virgin olive oil or nuts reduced CV events by 30% [6]. This magnitude of CV event reduction was compatible with those of statin trials, and importantly, it was achieved with small changes in LDL cholesterol, blood pressure, and blood glucose. The data in the PREDIMED study have clearly shed light on distinctive features of the power of diet therapy, which affects many aspects of not only classical risk factors but also other unknown biological processes modulating the pathophysiology of diseases.

3. Effects of dietary components on blood lipid

Major diet factors that affect blood LDL cholesterol include calories, three major nutrients (protein, fat, and carbohydrate), fat type, fiber, food sterol, etc. By modifying these factors, a Mediterranean diet and DASH diet are intended to improve cardiometabolic risk factors. These two diets ranked as top diets according to a US News and World report in 2018. They share many aspects beneficial for maintaining health. Especially, intake of healthy fats such as olive oil rather than saturated fatty acids (SFA) is a mainstay in the Mediterranean diet. The basic principle in diet is not to eat too much or too little of one component of foods, but rather to eat good balance of foods. Trials that change a single dietary factor have an advantage that makes them suitable to clarify the contribution of some specific component on diet parameters. Studies to evaluate effects of SFA or salt on LDL cholesterol or blood pressure are good examples. By contrast, the degree of efficacy and durability are, generally, greater in trials changing the entire diet style. Thus, this type of intervention trial, such as Mediterranean vs. typical western-style diet, is more suitable as a hard endpoint study.

3.1 Calories and plasma lipids

Optimization of intake of total calories is a foundation of maintenance of healthy life. Reducing food intake to induce undernutrition extends the life spans of multiple species, ranging from single-celled organisms to mammals [7]. By contrast, whether calorie restriction decreases CV events in human remains unclear except in bariatric surgery. The LookAHEAD study examined whether an intensive lifestyle intervention for weight loss for 10 years would decrease CV morbidity and mortality among 5145 obese patients with type 2 diabetes [8]. The intensive lifestyle intervention was aimed at achieving and maintaining weight loss of at least 7% by focusing on reduced caloric intake (calorie goal of 1200–1800 kcal per day, restricting fat calories to <30%) and increased physical activity. Although greater reductions in all CV risk factors was observed in the intervention group than in the control group, the rate of CV mortality and myocardial infarction was not different (**Figure 1a**). Rebound of weight in the intervention group (**Figure 1b**) increased the statin use in the control group, and the lack of instruction about saturated and unsaturated fats is suggested for reasons of the negative results in this study. Five years later, in the PREDIMED study [6], a Mediterranean diet loaded with high content of monounsaturated fatty acids (MUFA) and polyunsaturated fatty acids (PUSA) without calorie restriction and exercise recommendation reduced CV events significantly approximately by 30% compared to the control low-fat diet group (**Figure 2**). It is noteworthy that the reduction of CV events occurred in the Mediterranean diet groups that consumed about 200–250 kcal higher calories as fat than in the control group. The data of these two studies [6, 8] have strongly suggested that intake of unsaturated fat is more effective than a low-fat, low-calorie diet for reduction of CV events. However, weight reduction by the low-fat diet in the LookAHEAD study has brought in important health benefits other than CV event reduction. Patients in the low-fat group were more likely to have a partial remission of diabetes during the first 4 years of the trial [9], more improvement in terms of reductions in urinary incontinence [10], sleep apnea [11], and depression [12] and improvements in quality of life [12], physical functioning [13], and mobility [14] than were those in the control group. Calorie restriction by diet is effective in reducing body weight in obese subjects. Therefore, diet therapy should be individualized dependent on the treatment goal, patient's characteristics such as underlying disease, BMI, and daily diet habits.

The difference in LDL cholesterol in the two groups in the LookAHEAD study was 1 mg/dl at the end of study [8]. By contrast, the effects of bariatric surgery on plasma LDL cholesterol and CV events have been clearer, because bariatric surgery reduces body weight to a greater extent, 20–40% from baseline. In a study of registry data in Sweden, LDL cholesterol was reduced approximately 40% associated with a 30% decrease in all-cause mortality 15 years after the surgery [15].

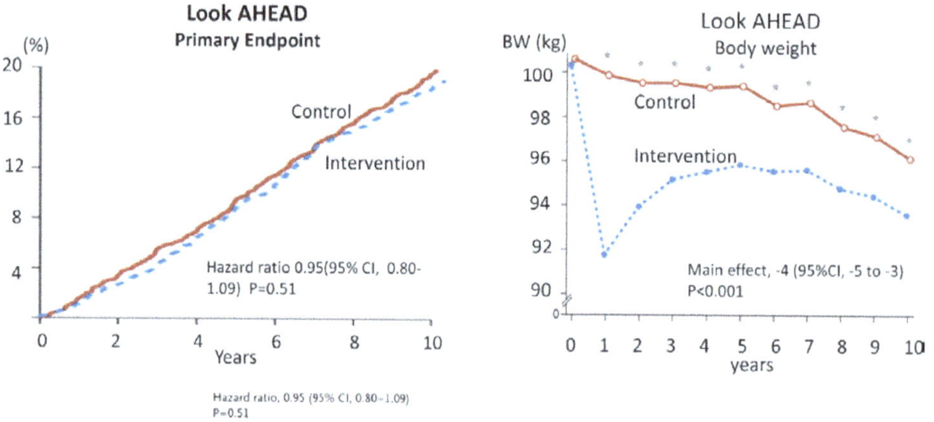

(a) (b)

Figure 1.
(a) Kaplan-Meier curves of the primary end point in look AHEAD study [8]. The primary outcome was a composite of death from cardiovascular causes, nonfatal myocardial infarction, nonfatal stroke, or hospitalization for angina. (b) Changes in body weight in the look AHEAD study [8].

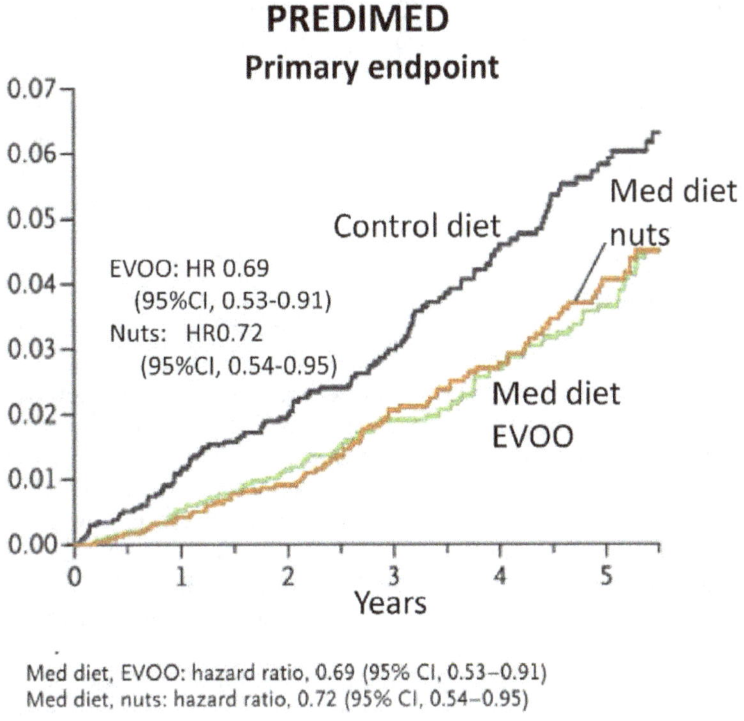

Figure 2.
Kaplan-Meier curves of the primary end point in the PREDIMED study [6]. The primary end point is a composite of acute myocardial infarction, stroke, and death from cardiovascular causes.

Bariatric surgery has also resulted in the remission of concomitant risk factors. A US cohort study in 2458 obese subjects showed that after gastric bypass surgery, the remission rate of was 62% for dyslipidemia, 38% for hypertension, and 68% for diabetes [16]. More than 150,000 bariatric surgeries had been performed in the US in 2013, which were almost one third of operations performed globally in 2013 [17]. Data from the bariatric surgery clearly indicate that it is important to provide substantial and sustainable body weight reduction for obese subjects in order to decrease CV events. If patients have difficulty maintaining calorie restriction, emerging evidence has been accumulating that a calorie-unlimited but well-balanced diet with MUFA/PUFA is a good choice.

3.2 Data and issues of low-carbohydrate vs. low-fat diet

In order to prevent muscle and bone wasting in aged people with sarcopenia, many scientific guidelines recommend that protein intake should be at least 1 g/kg/day of standard body weight unless renal function is abnormal. Thus, in limiting dietary calories, the requirement for protein usually cannot be changed. Much controversial data have been reported regarding whether the restriction of carbohydrate or fat is better in subjects with obesity or diabetes. Reduced carbohydrate diets are defined as having carbohydrate intake below the Dietary Guidelines for Americans (DGA) recommendation (45–65% of total energy intake). Regarding effects on body weight, several previous systematic reviews and meta-analyses [18–20] have shown that low-carbohydrate high-fat diets are just as effective, if not more so, than low-fat high-carbohydrate diets. Excess energy from carbohydrates stimulates the induction of lipogenesis in the liver via SREBP-1, resulting in accumulation of triglycerides (TG) in many organs [21], which induces obesity, dyslipidemia, and insulin resistance. Thus, the restriction of carbohydrates results in not only weight reduction but also improvement of dyslipidemia and insulin resistance.

Evidence has shown that under the controlled condition, both of the total calorie and the type of carbohydrate can affect body weight positively or negatively and plasma lipid profile as well. Even when receiving a high-calorie diet with increased fat content, obese subjects (BMI > 30) could reduce more weight with a low refined carbohydrate diet, compared with high-refined carbohydrate, low-fat, and energy-restricted diets in 1 year, based on a meta-analysis [22] and a 2-year intervention study [23]. One general consensus is that because refined carbohydrates are associated with high glycemic index, limiting intake of refined carbohydrates improves postprandial hyperglycemia, resulting in lower insulin release as well as decrease in body weight. In the period 1980–1990, calorie restriction by eating low-fat food was strongly recommended in many places in the US. The big issue of this nation-wide trend of low-fat diet was that most people were eating food containing refined carbohydrates with high glycemic index instead of fatty food (**Figure 3a**). An obesity epidemic in this period in the US coincided with the low-fat campaign. During the epidemic, the rate of obesity was almost triple, and the rate of diabetes doubled compared with three decades earlier [24, 25] (**Figure 3b**). It is ironic that people lost more money (low-fat food was generally more expensive) and gained weight while eating a low-fat diet.

In the OmniHeart study [26], the recommendation of fructose-sweetened beverages defined in the protocol could be one reason why the high-carbohydrate diets group showed the worst cardiometablic effects. Because of recent data showing fructose has worse effects on cardiometabolic risk markers than any other carbohydrates, the conclusion from the OmniHeart study cannot be extrapolated to all carbohydrates. Beverage makers in the US used to actively campaign by insisting that "over calories" was the reason for obesity rather than the type of sweetened carbohydrates included in beverages. However, each mono- and disaccharide has different effects on body metabolism. In a feeding study in overweight subjects, comparison of drinking_glucose- or fructose-sweetened beverages for 10 weeks showed that after fructose intake, fasting plasma glucose, insulin levels, and visceral adipose volume increased with a decrease in insulin sensitivity compared with the intake of glucose-sweetened beverages [27]. Glucose metabolism in blood and liver is tightly regulated by insulin and glucagon. On the other hand, because fructokinase does not play any role in the regulation of accumulation of fructose in the liver, the concentration of fructose in blood and liver increases with oral intake of fructose, which is called unregulated fructose uptake [28, 29]. Consequently,

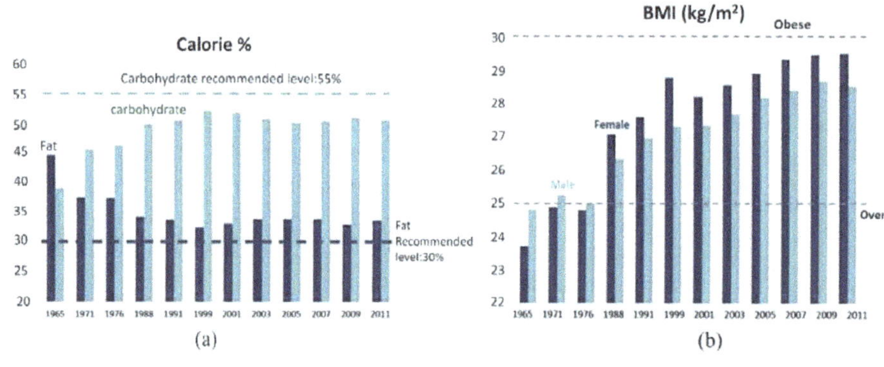

Figure 3.
(a) Changes in average fat and carbohydrate caloric consumption in adults from 1965 to 2011 [25].
(b) Changes in average BMI in adults from 1965 to 2011 [25].

accumulated fructose in the liver stimulates de novo lipogenesis and results in detrimental effects on glucose and lipoprotein metabolism [27].

Because of few reliable RCT, there have been many controversial results when comparing beneficial effects between low-fat and low-carbohydrate diet. It appears that the type of macronutrients replaced for fat or carbohydrate has significant effects on those results. A recent meta-analysis of studies with 432,179 subjects has shown that participants in low (<40%) and high (>70%) carbohydrate consumption groups had greater mortality than in moderate consumption groups, which is consistent with a U-shaped association [30]. The results varied according to the source of macronutrients. Namely, the mortality increased when carbohydrate was replaced with animal-derived fat or protein, and the mortality decreased when the substitutions were plant-based. This indicates that food source can be an important consideration for CV outcomes when one macronutrient is replaced with another macronutrient. It has been hypothesized that diets of lower plant carbohydrate with increased animal protein and fat stimulate inflammation, aging, and oxidative stress. On the contrary, nutrition based on low-carbohydrate and high-fat diet may have anti-inflammatory, anti-oxidative, and anticancer effects. A diet that contains reduced carbohydrate with higher fat or even a ketogenic diet, very low carbohydrate diet (<10% of carbohydrate calorie), slows down cancer growth and proliferation [31, 32]. Before instructing a patient to follow a low-fat or low-carbohydrate diet, clinical factors should be considered, including age, body weight, diet habits, underlying diseases, and kidney function. For example, a 75 y/o obese subject with diabetes who consumes a high-calorie diet with high content of fat from animal origin should decrease animal fat intake to reduce total calories for control of body weight. It makes sense to replace animal-fat with complex carbohydrates rather than plant-based unsaturated fat. This way would protect against the increase in total calories and let the glucose level decrease. If a subject has a history of myocardial infarction, partial substitution of animal fats with MUFA, such as found in olive oil, is another option, because of protection of CV disease by intake of olive oil. By considering many aspects of benefit and harm of carbohydrates and fat in this way, appropriate dietary composition should be individually fine-tuned based on patients' clinical characteristics and treatment goals.

3.3 Comparison of guidelines in Japan, the US, and Europe regarding fat content

Table 1 summarizes comparison of recommendations about dietary fat in several key scientific societies in the US, Europe, and Japan. Calorie intake from fat is restricted to 20–30% in guidelines of Ministry of Health, Labour and Welfare (MHLW) of Japan [33], Japanese Diabetes Societies (JDS) [34], and Atherosclerosis Societies (JAS) [35]. This value of 30% is classified as low-fat diet as defined by the 2014 the American Diabetes Association (ADA) guideline [36]. There are several reasons why restriction of calories from fat still remains in these recommendations in Japan. First, the LDL cholesterol level in Japanese is steadily increasing recently and at present it is higher among Japanese females than in American females [37]. A high-fat diet generally increases intake of SFA, resulting in increases in LDL cholesterol. Second, BMI in Japanese people is lower than in Caucasians. It is well known that thin Asian people are prone to develop diabetes with a mild increase in body weight. Therefore, because increases in fat calories are usually associated with increases in total calories and subsequently in body weight, restricting fat calories is often helpful to prevent worsening in blood glucose in diabetic subjects.

	Atherosclerosis/dyslipidemia			Diabetes			
	JAS (2017)	AHA/ACC (2013)	ESC/EAS (2016)	JDS (2016)	ADA (2014)	AACE (2013)	USDA (2015)
Total fat	20–25%	N/A[a]	N/R[b]	20–30%	N/R[c]	25–35%	N/R
MUFA	N/A[d]	N/A[d]	N/A	N/A	N/A[e]	<10%	N/A[d]
PUFA	N/A[d]	N/A[d]	<10%[e]	N/A	N/A	<20%	N/A[d]
Fish (n-3)	↑[f]	>Two times/week	↑[g]	↑[h]	>Two times/week	>Two times/week	>8 oz/ week
SFA	4.5–7%	<5–6%	<7%	<7%	<10%	<7%	<10%
Trans fat	<1%	↓[i]	<1%	↓[i]	↓[i]	<1%	↓[i]
Cholesterol	<200 mg	N/A[j]	<300 mg	<300 mg	<300 mg	<200 mg	N/A[j]

N/A: not available; N/R: no restriction; MUFA: monounsaturated fatty acids; and PUFA: polyunsaturated fatty acids.
[a]Recommendation for Mediterranean diet which usually has 32–35% as fat calorie.
[b]No restriction of fat intake, which is dependent upon individual preferences. However, fat intakes at >35% of calories are generally associated with increased intakes of both saturated fat and calories.
[c]No restriction of fat intake, inconclusive for an ideal amount of total fat intake for people with diabetes; therefore, goals should be individualized. Fat quality appears to be far more important than quantity.
[d]Not stated on intake of mono- and polyunsaturated fat. However, there are comments of improvement of LDL cholesterol by substitution of SFA with MUSA or PUFA.
[e]Intake of n-6 PUFAs should be limited to 10% of the energy intake in order to minimize the risk of lipid peroxidation of plasma lipoproteins and to avoid any clinically relevant HDL-C decrease.
[f]Recommend intake of fish. Increase in n-3 fat decreases plasma TG level with potential beneficial effects on CV events.
[g]Recommend intake of fish. Increase in n-3 fat decreases plasma TG level. Unknown for reduction of CV events.
[h]Recommend intake of fish. However, increase n-3 fat has no effects on prevention of diabetes and on CV events in diabetes.
[i]No upper limit defined. However, should decrease as much as possible.
[j]No upper limit.

Table 1.
Recommendations for intake of fat and cholesterol-related nutrients in major guidelines.

By contrast, in of the 2014 ADA guideline [36], lifestyle management by American Heart Association (AHA)/the American College of Cardiology (ACC, 2013) [38], European Society of Cardiology (ESC)/European Atherosclerosis Society (EAS, 2016) [39], and the Dietary Guidelines for Americans 2015–2020 [40], the upper limit in fat calories has been actually dropped, and they describe that it is advisable to determine it on an individual basis along with maintaining whole calories. Each of these guidelines stresses quality of fat rather than the total quantity of fat intake. There are a few important considerations for this major change. First, many people tend to often eat more refined carbohydrates as replacement for fat, and previous data have not shown clearly that this would reduce CV mortality and motility. A high-fat diet reduces body weight more than a high-refined carbohydrate diet [22, 23], which favors abandoning the upper limit of total fat intake from many guidelines. Second, limiting overall fat intake habitually carries the potential risk of reducing consumption of "good fat" such as MUFA/PUFA [36, 38–40]. All the guidelines have quoted data in the PREDIMED study, where a calorie-unlimited, fat-unrestricted Mediterranean diet reduced CV events about 30% compared with a low-fat diet [6]. It is noteworthy that fat calories in the Mediterranean intervention group was exceeded 40% in the PREDIMED study. The important message in removing the upper limit for fat calories from these guidelines is that to maintain consumption of an appropriate level of calories, one must include healthy high-quality fat in the diet.

3.4 Issues and limitations around nutritional trials

There have been several limitations of studies in nutritional science. Usually, a nutritional study lacks a double-blind design and a placebo for food. Without a placebo-controlled design, the study can provide no true evidence of either benefit or harm of the intervention. For example, if SFA were replaced by carbohydrate or protein, the isolated effect of SFA would be influenced by the changes in the composition of the other macronutrients to keep the diet calorie constant, which would make the isolated effect of SFA difficult to evaluate. Even in the subcategories of SFA, MUFA, and n-3, n-6 PUFA, there exists clear heterogeneity within each group that contributes to different biological effects. Furthermore, the food content within its SFA can have a significant impact on CV risk. The fermentation of dairy products provides a good example. The content of SFA in cheese is very high (20 g in 100 g of natural cheese compared with 3 g in 100 g of beef sirloin). A 10-year cohort study showed that the consumption of SFA from dairy products was associated with decreased risk of CV disease, and, by contrast, a higher intake of SFA from meat (including red and processed meat and poultry) was associated with greater CV disease risk [41].

Under- and over-reporting of dietary intake is common in nutritional studies. In contrast to easily countable items like coffee and sweetened beverages, the percentages of energy from fat and added sugar based on a food frequency questionnaire (FFQ) were underestimated [42]. Regarding longevity of habits of food intake, the protocol design in one cohort study had a diet assessment at baseline and approximately 36,000 participants were followed for 12 years [43]. This is a common type of study, in which a one time-point assessment can predict the occurrence of disease many years later.

The logic behind limiting the intake of SFA is derived from the risk factor model for coronary heart disease (CHD) causality, in which LDL cholesterol is a causal factor for CHD and a diet including SFA increases LDL cholesterol compared with other macronutrients. However, other biomarkers that predict CHD risk more have been proposed such as total cholesterol to HDL cholesterol ratio, small dense LDL cholesterol, apolipoprotein B, and others. Therefore, total CHD risk may be increased with elevations of these biomarkers even if LDL cholesterol does not change after the diet intervention.

Evidence coming from RCT is generally positioned above evidence from cohort studies in the research hierarchy. Findings in diet- and health-related RCTs are not necessarily more reliable than those from well-conducted cohort studies [44]. RCTs sometimes include subjects with underlying diseases and follow them up with a relatively short period. This means substantial limitation to extrapolate findings from RCTs to healthy persons, when CV events occur rarely over many years. Cohort studies also have their own sources of error, especially issues of confounding factors. For example, SFA intake is associated with behaviors indicating lower health consciousness, [45] whereas PUFA intake is either associated with behaviors indicating greater health consciousness [46], or is not related to health consciousness [47]. Therefore, confounding variables also often explain the inconsistent results regarding the replacement of SFA with PUFA for prevention of coronary heart disease. When reading manuscripts in nutritional studies, one must keep in mind these limitations and issues included in the studies.

3.5 Effects of replacement of SFA with PUFA

A high-SFA diet is quite palatable with weak effect on satiation, which results in potentially overconsumption and obesity [48]. There has been a tremendous amount of data showing that reducing SFA in food resulted in health benefit by lowering blood LDL cholesterol and CV events in RCT [49, 50], prospective cohort studies [51–53], and epidemiological studies [54]. Based on this evidence, AHA has recommended to decrease over-consumption of SFA since 1961. On the other hand, one RCT [55], a prospective cohort study [43], and meta-analysis [56] have reported that increases in SFA are not associated with increases in CV events. In the US where both myocardial infarction and consumption of beef are more than triple than that in Japan, whether the consumption of SFA in food results in health problems should be a serious issue [57, 58]. One recent article in the Annals of Internal Medicine in 2019 has concluded that red meat may have little or no effect on CV outcomes and cancer mortality based on low- to very-low-certainty evidence [59]. Just after this publica-tion, roughly 2000 emails, mostly caustic in tone, were sent to the inbox of an editor in the journal as a wave of backlash, including a push from one group attempting to have the guideline retracted even prior to publication.

The message from guidelines in major scientific societies reaches the same conclusion that limiting intake of SFA by replacing with MUFA and PUFA reduces LDL cholesterol and potentially reduces CV diseases. This conclusion was summarized in a position paper by the 2017 AHA presidential advisory board [60], which relied on four core randomized trials [61–64]. Results of a meta-analysis of these four core trials [60] are shown in **Figure 4**. The results showed that lowering calorie from SFA down to 7% and replacing them with vegetable oil rich in PUFA, primarily soybean oil, lowered blood cholesterol by 15% and the incidence of coronary heart disease (CHD) by 29%. The degree of efficacy by cutting this amount of SFA is compatible with that of statins [65].

Although it has become now widely accepted that the dominant dietary factor involving coronary heart disease is an excessive intake of SFA, recent new evidence has suggested that SFA may play a much less important role in coronary heart disease than was previously believed. As discussed previously, potential biases have been often included in diet studies, and earlier meta-analyses did not sufficiently account for major confounding variables. One study has shown different results in two meta-analyses of collecting only adequately controlled trials from collecting only inadequately controlled trials (**Figure 5**) [66]. These data clearly represent one typical example of difficulty in conducting well-controlled diet trials. The manuscript of the 2017 AHA presidential advisory board [60] that selected the 4 core RCTs may have had potential bias by excluding or including some studies from the

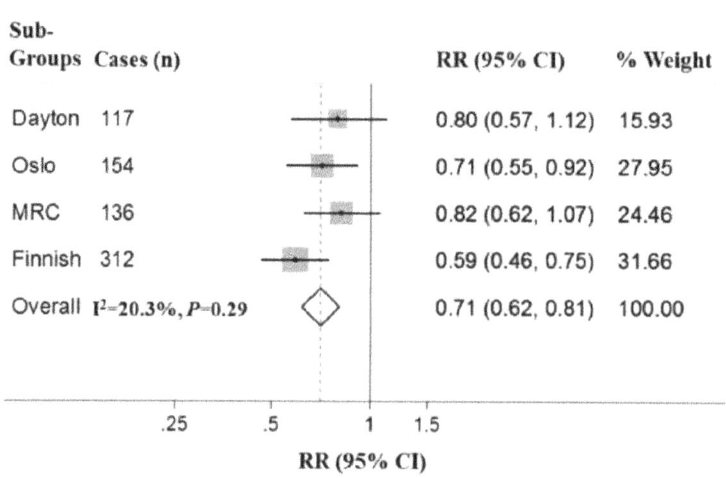

Figure 4.
Meta-analysis of core trials on replacing saturated with polyunsaturated fat [60].

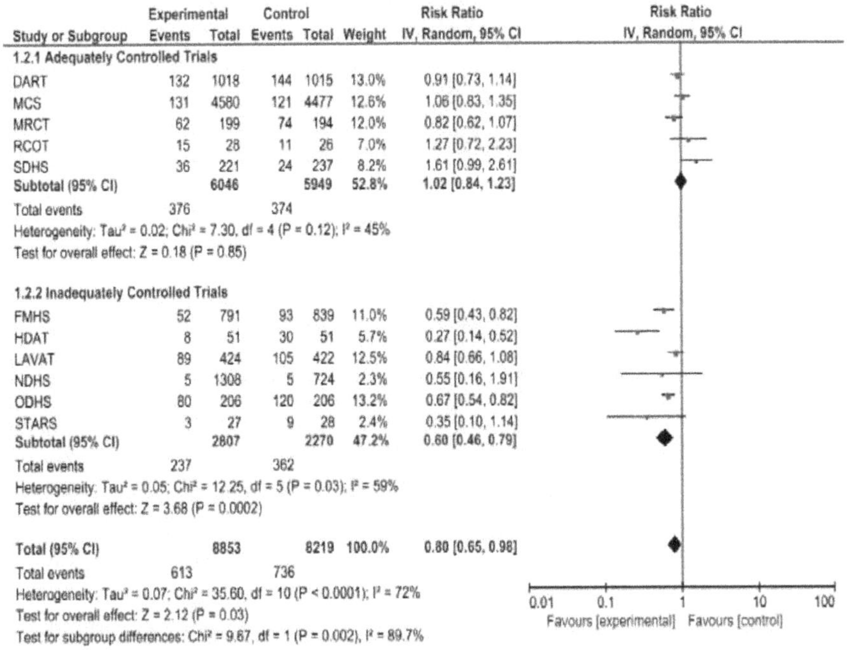

Figure 5.
Forest plot showing pooled RR with 95% CI for the number of total CHD events [66].

analysis. Notwithstanding apparently consistency of the description in many authoritative guidelines of harmful effects of SFA, some experts are insisting that there have been no solid evidence indicating that the consumption of SFA is related with higher incidence of CV disease [67].

It seems that one common key message in studies that the overestimated harmful effects of SFA is that other factors (e.g., increased refined carbohydrate/added sugar included in soft drinks, or trans fat; or decreased fish, fruit, and vegetables) play a more role in development of coronary heart disease than SFA [68]. However, previous data of substitution of SFA with PUFA have consistently shown improved blood lipid profile and blood pressure. Furthermore, increased intake of SFA from animal meat and butter generally is accompanied by more consumption of trans fat or other substances with potentially harmful effects on humans. The Mediterranean and DASH diets, which include high amount of MUFA and PUFA with low contents of SFA, have constantly shown health benefits. Based on all these data, as in the authorized opinions, restriction of SFA is a reasonable strategy.

3.6 Effects of replacement of SFA with MUFA

Compared with PUFA, less data have been available evaluating benefits of MUFA [69]. In human cohort studies, the replacement of SFA with MUFA yielded smaller reduction of LDL cholesterol [70] and incidence of CHD [71–73], compared with PUFA. One huge cohort study in 127,536 subjects combining the Nurses' Health Study and the Health Professionals Follow-up Study has shown that replacing 5% of energy intake from SFAs with equivalent energy intake from PUFA or MUFA was associated with a 25 and 15% lower risk of CHD, respectively (**Figure 6**) [73]. A review of the Cochran database in 2015 has concluded that replacing the energy from SFA with PUFA appears to be a useful strategy and that, by contrast, effects of replacement with MUFA were unclear due to inclusion of only one small trial [69].

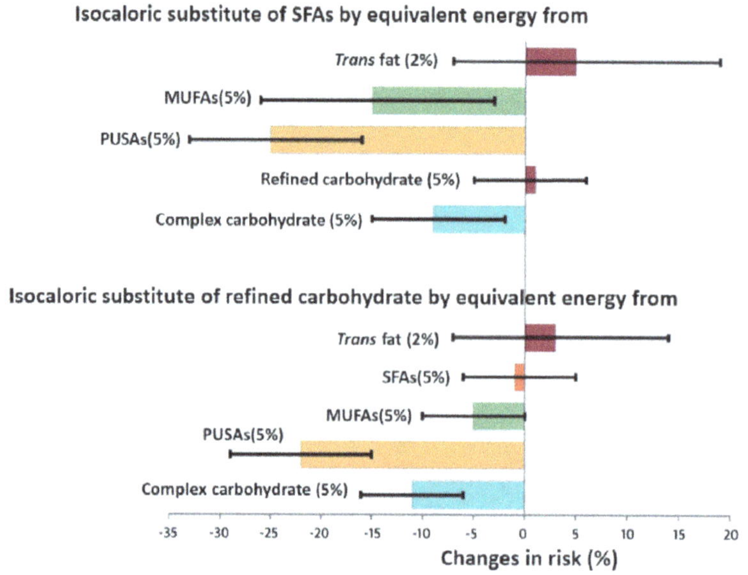

Figure 6.
Estimated percent change in the risk of CHD after isocaloric substitute of SFA (upper half) or refined carbohydrate (lower half) by other nutrients [73].

The source and origin of MUFA within a specific diet may explain the inconsistent previous results with MUFA [74]. One huge meta-analysis including 32 cohort studies in 840,000 subjects has shown data that effects of MUFA on CV disease and its mortality varied depending on the different dietary sources of MUFA. Whereas MUFA of mixed animal and vegetable sources per se did not yield any significant effects on major CV outcomes, importantly, significant associations could only be found between higher intake of olive oil and reduced risk of CV events. It is of note that all studies which showed benefit for CV risk were conducted in the Mediterranean nations where extra-virgin olive oil is the most dominant source of this type of fatty acid [75]. The amounts of olive oil in the highest consumption group used in those studies were > 30 g/day in the EPIC cohort (in Spain), 48 g/day in the EPIC cohort in Greece [76], 52 g/day in a case-controlled study in Spain [77], and 56 g/day in the PREDIMED study [78]. Although mean olive oil consumption in the US is increasing, it is still very low at 4.2 g/day in 2010 compared with those in the Mediterranean areas (**Figure 7**) [79]. Another study in Spain has shown clearly different effects on cardiometabolic parameters between olive oil and sunflower oil (11% for MUFA and 60% for PUFA) [80]. With a slight increase in LDL cholesterol in the olive oil group, olive oil improved other risk factors such as glucose, TG, and body weight to a greater extent than in the sunflower oil group. The amount of olive oil in this study was expected to be more than 40 g/day, based on data showing that Spanish diet usually includes olive oil accounting for 18% of calorie intake [81]. All of these findings indicate that a large amount of olive oil (probably > 30 g/day) has distinctive effects compared with other oils from plant or animal origin.

Along with firm evidence of CV event reduction in two RCTs (Lyon Diet Heart study [82, 83] and PREDIMED [6]), olive oil should be viewed not only as "better" MUFA but also as a nutrient including many biologically active ingredients such as polyphenol. In 2018, the FDA approved a qualified health claim for consuming oils with high levels of oleic acid (major MUFA in olive oils) to reduce risk for coronary heart disease [84]. This new claim allows manufactures of olive oils to state that "supportive but not conclusive scientific evidence" suggest that daily consumption of one and half tablespoon (20 g) of olive oil may reduce CHD risk.

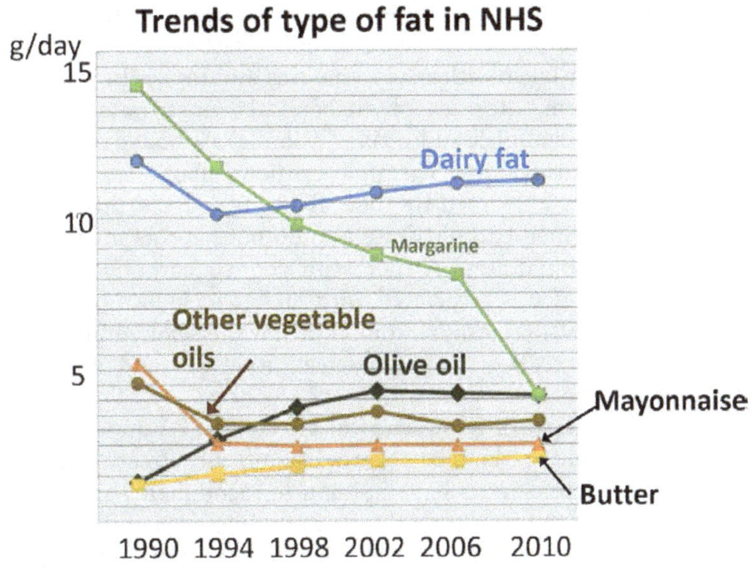

Figure 7.
Trends of types of fat intake from 1990 to 2010 in Nurses' Health Study (NHS) [79].

3.7 Effects of replacement of saturated fat with carbohydrate

In many studies which replaced SFA with carbohydrate, total calories from fat was roughly reduced from 40% to 20–30%, and this has affected diet adherence in subjects who are accustomed to eating oily food. In the Women's Health Initiative Study [85], the protocol intended originally to reduce fat calories from 37 to 20% in the low-fat/high carbohydrate group. In 8 years, the fat calories increased to 37% in this group, which was higher than the fat calories in the control group (35%) because of poor compliance. In the low-fat/high carbohydrate group, although LDL cholesterol decreased by 3 md/dl, CV events were not reduced significantly. One meta-analysis including 15 randomized controlled trials with 59,000 participants [69] concluded that the replacement of SFA with carbohydrates reduced LDL cholesterol mildly (5%) without affecting CV events. In most of the studies used in this meta-analysis, it is noteworthy that refined carbohydrates were incorporated as replacement for SFA. A growing weight of authoritative opinion is to recommend intake of complex carbohydrates including much fiber and minerals. Two recent studies [56, 86] have also shown the same results that the CV benefit by reduced SFA tends to be neutralized by increasing intake of refined carbohydrates.

Combined analysis of two prospective, cohort studies [73] in the Nurses' Health Study (84,628 women) and the Health Professionals Follow-up Study (42,908 men) has the advantage of investigating effects of different sources of carbohydrates, refined or complex, on CHD risk for long periods up to 30 years. **Figure 6** shows that when 5% of energy from SFA was replaced with 5% of energy from carbohydrates, the risk of CHD decreased by 9%. By contrast, when replaced with refined carbohydrates/added sugars, the risk of CHD did not decrease. This study has also shown change of CHD risk when refined carbohydrates/added sugars were replaced with other nutrients. Replacing refined carbohydrates/added sugars with MUFA, PUFA, or complex carbohydrates was significantly associated with a lower risk of CHD (5, 21, and 12%, respectively). However, there was no change in the risk of CHD when refined carbohydrates/added sugars were replaced with SFA. Results of this cohort study provide additional evidence that effects of refined carbohydrates on CV risk are at least equipotent to those of SFA.

At present, intact or minimally processed carbohydrates where fiber, bran, and germ content is high are generally called complex carbohydrates. Bran of whole grain is fiber-filled outer layer with many vitamins and minerals, and germ, which is a nutrient-packed core, includes phytochemicals, unsaturated fat as well as vitamins. Differences in complex and refined (simple) carbohydrates are shown in **Table 2**. The mechanisms for harmful cardiometabolic effects of refined carbohydrates are mostly explained by their ability to increase insulin release and shorten satiety [87]. Refined carbohydrate also do not have as much vitamins and fibers as complex carbohydrates. A diet with refined carbohydrates with high glycemic index such as rice is associated with higher incidence of coronary heart disease and diabetes [88–91]. Reduction of refined carbohydrates in food has decreased blood pressure, TG, and high-sensitivity CRP, and improved insulin resistance [92, 93].

Emerging evidence regarding the harmful effects of SFA and refined carbohydrates on cardiometabolic markers has exerted significant effects on the food label authorized by FDA. Some experts have opinion to recommend on leaving percent daily value of SFA with dropping % total fat, and adding on % refined carbohydrate instead of % carbohydrate against the daily value of these nutrients [94]. Because of data showing that refined carbohydrates with high glycemic indices worsen diabetic status, the FDA changed the nutrition facts section of the food label in 2019 to require listing the amount of and percent daily value for added sugars (**Figure 8**, arrow 1). Furthermore, "Calories from Fat" was removed, because abundant data show that the type of fat is more important than the amount (**Figure 8**, arrow 2).

Foods and drinks that contain no significant nutrients but are high in calories are said to have "empty calories." Drinks with added sugar are a typical example of empty calories. Sugar-sweetened beverages are the largest source of added sugar in the diet. In the US, the consumption of sugar-sweetened beverages has decreased modestly since around 2009; however, the intake level is still high (**Figure 9**) [95]. The Dietary Guidelines for Americans [40] and WHO [96] recommend no more than 10% of daily calories from all added sugars. As shown in **Figure 9**, adults in the US consumed an average of 160 kcal/day from sugar-sweetened beverages in 2014. This means that sugar-sweetened beverages alone correspond to 8% of total calories. To date, a large body of evidence supports a strong link between intake of sugar-sweetened beverages and weight gain [97], risk of type 2 diabetes [98], and CV diseases [99–101]. Sugar-sweetened beverages, as well as saturated fat, present a clear target for health policy.

	Complex	Simple (or refined)
Structure	Polysaccharides	Mono, disaccharides
Taste	No taste	Sweet
Digestion	Slow	Easy
Blood sugar	Slowly increases	Rapidly increases
Insulin response	Low	High
Glycemic index	Low	High
Satiety	Longer	Shorter
Fiber	High	Low
Body weight	Loss	Gain

Table 2.
Differences in two types of carbohydrate: complex vs. simple (refined).

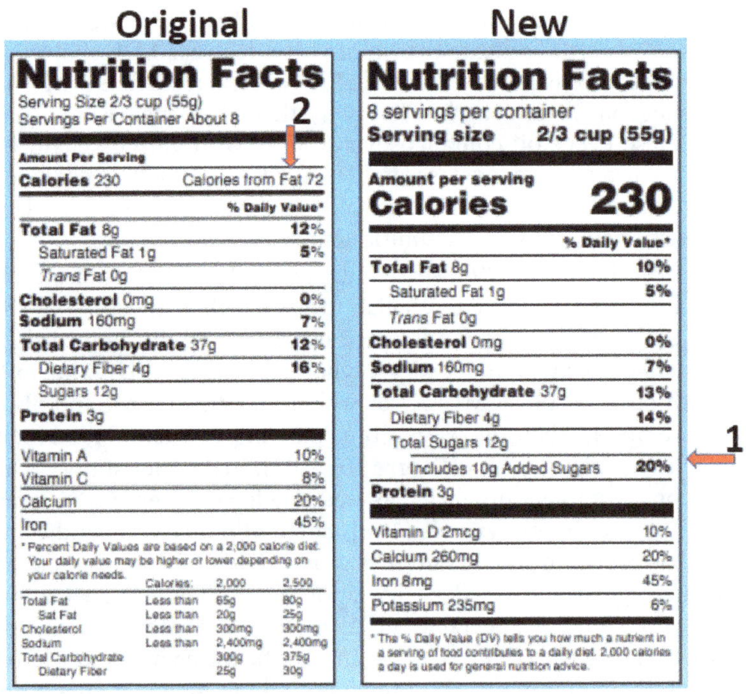
Original
Nutrition Facts
Serving Size 2/3 cup (55g)
Servings Per Container About 8
2
Amount Per Serving
Calories 230 Calories from Fat 72
% Daily Value*
Total Fat 8g 12%
Saturated Fat 1g 5%
Trans Fat 0g
Cholesterol 0mg 0%
Sodium 160mg 7%
Total Carbohydrate 37g 12%
Dietary Fiber 4g 16%
Sugars 12g
Protein 3g
Vitamin A 10%
Vitamin C 8%
Calcium 20%
Iron 45%
New
Nutrition Facts
8 servings per container
Serving size 2/3 cup (55g)
Amount per serving
Calories 230
% Daily Value*
Total Fat 8g 10%
Saturated Fat 1g 5%
Trans Fat 0g
Cholesterol 0mg 0%
Sodium 160mg 7%
Total Carbohydrate 37g 13%
Dietary Fiber 4g 14%
Total Sugars 12g
Includes 10g Added Sugars 20%
1
Protein 3g
Vitamin D 2mcg 10%
Calcium 260mg 20%
Iron 8mg 45%
Potassium 235mg 6%

Figure 8.
Changes in the format of the nutrition label of the original and the new version on Jan 2020.

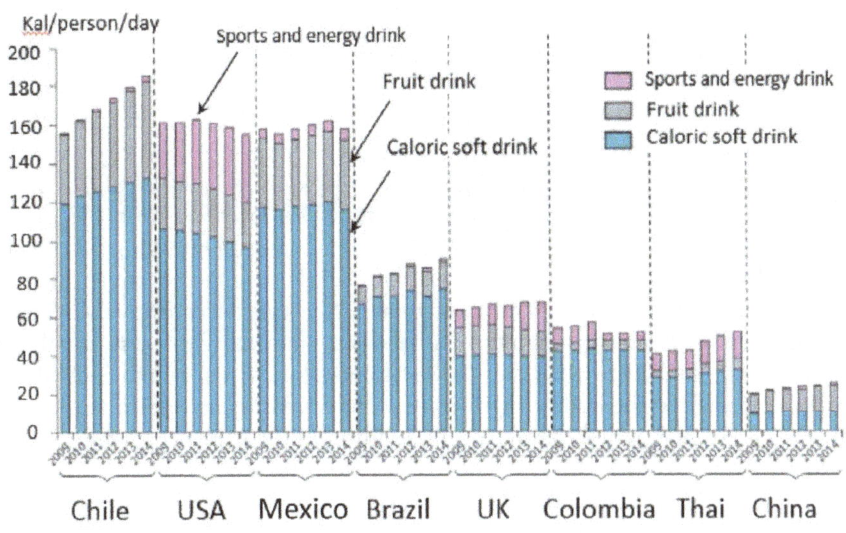

Figure 9.
Sales of sugar-sweetened beverages (SSBs) in kcal/person/day by beverage type in 2009–2014 in some selected countries [95].

3.8 Effects of replacement of SFA with other nutrients on plasma lipids, blood pressure, and other risk markers

Replacing 1% of energy from SFA with 1% of energy from PUFA, MUFA, or complex carbohydrates decreased plasma LDL cholesterol by 2.1, 1.6, and 1.3 mg/dl, respectively [102]. HDL cholesterol decreased by 0.2, 0.2, and 0.4 mg/dl after substitution of SFA by PUFA, MUFA, or complex carbohydrate. The change in TG was −0.9, −0.4, and +1 mg/dl by substituting with PUFA, MUFA, or complex carbohydrates. These data indicate that in order to decrease LDL cholesterol or TG, the best strategy is to reduce the intake of SFA. SFA exert different LDL increasing ability depending on chain length. However, this difference is not clinically so important, because every oil contains several SFAs with various chain lengths. In general, there are progressive increases in LDL-C with diminishing chain length. The potency of the LDL-raising effects of individual SFAs is lauric acid (C12:0) > myristic acid (C14:0) > palmitic acid (C16:0) [103].

SFA may affect the risk of CV disease independently of LDL cholesterol, through the effects on inflammation, endothelial function, thrombosis, and ventricular arrhythmias [104]. One ex vivo randomized cross-over study showed that a breakfast with butter (35% SFA) induced a higher increase in TNF-alfa mRNA than breakfasts with olive oil (36% MUFA) or walnuts (16% PUFA), and also a higher response in IL-6 mRNA than the walnut breakfast in peripheral blood mononuclear cells (PBMCs) in healthy subjects (**Figure 10**) [105]. In another study, LDL-induced adhesion of monocyte to endothelial cells was also lower after MUFA consumption than after SFA in healthy individuals [106]. Some other ex vivo studies in humans have shown that consumption of butter was associated with more activated genes involved in the regulation of cell proliferation and inflammation compared with consumption of olive oil or vegetable oil [107, 108]. In these studies, activation of inflammatory markers has occurred without significant changes in the blood lipid profile [106, 108]. In summary, the previous findings strongly suggest that saturated and unsaturated fats have unique biological effects on vascular walls which are independent on the reduction in LDL cholesterol, which is like the effects of statins.

3.9 Guideline recommendations for dietary intake of SFA

Guidelines of authoritative opinions in Japan, the US, and Europe including cardiology, diabetes, and atherosclerosis societies except ADA [36] recommend less than 7% of calorie from SFA in subjects with background diseases (**Table 1**). In healthy subjects, the recommended upper limit of SFA is 7% in Japan [33] and 10% in the US [109]. Restriction of SFA to <10% rather than 7% in diabetic subjects as recommended by the ADA [36] may sound a little strange, because diabetes is associated with high CV risk, and on-target LDL cholesterol criteria is generally more stringent. This recommendation is based on the data from one small 3-week study that compared a low SFA diet (8% of total calories) vs. a high SFA diet (17% of total calories), and showed no significant difference in glycemic control and most CVD risk measures [110]. Therefore, there is limited research regarding effects of

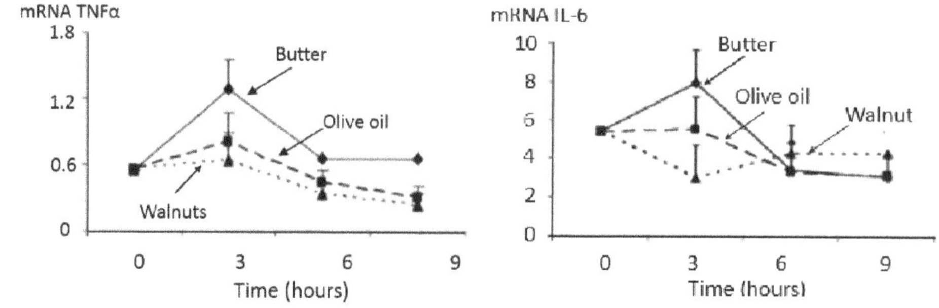

Figure 10.
Response of mRNA TNFα (left) and IL-6 (right) in breakfast with butter, olive oil, and walnuts measured in peripheral blood mononuclear cells (PBMCs) [105].

SFA on diabetic control, and the ADA nutrition position paper recommends people with diabetes follow the guidelines for the general population, which is 10% according to USDA [109]. Despite insufficient data about effects of SFA on glycemic control, the evidence in many review manuscripts or meta-analyses so far accumulated has indicated that a Mediterranean diet helps prevent type 2 diabetes and causes HbA1c reduction in persons with established diabetes [111–115]. Therefore, food habits to restrict intake of SFA as in the Mediterranean diet is a very reasonable strategy in diabetic subjects.

Three Japanese cohort studies have shown that the incidence of brain hemorrhage is inversely related to intake of SFA [116–118], and this moved the JAS to define the lower limit (4.5%) of intake of SFA [35]. This relation has not been demonstrated in meta-analysis of subjects in the US and Europe. There have been no data showing high incidence of stroke in vegetarians who consume very little SFA. Therefore, none of the guidelines in the rest of the world have incorporated the lower limit of intake of SFA. One has to be cautious that limiting SFA in the diet tends to decrease intake of good fat, as PUFA, fish oil, or olive oil.

Intake of 7% of calories as SFA is equivalent to about 15 g of SFA in a person who needs 2000 cal/day. Average intake of SFA is 15.2 and 13.8 g/day for Japanese men and women at the age of 30–49 years old [119], and 31.4 and 20.3 g/day for American men and women at the age of 31–50 years old [120]. It is reasonable that refraining from red meat, processed meat, butter, or SFA-loaded snacks is a simple way to cut SFA in daily food habits. In the US, only approximately 5% of the population consumes less than 7% of their calories from saturated fat [120].

3.10 Guideline recommendations for dietary intake of PUFA and MUFA

Beneficial effects of PUFA and MUFA seem to be fully recognized in guidelines in the US and Europe (**Table 1**). Guidelines from ADA, ACC/AHA, NLA, and USDA strongly recommend the Mediterranean and DASH diets. Regarding efficacy of decreasing blood glucose, the ADA provides the same recommendation for both PUFA and MUFA [36]. The 2013 AHA/ACC Guideline on Lifestyle Management [38] states that PUFA or MUFA should be used for reducing LDL cholesterol instead of SFA at the same recommendation level.

Literature has emerged that the biological effects of olive oil differ from those of plant-based MUFA or PUFA. Incorporating data from the PREDIMED study [6], the 2016 Canadian Cardiovascular Society Guidelines for the Management of Dyslipidemia [121] concretely recommend olive oil (>60 ml/day) and nuts (>30 g/day) rather than using general terms for MUFA. An authoritative review of dietaries and policies for cardiovascular diseases in 2016 [122] has also listed its daily recommended doses of MUFA and PUFA, such as 10–30 ml/day of soybean oil (MUFA: 22%, PUFA: 56%, and SFA: 15%), extra virgin olive oil (MUFA: 74%, PUFA: 7%, and SFA: 13%), and canola oil (MUFA: 64%, PUFA: 28%, and SFA: 7%). These guidelines provide data of effects on plasma LDL cholesterol and CV events by substitution of SFA with PUFA and MUFA.

The differences in guideline recommendations of the fat intake appear to reflect the differences in food habits and in recognition of the benefits of healthy fats between countries. In 2010, nonoptimal intake of n-6 PUFA, SFA, and trans fat resulted in 710,000, 251,000, and 537,000 deaths from CHD per year worldwide [123]. In 80% of nations, including Japan, China, and other many Asian nations, CHD burdens attributable to n-6 PUFA were 2-fold higher than the SFA-attributable burdens. These data indicate that it is more important to focus on increasing healthful n-6 rich vegetable oils in the diet than to focus on replacement of SFA and carbohydrates for public health benefits.

4. Cholesterol

4.1 Relation of plasma LDL cholesterol and dietary intake of cholesterol

Plasma LDL cholesterol value changes depending on oral intake of cholesterol. One meta-analysis of 17 studies reported that a 100 mg increment in dietary cholesterol from eggs elevated plasma total cholesterol by 2.2 mg/dl [124]. On the contrary, many studies have brought into question the apparent association between dietary cholesterol consumption and blood cholesterol [38]. Plasma cholesterol undergoes a highly degree of regulation to balance absorption in the intestine and synthesis in the liver [125]. Low dietary cholesterol intake is compensated for by an increase in absorption. These mechanisms explain the inter-individual variability in absorption (20–80%) in humans. Thus, there are responders and nonresponders to intake of cholesterol in terms of plasma cholesterol levels. Interestingly, repeated cholesterol loading has changed some nonresponders to responders [126, 127]. The presence of two types of cholesterol response may reflect just day-to-day variation of cholesterol absorption from the gut in a single person rather than a true difference between responders and nonresponders. In responders, both LDL and HDL cholesterol increased with no change in ratio of LDL to HDL. A gene of ABCG5/8 regulates absorption of dietary cholesterol and sterol from gut [128]. People carrying polymorphisms of ABCG5/8 have a higher absorption rate of cholesterol. In these subjects, the effects of manipulation of intake of cholesterol in food on plasma LDL cholesterol levels have been very significant.

The possible link between dietary cholesterol and CHD risk is potentially distorted by confounding factors from other features in the diet, especially SFA [129]. A previous recommendation of less than 300 mg of dietary cholesterol has been removed from the 2013 AHA/ACC Guideline on Lifestyle Management to Reduce Cardiovascular Risk [38], stating that there is insufficient evidence to determine whether lowering dietary cholesterol reduces LDL-C. The same action was taken in the 2015 Dietary Guidelines of USDA [40] and the 2015 Japanese dietary intake standards by Ministry of Health, Labor and Welfare [33]. By contrast, other guidelines still restrict the dietary cholesterol intake, for instance, 200 mg/day in JAS [35] and AACE [130] guidelines, or 300 mg/day in ESC/EAS [39], ADA [36], and JDS [34] guidelines. These guidelines engender the risk of potentially increasing intake of SFA by abandoning the recommendation for dietary cholesterol intake. However, all of these, in common, stress risk evaluation of atherothrombotic diseases and execution of comprehensive management to reduce the risk. Even the guideline from JAS, which limits dietary cholesterol intake at 200 mg/day, states very clearly that only restricting dietary cholesterol intake is hardly efficacious in reducing plasma LDL cholesterol, and rather more attention should be paid to reducing SFA in food.

5. Polyunsaturated fat

5.1 n-3 and n-6 PUFA

Every cooking oils or foods generally include several kinds of fatty acids. **Table 3** shows the amounts of different fatty acids in several commercially available oils and foods. In the US, people use soybean oil very frequently for cooking, and its dominant fatty acid is n-6 PUFA (50%), along with MUFA (25%). Olive oil, a very popular oil in the Mediterranean Sea area, is a well-known representative with

	Fat	SFA	MUFA	PUFA n-3	PUFA n-6
Rapeseed oil 100 g	100 g	7.4 g	63 g	9 g	18 g
Soybean oil 100 g	100 g	16 g	23 g	6.8 g	50 g
Olive oil 100 g	100 g	14 g	73 g	0.8	9.8 g
Mackerel 100 g	17 g	4.6 g (27%)	5 g (8.5%)	2.1 g (12%)	0.4 g (2.4%)
Butter 100 g	81 g	51 g (63%)	21 g (26%)	0.3 g (0.3%)	2.2 g (2.7%)
Peanuts 100 g	56 g	11 g (20%)	26 g (46%)	0 g (0%)	17 g (30%)

Figures in parenthesis (%) are the percent of calories from each fatty acid compared to the total amount of fat.

Table 3.
Amounts of different fatty acids contained in several cooking oils, butter and foods.

MUFA making up more than 70% of all fatty acids. Both soybean oil and olive oil include SFA at about 15% of all fat. It should be noted that mackerel, which people believe is a very rich source of fish oil (=n-3 PUFA), contains more than twice as much SFA and MUFA compared to n-3 PUFA. Bluefin tuna (nonoily tuna) and salmon contain only one-tenth and one-third the amount of n-3 PUFA compared with that in mackerel, respectively.

From this table, it is easily understandable that saturated fat is not synonymous with fat from animal food and likewise unsaturated fat is not synonymous with plant food. When compared gram for gram, olive oil has 7 times SFA of the trimmed beef sirloin. Furthermore, the oily fish, mackerel, which are advised to eat, has more than two times SFA of the beef sirloin. Therefore, it is not unexpected that results in clinical studies with pharmaceutical drugs with highly purified EPA differ from those of epidemiological studies with variable fish consumption. When reading manuscripts of nutritional studies with interventions involving fatty acid(s), it is important to consider which oils or food stuffs are added to modify the specific fatty acids.

The ratio of n-6 to n-3 fatty acids in the diet of early humans was estimated to be 1:1 [131]. The ratio in the diet of the US today has risen to 10:1 because of the combination of reduced n-3 fatty acid intake and the widespread use of vegetable oils rich in linoleic acid (n-6). As shown in **Table 3**, all listed foods and oils have much higher content of n-6 compared with that of n-3 except mackerel. It has been proposed that while n-3 fatty acids have anti-inflammatory effects, n-6 fatty acids have pro-inflammatory effects. This is based on data that oxylipins synthesized from n-6 PUFA have more inflammatory, vasoconstrictive, and proliferative effects compared with a metabolite derived from n-3 PUFA, although there are notable exceptions [132]. Because enzymes generating inflammatory metabolites from n-6 PUFA are inhibited by EPA and DHA from n-3 PUFA, increases in tissue concentration of EPA and DHA tend to shift the activity toward anti-inflammatory status. This is the rationale for using the ratio of n-6 to n-3 PUFA (n-6/n-3) in the blood as a potential risk marker for CV diseases, cancer, and some other chronic inflamma-tory diseases such rheumatoid arthritis, and bronchial asthma [133]. However, it is difficult to predict the appropriate cut-off value of n-6/n-3. Furthermore, blood concentration of n-6/n-3 does not reflect the amount of oral intake of n-3 and n-6 PUFAs [134–136]. At present, a general consensus is that high linoleic acid (n-6 PUFA) in the diet or circulation is not associated with higher in vivo or ex vivo pro-inflammatory responses, and that those individuals consuming the highest level of α-linolenic acid (n-3 PUFA) had the lowest inflammatory status [136]. Therefore, the oral intake of linoleic acid should not be restricted and it is unnecessary to consume more n-3 PUFAs.

Instead of ratio of n-6 to n-3, ω-3 index, based on measurements of EPA and DHA in red blood cells, was proposed as a marker for previous consumption of fish for last 120 days [137, 138]. The ω-3 index >8% has been proposed as optimal for cardioprotection. The average ω-3 index in Japanese is 9–11%. By contrast, the average in the US people is 4–5% and only <10% of individuals have the ω-3 index >8% [139], which reflects well the difference of fish consumption between Japan and the US.

5.2 Epidemiology and history regarding health benefits of fish oil (n-3 PUFAs)

As shown in **Table 1**, the guidelines from AHA/ACC, ADA, and AACE recommend 2 servings of fatty fish per week for the general population. A typical serving of fish can range from 3 to 6 ounces (about 85–170 g), depending on the type of fish and its preparation. Most adult Americans eat only 7–13 g/day of fish, and Japanese who are 20 years and older eat 73 g/day of fish, based on a 2013 national survey [140]. Because of the difference of daily intake of fatty food, the percent of calorie from total fat is higher among Americans than Japanese, except for n-3 PUFA, which is only 30% higher in Japanese [119, 141]. Reason for the relatively small difference in fat calorie from n-3 FUFA is that in Americans, the intake of red meat and poultry as a source of n-3 PUFA is much higher among Americans. When comparing percent of calories from EPA and DHA between Japanese and Americans, this parameter is almost four times higher in Japanese [140, 141]. The percent of calories from EPA and DHA and their concentration in the blood reflects baseline consumption of fish intake in diet.

Epidemiological data of Greenlanders from almost half century ago [142] and WHO study [143] have shown that fish consumption was independently, significantly, and inversely associated with all-cause and CHD mortality. In 1999, the GISSI-P study, the first RCT of dietary supplementation with n-3 fatty acid, showed significant reduction in the risk of the major CV events by 10% [144]. Based on the results of this RCT and positive observational studies, since 2000, the European Medicines Agency (EMA) has authorized n-3 fatty acid medicines for use after a heart attack in several EU countries, at a dose of 1 g per day. In 2002, the second AHA Science Advisory "Fish Consumption, Fish Oil, Lipids, and Coronary Heart Disease" concluded that individuals at risk for CHD benefit from the consumption of plant- and marine-derived n-3 fatty acids (1 g of EPA + DHA per day) [145].

However, since the 1990s at almost the same time as US and EU recommendations, conflicting data have been substantially reported showing no correlation between n-3 fatty acid consumption and CV events [146–154]. The Cochran meta-analysis in 2004 including 48 RCTs (36,913 participants) and 41 cohort analyses has concluded that consumption of n-3 fats did not show a reduction in the risk of total mortality or combined CV events [155]. Until the positive results in the REDUCE-IT study in 2019 [156], all major RCTs with n-3 fatty acids [157–162] except JELIS study (**Table 4**) [163], which were conducted in Japan with open-blind design. These negative results in observational studies and RCTs were enough to result in label changes in for n-3 supplements in Europe. In 2016, the ESC/EAS guidelines concluded that it was unclear whether n-3 fatty acids had beneficial effects on CV events [39]. Furthermore, 2 years later in 2018, EMA concluded that omega-3 fatty acid medicines are not effective in preventing further CV events in subjects with a history of myocardial infarction and that n-3 fatty acid supplements would no longer be authorized for secondary prevention [164]. Results of the ASCEND study [162], which was published several months before this recommendation, had substantially affected this EMA decision. The ASCEND study, which has been the largest double-blind omega-3 RCT, evaluated MACE for 7.4 years in 15,480 subjects

Study	Year	Inclusion	Statin	Follow up	Regimen	Baseline TG	Primary EP	Results
EPA/DHA study								
GISSI-P	1999	11,324 Post MI	BL = 5% EOS = 46%	3.5 y	850 mg EPA + DHA	162 mg/dl	MACE	HR = 0.85 (0.74–0.98)
GISSI-HF	2008	6975 HF	22%	3.9 y	850 mg EPA + DHA	126 mg/dl	Death + Hosp	HR = 0.91 (0.83–0.99)
OMEGA	2010	3851 Post MI	94%	1 y	840 mg EPA + DHA	121 mg/dl	Sudden death	OR = 0.95 (0.56–1.6)
Alpha-OMEGA	2010	4837 Post MI	85%	3.3 y	400 mg EPA + DHA	144 mg/dl	eMACE	HR = 1.01 (0.87–1.17)
SU.FOL.OM3	2010	2501 Post MI	85%	4.7 y	600 mg EPA + DHA	115 mg/dl	MACE	HR = 1.08 (0.79–1.47)
ORIGIN	2012	12,536 dyslipidemia + CVD	53%	6.2 y	840 mg EPA + DHA	140 mg/dl	CV death	HR = 0.98 (0.87–1.1)
Risk & Prevention	2013	12,513 High risk + CVD	41%	5 y	850 mg EPA + DHA	150 mg/dl	CV death	HR = 0.97 (0.88–1.08)
ASCEND	2018	15,480 Dm	75%	7.4 y	850 mg EPA + DHA	NA	MACE	HR = 0.9 (0.87–1.08)
Pure EPA study								
JELIS	2007	18,645 dyslipidemia	100%	4.6 y	1.8 g EPA	151 mg	eMACE	HR = 0.81 (0.69–0.95)
REDUCE-IT	2018	8179 CVD+ High risk	100%	4.9 y	4 g EPA	216 mg/dl	eMACE	HR = 0.74 (0.68–0.83)

DHA: docosahexaenoic acid, EPA: eicosapentaenoic acid, BL: baseline, EOS: end of study, EP: end point, MACE: major CV event (death, myocardial infarction, stroke), eMACE: expanded major CV event (MACE + revascularization).

Table 4.
Comparison of RCTs of n-3 PUFA [156–163].

with diabetes living in England. The n-3 supplements had no effects not only on CV events but also on mortality of other chronic diseases such as cancer and COPD. The authors also commented on the issue of cost of n-3 supplements, because up to 31% of all British people were using them. The authors clearly concluded that the recommendation of n-3 in guidelines in major meetings should be drastically corrected [162].

Compared with the clear negative opinion against effects of n-3 fatty acids from EMA, the USFDA has accepted the potential medical benefit of n-3 fatty acids for secondary prevention. In 2017, the most recent AHA Science Advisory still concluded that treatment with omega-3 PUFA supplements is reasonable for secondary prevention, stating that a potentially modest reduction in CHD mortality (10%) in this clinical population would justify treatment with a relatively safe therapy [165]. The Cochran review in 2018 (included 79 RCTs, 112,059 participants) concluded that increasing n-3 saturated fat intake made little difference to all-cause mortality and CHD mortality, which did not support the recommendation in the 2017 AHA Science Advisory of the use of n-3 fat supplements for patients with CHD [166].

Despite the inconsistent recommendation between EMA and FDA, all guidelines support an indication for reducing TG by n-3 supplements. Furthermore, they positively advise intake of fish, a rich source of marine- or plant-derived omega-3 fatty acid. The positive effects of fish consumption on CHD have been mostly attributed to n-3 PUFA (EPA and DHA); however, fish is also an excellent source of bioactive peptides which have shown beneficial activities for cholesterol-lowering, hypotensive effects through ACE inhibition, or inhibitory action for atherosclerosis, inflammation, or oxidation [167]. Supplements containing fish oil are very popular among people living in the US, being used by 7.8% of the population [168]. The reason for the popularity of n-3 supplements in the US reflects a typical lifestyle not to eat fish often (one serving of fish/week) as well as a general belief in beneficial effects of omega-3 oil for health. The commercially available n-3 supplements do not contain fish peptides but usually include at least some amount of other ingredients that are potentially harmful for health such as SFA, mercury, etc.

5.3 Reasons for inconsistent data of omega-3 fatty acids for coronary heart disease

Most of the RCTs with n-3 supplements generally have not shown a significant reduction of CV events so far. **Table 4** shows comparison of previous RCTs [144, 156–163, 169]. Inconsistent data in RCTs as well as observational studies of n-3 supplements could be attributed to statin use, dose of n-3 fatty acid, or TG and HDL values at baseline. The statin use was very low in two positive studies (GISSI-P [144] and GISSI-HF [169]), which mainly recruited subjects two decades ago, before the wide-spread use of stains. One study showed that although among statin-users coronary vascular events were not reduced with n-3 fatty acid supplements, the events significantly decreased in statin nonusers [170]. This suggests that statin treatment modified the effects of n-3 fatty acids on the incidence of major cardiovascular events.

The dosage is another important factor. Findings in two Cochran review manuscripts showed no dose dependency of n-3 fatty acids [155, 166]. It is of note that the absolute amount of fish intake was very small in some studies, which tends to make the correlation between n-3 fatty acids and CV events less clear. In some studies in cultures where eating fish is not common, the participants who belonged to the group with the highest intake of fish consumed just 2–3 servings/week, and one extreme example is a study to compare subjects who consumed no fish to subjects who ate fish once a week [148]. The JPHC study, conducted in Japan, showed clear dose-dependency between n-3 fatty acids and CV events even in the primary prevention population [171]. Incidence of myocardial infarction was reduced by 56% in the comparison of highest (8 servings per week, or 180 g/day) vs. lowest quintiles (once a week, or 23 g/day) of fish intake. Generally speaking, a small gradient of fish consumption is associated with negative results in observational studies.

Because consumption of omega-3 fatty acids is evaluated based on self-report or food surveys by questioners, the issue of reliability about how much n-3 fatty acids was consumed has always existed. Furthermore, variability of n-3 fat content among fish species makes estimation of EPA + DHA consumption more difficult. For instance, EPA + DHA ranges from 200 to 300 mg in 3 pounds of wild tuna to more than 1500 mg in the same amount of wild mackerel.

Dose dependency of n-3 fatty acids appears to be clear in results of RCTs. As shown in **Table 4**, whereas doses of EPA/DHA used in recent negative studies were generally less than 1 g, the JELIS [163] and REDUCE-IT [156] studies, which showed significant CV risk reduction, used larger doses of EPA (see Sections 4 and 5 REDUCE-IT study). Finally, baseline TG value was suggested to affect the effects of n-3 supplements. Three positive studies, GISSI-P [144], JELIS [163], and REDUCE-IT [156] studies recruited subjects with higher baseline TG values of more than 150 mg/dl compared with the levels in other studies with negative results. In the JELIS study, whereas 1.8 g EPA reduced CV events in the whole population by 19%, the CV reduction was 53% in the subgroup with high TG (>150 mg/dl) and low HDL cholesterol (<40 mg/dl) at baseline [172] (**Figure 11**). A similar trend toward greater efficacy in subjects with higher TG and lower HDL-cholesterol at baseline was also observed in the REDUCE-IT study (**Figure 12a** and **b**) [156]. In subjects with high TG (>200 mg/dl) and low HDL cholesterol (<40 mg/dl) in the REDUCE-IT study, the percent reduction of primary endpoint by 4 g EPA was almost double (38%) compared with that in subjects with normal TG and HDL-cholesterol (21%, P for interaction = 0.04). In two fibrate studies, the BIP study (bezafibrate) [173] and the ACCORD study (fenofibrate) [174], no significant reduction of CV events reported despite the greater decrease in TG (21% in BIP and 26% in ACCORD) with higher

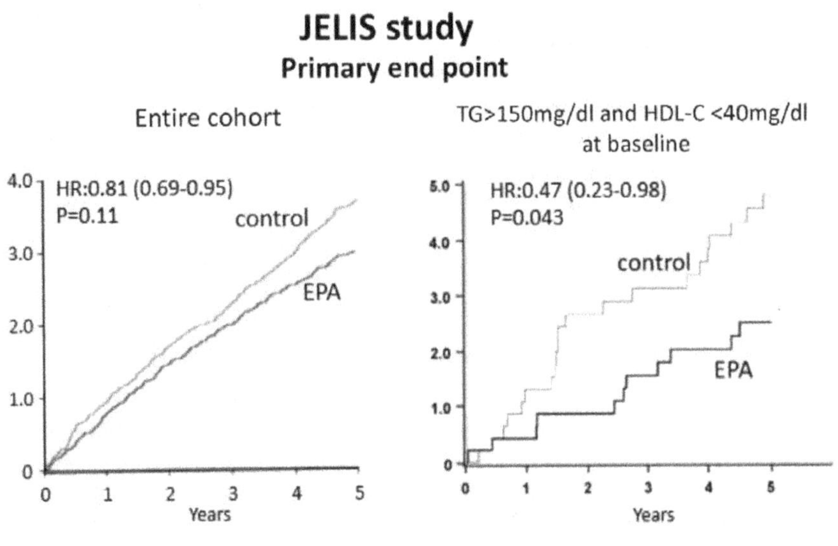

Figure 11.
Kaplan-Meier event curves for the primary end point in the entire cohort (left) and the subgroup with high TG and low HDL (right) in the JELIS study [163]. The primary end point is a composite of sudden cardiac death, nonfatal myocardial infarction, nonfatal stroke, unstable angina, and coronary revascularization.

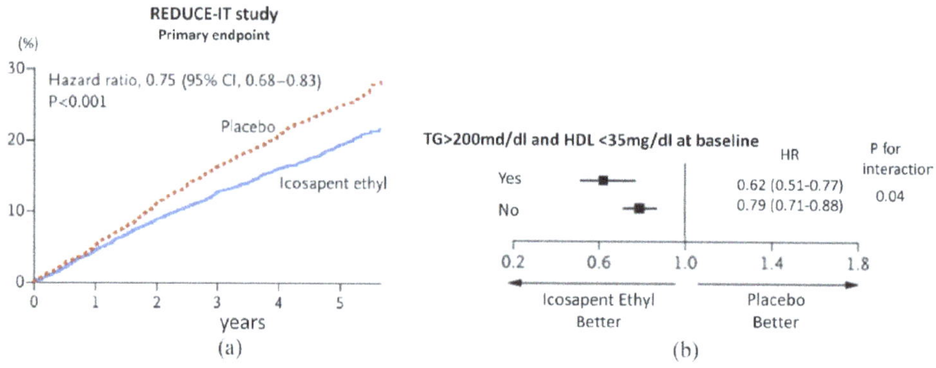

Figure12.
(A) Kaplan-Meier event curves for the primary end point in the entire cohort in the REDUCE-IT study [156]. The end point is a composite of CV, nonfatal myocardial infarction, nonfatal stroke, coronary revascularization, or unstable angina. (B) The hazard ratios and 95% CI in the subgroup according to the baseline TG and HDL for the primary efficacy end point in REDUCE-IT study [156].

increases in HDL cholesterol (18% in BIP and 6% in ACCORD) compared with the REDUCE-IT study (18% decrease in TG and 3% increase in HDL). However, like the JELIS [163] and REDUCE-IT [156] studies, there was a significant reduction in CV events in subjects with higher baseline TG at >200 mg/dl [173, 174]. These data suggest that with greater abnormalities of baseline TG and HDL cholesterol, the two different dyslipidemic drugs, EPA and fibrates, tend to show greater CV events reduction. However, from the comparison of efficacy size on CV events in studies with EPA and fibrates, although at least some of the beneficial effects in the EPA studies could be explained by changing the plasma lipid, effects other than improvement of dyslipidemia are at work in the reduction of CV events by EPA.

5.4 Antithrombotic effects of n-3 fatty acids

Reduction of CV events by consumption of fish is mostly attributable to beneficial effects of n-3 fatty acids (EPA/DHA). Potential effects include antiplatelet, activity, inhibition of life-threatening arrhythmia, decrease in LDL cholesterol and TG, increase in HDL cholesterol, decrease in blood pressure, stabilization of inflammation in lipid-rich plaque, and antioxidation. Although n-3 fatty acid products are generally approved for TG lowering, this class of drugs has only modest TG lowering. Based on the modest changes in non-HDL cholesterol, reduction of CV events is calculated to be only 6–8% [175]. Therefore, changes in lipid profile alone cannot explain why EPA in the REDUCE-IT study reduced CV events by 25%.

Previous data have indicated that inhibition of platelet aggregation by n-3 fatty acids at pharmaceutical doses is insufficient for reduction of CV events. Compared with the reported value of inhibition of platelet aggregation by aspirin, prasugrel, or ticagrerol, all of which have been proven effective for reduction of CV events, antiplatelet efficacy of omega-3 fatty acids appears to be relatively small [176]. Supplementation with omega-3 fatty acids had no effect on platelet activation in the presence of aspirin [177] or clopidogrel [178]. A high level of dietary EPA + DHA (4.5, 9.5 g) or estimated biologically equivalent amounts of alpha-linolenic acid did not affect coagulation factors, fibrinogen, plasminogen activator inhibitor-1, or tissue plasminogen activator activity compared with the control [179]. All of these data suggest that antithrombotic efficacy via platelets, coagulation, and fibrinolysis does not play a major role in n-3 fatty acid-induced decrease in CV events in the positive previous studies.

5.5 REDUCE-IT study

5.5.1 Results of REDUCE-IT study

The REDUCE-IT trial has shown that use of highly purified icosapent ethyl (EPA) 2 g twice daily reduced CV events by 33% compared with placebo among patients with high TG and either known CV disease or high risk for CV disease (**Figure 12A**) [156]. The absolute reduction of the primary endpoint was 4.8%, and number needed to treat (NNT) was 21 persons/5 years (105 persons/year). This number is very excellent compared to other clinical trials recently conducted. There have been two other positive classes of drugs in addition to statins which showed significant reduction in CV events, ezetimibe and PCSK9 inhibitor. The absolute risk reduction in ezetimibe study was only 2% for 7 years (34.7–32.7%) [180]. NNT was 50 persons/7 years (350 persons/year). In the two PCSK9 inhibitors, evolocumab [181] and alirocumab [182], NNT value was 67 persons/2.2 years (147 persons/year) and 63 persons/2.8 years (176 persons/year), respectively.

5.5.2 Success factors in the REDUCE-IT study

This study had three distinctive features, compared to the previous n-3 studies that are considered to be responsible for the positive results; dose, formulation, and baseline TG. The daily dose of EPA used in the REDUCE-IT study was 4 g, more than four times higher than the doses used in previous studies. The daily dosage of n-3 supplements is usually 2 capsules containing the combination of 180 mg EPA and 120 mg DHA (=0.6 g/day of n-3), and no more than 2 g/day as dietary n-3 supplements in the FDA recommendation of 2014 [183]. The rationale of 4 g EPA in REDUCE-IT was that the blood concentration at this dose (183 μg/ml) was similar to that in Japanese subjects in JELIS study who received 1.8 g of EPA (170 μg/ml) [156, 185]. This occurred because Japanese people have much higher background intake of fish and thus have higher EPA and DHA blood concentrations than seen in Western populations. These data suggest that there may be some threshold dose to show reduction of CV events despite abundant in vitro and ex vivo data of various biological effects at smaller doses of n-3 fatty acid.

The entry criteria for TG initially was 150 mg/ml and later was changed to 200 mg/ml to increase the enrollment of patients with more significant TG elevations. Therefore, the participants' TG level at baseline was the highest (TG = 216 mg/dl) among all omega-3 studies. The ongoing STRENGTH trial, which aims to assess the efficacy and safety of a 4 g EPA/DHA combination drug, will help to clarify the influence of different formulations and dosages on CV outcomes. In January 2020, following the recommendation from DSMB, the sponsor for this study decided to close the Phase III STRENGTH trial due to its low likelihood of demonstrating a benefit to patients with mixed dyslipidemia [184]. DHA plus EPA raises LDL levels, whereas EPA alone does not raise LDL levels. The inclusion criteria for lipids were different in the two studies. REDUCE-IT had a mineral oil placebo, whereas STRENGTH had a corn oil placebo. An in vitro study has shown that EPA has direct antioxidant benefits in various apoB-containing particles that are more pronounced than those of DHA and other TG-lowering agents [185]. Although all these differences may explain partially the inconsistent results in the two studies, it appears most plausible that EPA may have different biological effects on CV events compared with those of DHA.

5.5.3 Role of EPA in management of CV disease in the future

The REDUCE-IT study is actually the first study to demonstrate significant reduction of CV events by purified EPA among Caucasians in the strong statin era.

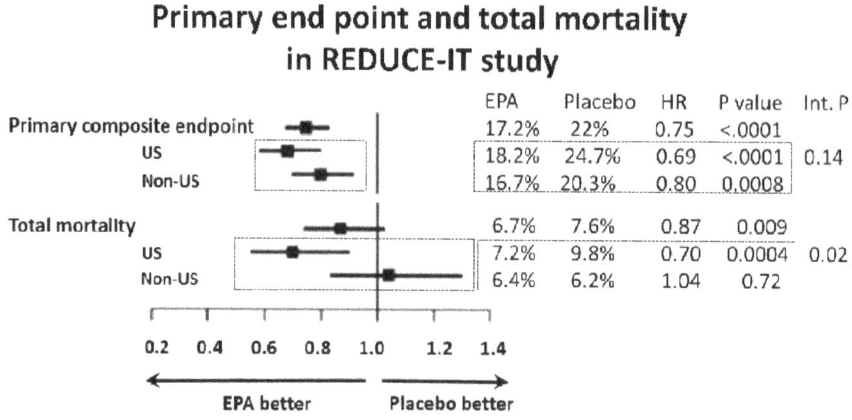

Figure 13.
The hazard ratios and 95% CI in the US and non-US population for the primary efficacy end point in REDUCE-IT study [186].

Recently, a subgroup analysis of REDUCE-IT study was conducted to determine the degree of benefit of EPA in the 3146 patients in the United States [186]. As shown in **Figure 13**, the US subgroup in REDUCE-IT demonstrated more robust risk reduction. The primary endpoint was reduced by 31% in the US cohort compared with 20% in the non-US cohort. Especially, whereas total mortality was numerically increased after 5 years in the non-US cohort, EPA reduced total mortality by 30% from 9.8 to 7.2% in the US cohort. In the current era when many clinical CV event trials have failed to show mortality benefit, this magnitude of the decrease in total mortality in the US cohort is very amazing.

Independent analysis showed that this regimen was a very rare case of high cost-effectiveness, and that EPA at $4.16/day offered better outcomes at lower health care costs for payer-eligible patients in the REDUCE IT trial [187]. Cost-performance results in clinical trials are, generally, very persuasive for obtaining regulatory approval for FDA and EMA. In December 2019, EPA became the first FDA approved drug with an indication for reduction of CV risk among patients with elevated TG levels as an add-on to maximally tolerated statin therapy [188].

A recent analysis of the REDUCE-IT study with the measurement of blood concentration of EPA has clarified the more important role of pleiotropic effects of EPA rather than lowering TG as potential mechanisms to reduce CV events [189]. The blood concentration of EPA at baseline was in a relatively narrow range and the administration of 4 g icosapent ethyl raised the blood levels by 400%. Importantly, the reduction in CV events seen in the REDUCE-IT trial was directly related to on-treatment serum levels of EPA [189]. The reduction in TG levels contributed just 2 percentage points to the overall 25 percentage points reduction in CV events in the study. This means that TG-lowering effect by EPA was not a major reason for the reduction of CV events in the REDUCE-IT study.

6. Monounsaturated fat

Compared with clinical studies on PUFA, fewer studies focusing on MUFA have been published in the literature. Whereas the replacement of SFA in the diet with MUFA increased CV events in some studies [74], other studies showed reduction [190] or no change [56, 191] in CV events. As already described, one plausible reason for this inconsistency is the type of MUFA in the studies. It seems clear that substitution of SFA with olive oil consistently reduced CV events, meaning that it is necessary to recognize the different metabolic effects between olive oil and other oils that contain MUFA.

6.1 Lyon Diet Heart study

6.2 Results of the Lyon Diet Heart study

Despite the small decreases in LDL-cholesterol (usually <5%) with the Mediterranean diet food, in meta-analysis of many cohort studies, the magnitude of decreases in CV events was to the same extent or even larger than in statin studies [192–194]. Effects on CV events beyond LDL-cholesterol reduction with the Mediterranean diet has been demonstrated in two RCTs, the Lyon Diet Heart study and the PREDIMED study [6]. The Lyon Diet Heart study [82, 195], which was the first RCT of the Mediterranean diet before the statin era, randomized 605 patients with history of myocardial infarction to compare that diet with a French style diet. The Mediterranean diet reduced the primary endpoint by 73% (CI: 0.12–0.59, $P = 0.001$). The overall mortality was also reduced by 70% (CI: 0.11–0.82, $P = 0.02$). Although the study was originally planned to follow CV events for 5 years, it was terminated early, 2 years and 3 months after the study initiation, due to the high mortality rate in the control group. There were no significant differences in body weight, blood pressure, LDL and HDL cholesterol, and blood glucose levels between the two diet groups at the end of the study. Therefore, the marked differences in rates of CV events were not due to improvement of these classical surrogate risk markers. The investigators presented results of an extended follow-up, and the striking reduction of CV evens was maintained for up to 4 years [195].

6.2.1 Nutritional data in the intervention and control group

Table 5 shows the comparison of nutritional data in the intervention and control groups at the end of the study (27 months after the randomization) [82, 195, 196].

	Control	**Intervention**	***P***	**To maintain desirable BW**	
				Step 1	**Step 2**
Energy, cal	2088	1947	0.033		
Total lipids, *E*%	33.6	30.4	0.002	<30	<30
SFA, *E*%	11.7	8.0	0.0001	8–10	<7
PUFA, *E*%	6.1	4.6	0.0001	up to 10	
Linolenic (n-3), *E*%	0.29	0.84	0.0001		
Linoleic (n-6), *E*%	5.3	3.6	0.0001		
Oleic (MUFA), *E*%	10.8	12.9	0.0001	up to 15	
Carbohydrate, *E*%	49.8	53.4	N/A		
Protein, *E*%	16.6	16.2	0.3		
Fiber, g	15.5	18.6	0.004	20–30	
Cholesterol, mg	312	203	0.0001	<300	<200

Table 5.
Comparison of nutritional data in the intervention and control groups in the Lyon Diet Heart study at the end of the study (27 months after the randomization) [82, 195, 196].

In order to show the uniqueness of the intervention group in this Lyon Diet Heart study, the nutrient profiles of the NECP/AHA step 1 and step 2 are also presented. Because the intake of calories and the percentages of energy (*E* %) of three major nutrients were relatively similar, it appears that the differences in fat components had substantial effects on CV events. In the Mediterranean diet group, SFA was 32% lower (8.0 vs. 11.7%), oleic acid (MUFA) was 20% higher (12.9 vs. 10.8%), and α-linolenic acid (n-3 PUFA) was 190% higher (0.84 vs. 0.29%). Because there was no restriction of butter, fatty red meat, or snacks (rich sources of SFA) in the control diet group, and animal meat has also high content of MUFA, the energy percentage of SFA was high in the control diet group and the total unsaturated fat (MUFA + PUFA) was not different between the two groups (control vs. Mediterranean: 16.9 vs. 17.5%). The change in fat components in the Mediterranean diet group was not in accord with the current general recommendations regarding SFA and PUFA. The group had relatively high intake of SFA (8%) and lower intake of PUFA than in the control group (4.6 vs. 6.1%, **Table 4**), which could explain the small change in LDL cholesterol by the intervention. The findings in this study clearly illustrate the importance of the risk factors beyond lipids and lipoproteins.

Compared with data in PREDIMED study [6], conducted two decades later, which was loaded with extra-virgin olive oil and nuts with less refined carbohydrate, the percentage of energy of MUFA was almost half (12.9 vs. 22.1%), fat calorie was 10.8% lower (30.4 vs. 41.2%), and inversely, carbohydrate calories were 12.2% higher in the Mediterranean diet group in the Lyon Diet study (53.4 vs. 41.2%). Furthermore, the percent of calories from n-3 PUFA was low compared with those values in the REDUCE-IT [156] and JELIS [163] studies where highly purified marine-derived n-3 EPA was given. Therefore, it is unlikely that the beneficial, biological effects of n-3 PUFA or MUFA on CV risk reduction were maximally utilized for the reduction of CV events in the Lyon Diet Heart study. The very high value of SFA in the control group (11.7%) may be another factor contributing the exaggerated CV event reduction in this study. In one cohort study with 2.96 million person-years of follow-up which evaluated effects of red meat consumption on risk of CV diseases [197], the total mortality in the top quintile was 40% higher than in the bottom quintile. SFA consumption in the control group in the Lyon Diet Heart study was almost identical to that in the top quintile in that cohort study. At present, as SFA is well known to increase in LDL cholesterol, it is nearly impossible to conduct any diet trials with more than 8% intake of SFA for ethical reasons.

6.3 PREDIMED study

6.4 Protocol and results

The second RCT of the Mediterranean diet was the PREDIMED study [6]. There are several distinctions between the Lyon Diet Heart and PREDIMED studies. First, the PREDIMED study had much more participants (605 vs. 7447 subjects). Second, the Lyon Diet Heart study enrolled subjects with a history of acute myocardial infarction, and by contrast, the target is primary prevention with a high CVD risk in the PREDIMED study. Third, the Mediterranean diets were substantially different in the two studies. In the Lyon Diet Heart study, the Mediterranean diet was enriched with alpha-linolenic acid (n-3 PUFA), because margarine was provided freely in substitution for butter and cream, but not olive oil, and, by contrast, in the PREDIMED study, the diet for participants assigned to be the Mediterranean groups was loaded with extra-virgin olive oil or nuts. Finally, regarding the fat content in the control group diet, a high-fat diet was used in the Lyon Diet Heart and a low-fat diet in the PREDIMED study.

After the original version of the PREDIMED study was protocol was published in 1993 [198], statistical issues and randomization errors had been corrected, and then a revised version was published in 2018 [6]. Participants were randomized into one of three interventions: Mediterranean diet supplemented with extra-virgin olive oil (EVOO, a minimum of 50 ml/day for participants), or Mediterranean diet supplemented with nuts (30 g/day: 15 g walnuts, 7.5 g almonds and 7.5 g hazelnuts) or control diet (advice to follow a low-fat diet). The reasons for recommending EVOO was that the content of polyphenol is quite variable among olive oils, and that EVOO has reduced CV events to a greater extent compared with non-EVOO (HR 0.84 vs. 0.97) [199]. All participants were Spanish people living in the Mediterranean area. Olive oil is a rich source of MUFA (usually more than 70% of all fat) as well as phenolic antioxidants. Walnuts contain much more PUFA (n-3: 14%, n-6: 58%) than MUFA (14%) compared with EVOO (PUFA: 13%, MUFA: 70% or more). The other half of the nut allowance was almonds and hazelnuts, both rich in MUFA (80%) and polyphenols. Thus, although having the same general food pattern as the Mediterranean diet, the EVOO group was enriched in MUFA and polyphenols and the nuts group was enriched in MUFA and (n-3, n-6) PUFA as well as polyphenols.

Figure 14 shows the daily intake of EVOO and nuts in the three groups in the PREDIMED study compared with that of Japanese aged of >60 y/o in 2015. Consumption of EVOO and nuts was very high in subjects who followed the Mediterranean diet with EVOO or nuts, respectively. It is noteworthy that even the control group had much higher consumption of EVOO than in Japanese (data on average consumption is not available; however, based on amounts of import and domestic production of olive oil in Japan, this value is very likely to be in the low single digits) and in the US population (4.2 g/day/person) [79]. Consumption of nuts was also high in the two Mediterranean groups and substantially higher in the control low-fat group than in Japanese, and probably in Americans, because according to statistical data in a US national survey in 2009–2010, 63.3% of men and 60.5% of women in the US did not consume any nuts on a given day [200]. These data indicate that all participants including those in the control cohort in this study had, to some extent, Mediterranean-style diet.

The primary endpoint (MI, stroke, and CV death) was significantly reduced, with an adjusted hazard ratio of 0.69 (CI, 0.53–0.91) for the EVOO group and 0.72 (9CI, 0.54–0.95) for the nuts group, as compared with the control diet (**Figure 2**). The Kaplan-Meier curves for the primary end point diverged soon after the trial started. The average age of participants in this study was 67 years old and a subgroup analysis showed that CV events were reduced by 30% in people more than 70 years old, similar to the value in younger people, indicating that it is never too

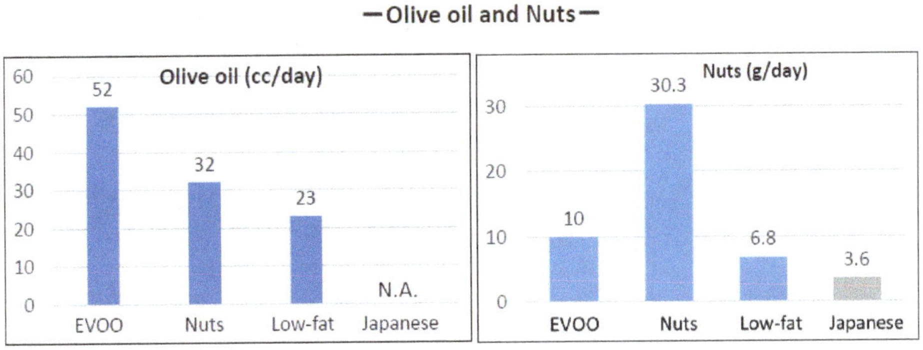

Figure 14.
Daily consumption of olive oil and nuts in the PREDIMED study at the end of the study compared with those in Japanese in their 60s [6, 140].

late to change dietary habits to improve CV health. It should be stressed that the two Mediterranean diets decreased systolic blood pressure by 5–6 mmHg, LDL- cholesterol by 5% or less, and fasting blood glucose by 2–4 md/dl, and that these small changes of risk factors alone can hardly explain the very early and significant 30% risk reduction of the primary end point.

6.4.1 Comparison to other CV studies to intervene in traditional CV risk factors

Although the primary end point was positive in the entire cohort of subjects including those in primary and secondary prevention studies, of the CANVAS program (canagliflozin) [201], the DECLARE-TIMI58 study (dapagliflozin) [202], or the LEADER study (liraglutide) [203], the subgroup analyses have shown a very small reduction in primary endpoint in subjects without established atherosclerotic diseases (**Figure 15**).

The absolute and relative risk reduction by aspirin was 0.06%/year and 12% in primary prevention group [204] and thus, because of increased bleeding complications, aspirin has not been indicated in subjects without CV diseases. What is remarkable in the PREDIMED study is that the huge reduction in CV events was

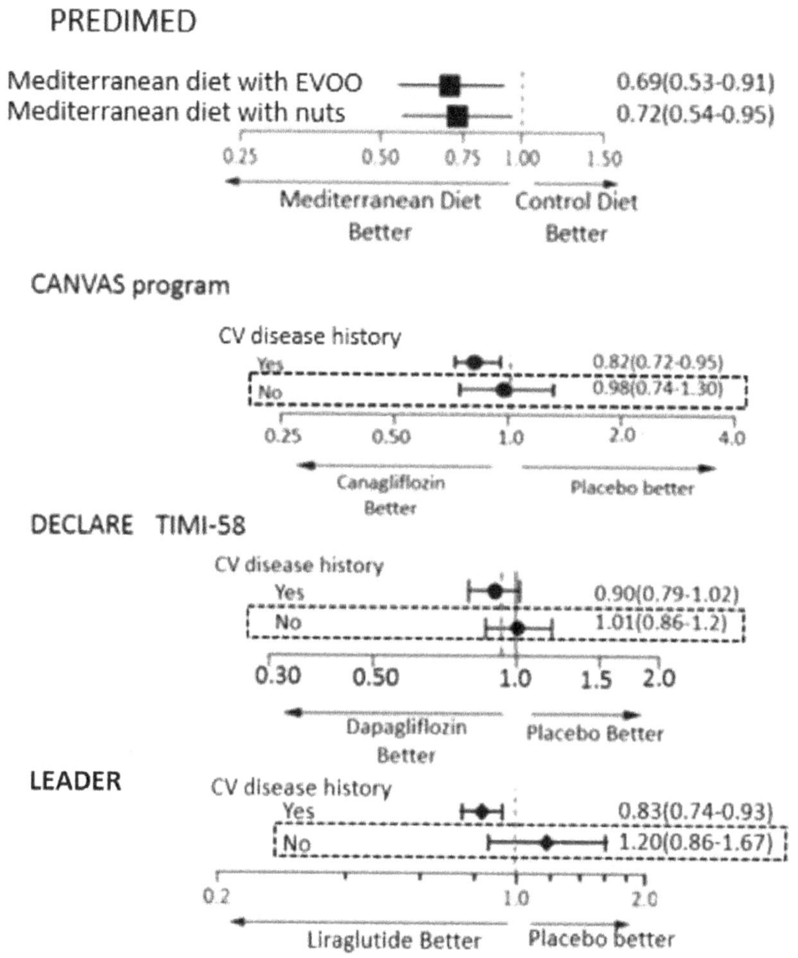

Figure 15.
The hazard ratios and 95% CI in the PREDIMED, CANVAS, DECLARE, and LEADER studies according to presence or absence of established CV diseases [6, 201–203].

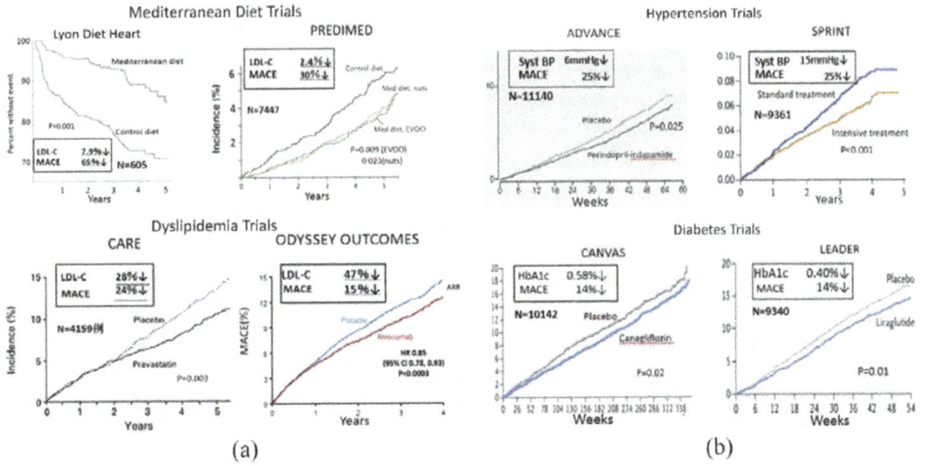

Figure16.
(a) Kaplan-Meier event curves for the primary end point in the Lyon Diet Heart, PREDIMED, CARE, and ODYSSEY OUTCOMES studies [6, 201–203]. (b) Kaplan-Meier event curves for the primary end point in the ADVANCE, SPRINT, CANVAS, and LEADER studies [201, 203, 206, 207].

observed in the primary prevention cohort (**Figure 15**), where rates of CV events are usually low and historically, effects of drugs are rarely observed in pharmacological trials. The absolute risk reduction was almost five times higher in the PREDIMED study (0.32%/year) than that of aspirin (0.06%/year) [204].

The rapid onset of reduction in CV events should also be addressed. **Figure 16a** and **b** shows the Kaplan-Myers curves of the Lyon Diet Heart, PREDIMED, dyslipidemia (CARE [205] and ODESSEY OUTCOME [181]), hypertension (ADVANCE [206] and SPRINT [207]), and diabetes (CANVAS program [201] and LEADER [203]) studies. Whereas it takes 6 months to 2 years before the decline in CV events in most of these studies, the Kaplan-Myer curves of the two Mediterranean diet studies were separated early in the course, less than half a year. Previous studies have shown that it takes years for imaging parameters to significantly change during antihypertensive agents with carotid ultrasound [208], statin therapy [209] or an antidiabetic drug [210] with coronary intravascular ultrasound (IVUS). Considering that process in regression of plaque size needs years from studies with these image modalities, the Mediterranean diet in the PREDIMED study may be associated with early changes in plaque component, causing more stable atherosclerotic plaque which results in reduction of CV events.

6.4.2 Comparison of macronutrients between groups in PREDIMED study

Figure 17 shows comparison of total calories and percent energy from protein, fat, and carbohydrate (**Figure 17a**), and percent energy from each fatty acids (**Figure 17b**) in the PREDIMED study at the end of the study. For comparison with residents in non-Mediterranean diet cultures, data for Japanese in their 60s in 2015 [140] and US adults at age > 60 years old (total calories) and >20 years old (3 major nutrients) in 2011 [120] are also shown. In the two Mediterranean diet groups, high fat food was allowed, as long as the fat was derived from vegetable sources, particularly olive oils and nuts, and also from fatty fish. As a result, the total calories reached approximately 2200 kcal/day with fat calories exceeding more than 40% of total calories, and both of them were higher than in the low-fat control diet group (1960 kcal/day and 37%). Clearly, this was a calorie-unrestricted, high-fat diet, which is usually not recommend in obese subjects.

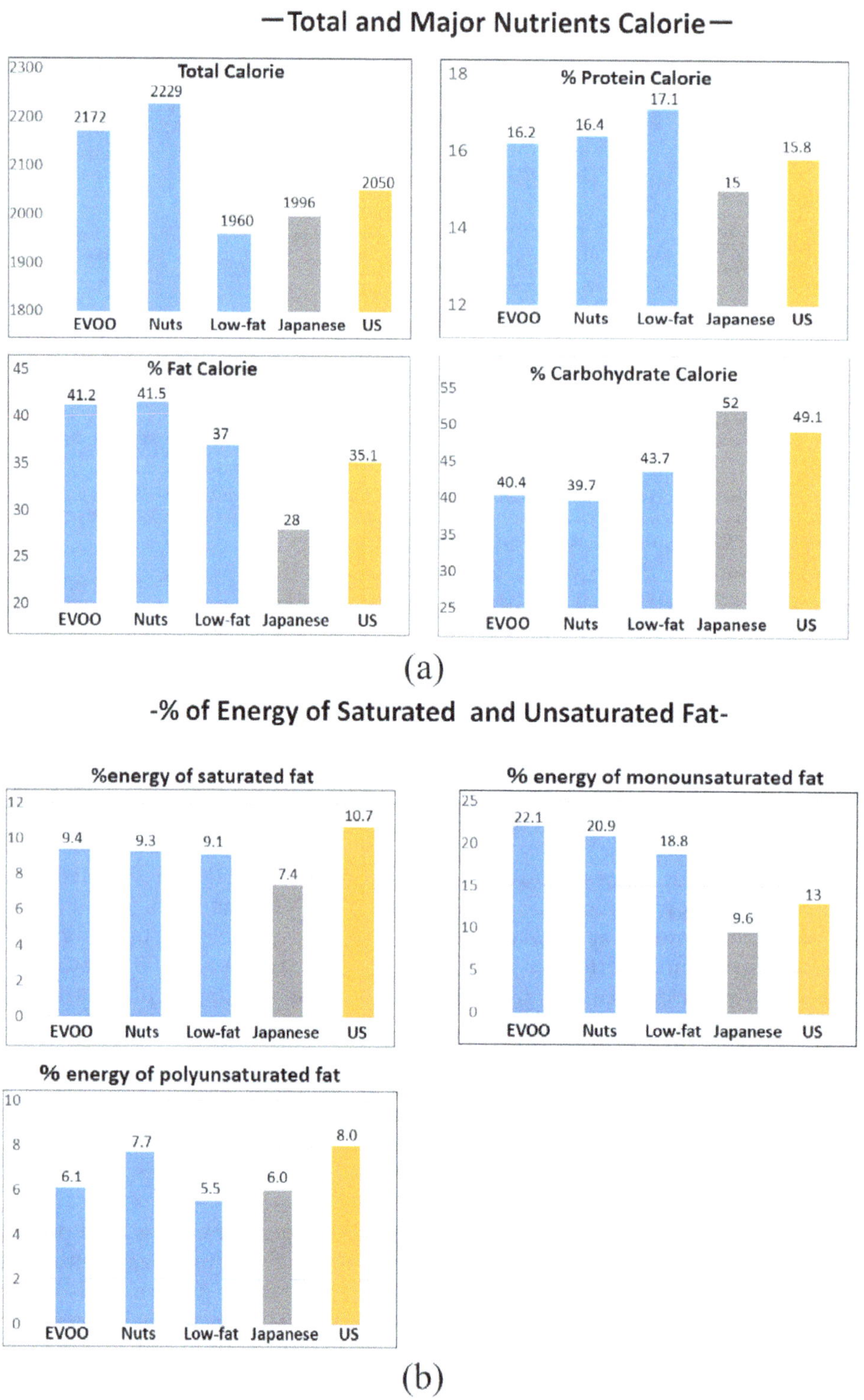

Figure17.
(a) Total calories and percent energy from protein, fat, and carbohydrate in the PREDIMED study at the end of study [6] compared with those of Japanese in their 60s in 2015 [140] and those of US adults at age > 60 years old (total calories) and >20 years old (protein, fat, and carbohydrate) in 2011 [120]. (b) Percent energy from SFA, MUFA, and PUFA in the PREDIMED study at the end of the study compared with those of Japanese in their 60s in 2015 [140] and those of US adults at age > 20 years old in 2011 [120].

Average BMI of participants at baseline was approximately 30 and half of them fell within the class 1 obesity category (BMI > 30). A calorie-restricted diet with limited fat consumption (<30–35% of calories as fat) is usually recommended for these subjects. In the control diet group, although the focus was to reduce all types of fat and they were advised to avoid fatty foods, fat calories was elevated at 37%. This value is actually higher than in the standard low-fat diet (<30%), and higher than in Japanese and even the US adults. Therefore, all participants in the PREDIMED study represent people receiving a high fat diet. Regarding carbohydrates, in the control group, low-fat dairy products, refined carbohydrates, fruits, and vegetables were recommended as substitution for high-fat foods Therefore, a decrease in fat calories in the control group was compensated with an increase in carbohydrate calories, which was higher than the two Mediterranean diet groups. However, the level of carbohydrate calories in the control group was still lower than in Japanese and US adults.

Percent calories from fat type after 5 years of treatment in the PREDIMED study deserve attention (**Figure 17b**). The participants of all three groups were to restrict intake of red and processed meat, commercial bakery goods, sweets, and pastries, all of which are abundant sources of SFA, and were advised to select white meats (poultry without skin or rabbit). However, white meat contains a high content of SFA (30–40% of all fat). Olive oil (15%) and nuts (40% in walnuts, 7% in hazelnuts and peanuts) also contain significant amounts of SFA. As a result, the SFA was equally increased to 9% in each group, which is beyond the recommended level of SFA (<7%) in authoritative opinions. The percent SFA calories in the participants in the PREDIMED study was higher than in Japanese (in their 60s) and less than in US adults (>20 y/o).

Because of increased consumption of EVOO or nuts, MUFA was substantially higher in the EVOO and nuts group (22.1, 20.9 vs. 18.8% in control group) than in the control group. Compared with intake of MUFA in Japan (9.6%) and the US (13%), the very high percent of calories from MUFA is the most distinctive feature that characterizes the changes in nutrition in the two intervention groups. The daily recommend dose of MUFA is not defined in many guidelines except the AACE 2017 guideline which defines it as less than 10% of calories. Even in the control group, the percent of calories from MUFA (18.8%) was much higher than in subjects assigned to the Mediterranean diet in the Lyon Heart Diet study (12.9%) [82, 195]. This is because, in addition to daily intake of olive oil and nuts, many foods in Mediterranean diets are rich in MUFA, and are lower in SFA. The percent energy of PUFA was similar between the three groups and was not very different from in Japan and US. Furthermore, because the consumption of important food components for Mediterranean diet, such as fish, fruits, and vegetables (**Figure 18**), was maintained at high levels during the course of the study, the compliance in diet as described in the protocol was excellent in most participants in the PREDIMED study.

6.4.3 Potential mechanisms of reduction of CV events by olive oil and nuts

The Mediterranean diet protects against CV disease via numerous mechanisms, including reduction of blood pressure, LDL cholesterol, and blood glucose, improvement of vascular endothelium, vasodilation, anticoagulation, anti-inflammation, and antioxidant activity [192, 211]. Although components of the Mediterranean diet, which consists of fish, olive oil, vegetables, fruits, whole grains, legumes/nuts, and moderate red wine consumption, have been found to reduce CV disease risk, the general consensus is that a Mediterranean diet offers benefit against CV disease in aggregate rather than considering the effects of individual

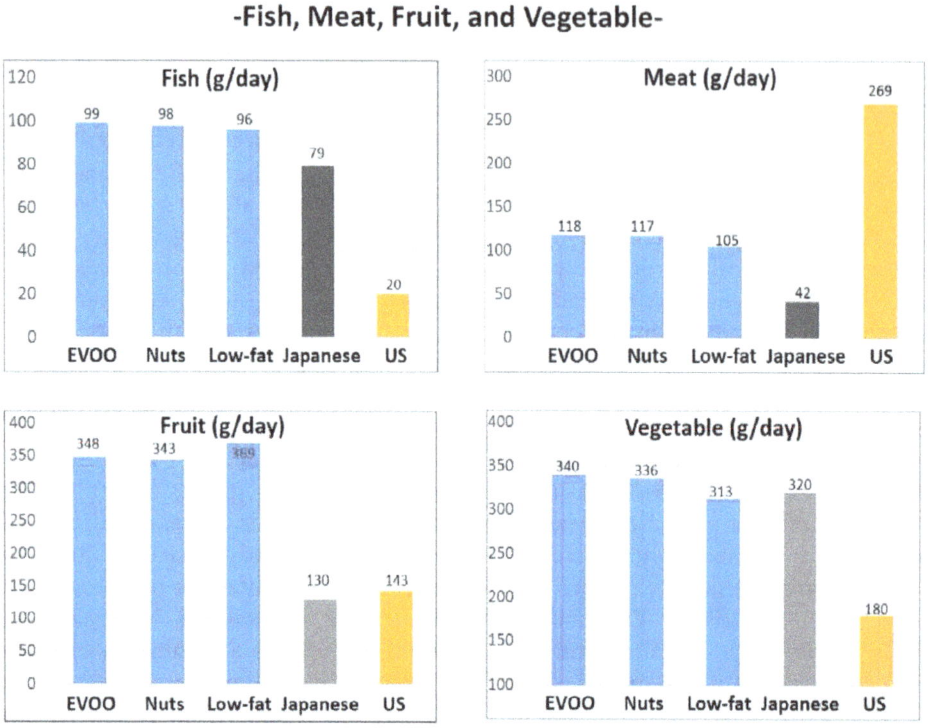

Figure 18.
Daily consumption of fish, meat, fruit, and vegetable in the PREDIMED study at the end of the study compared with those of Japanese in their 60s in 2015 [140] and those of US adults at age > 20 years old in 2011 [120].

constituents [211, 212]. This is further supported by data that the reduction of CV disease is correlated with rating for overall adherence of the Mediterranean diet [193, 213, 214]. The control group in the PREDIMED study did not consume a typical low-fat diet but rather a Mediterranean diet with mild restriction of olive oil or nuts. The subjects in the control group consumed food constituents affecting CV disease risk such as fish, vegetables, and fruits to the similar extent as in the Mediterranean diet groups except for EVOO and nuts (**Figures 14** and **18**). These findings indicate that, contrary to the previous concept of beneficial effects by synergy of all nutrients in the Mediterranean diet, extra-loaded EVOO and nuts play a critical role in the reduction of CV events in the PREDIMED study.

The key message in the PREDIMED study is that only adding EVOO or nuts to calorie-unrestricted Mediterranean diet has cut CV events by approximately 30%. High-sensitive CRP (hsCRP) in blood reflects systemic vascular inflammation. In the PROVE-IT study, 80 mg atorvastatin decreased hsCRP by 36% along with reduction of CV events by 16% [215]. In the PREDIMED study, hsCRP decreased by 50 and 40% in the EVOO and nuts groups compared with the control group [6, 198]. The magnitude of changes in hsCRP and CV events were numerically greater in the PREDIMED study than in the stain trials. These data indicate that the diet interventions have resulted in substantial improvement of vascular inflammation resulting in 30% CV event reduction. The mechanism(s) responsible for stabilization of vascular inflammation with the Mediterranean diet remains still unclear.

How about the magnitude of the well-known antioxidant effects of EVOO and nuts in the two Mediterranean diet intervention groups? The difference in amounts of polyphenol, a representative antioxidant in EVOO and nuts in the intervention groups vs. the control group, is estimated to be around 10 mg/day. Polyphenol is very abundant in other foods, such as red wine (200–400 mg/100 ml), beans (500–

1500 mg/100 g), vegetables, and fruits, and more than 1000 mg/day is usually consumed in a typical dinner on the Mediterranean diet. Furthermore, although laboratory experiments have shown beneficial effects of many antioxidants (vitamin A, C, E, NAC, polyphenol) on vascular atherosclerosis, results of human studies have generally been negative [216]. All of these data strongly suggest that the anti-oxidant effects of EVOO or nuts alone is unlikely to explain reduction in CV events observed in the two Mediterranean diet groups in the PREDIMED study.

In human, two cohort studies have shown that there was an inverse association between the dose of olive oil and CV risk [199, 217]. In the EPIC-Spain cohort study, the highest quartile of olive oil consumption (>30 g/day) was associated with a 26% reduction in risk of overall mortality and a 44% reduction in CVD mortality in comparison with non-consumers. For each increase of 10 g/day in olive oil, there was a 7% decreased risk of overall mortality and a 13% decreased risk of CVD mortality. In the PREDIMED study, the highest tertile group of mean intake of total EVOO (56.9 g/day) showed 48% reduced risk of CV mortality compared with those of the lowest tertile (21.4 g) [78]. As in previous study [21], for each 10 g/day increase in EVOO consumption, CV disease and mortality risk decreased by 10 and 7%, respectively, in the PREDIMED study. Results of all these data suggest that more CV benefit is expected for higher intake of EVOO up to 30–60 g/day.

In contrast to olive oil, the beneficial effects of nut consumption on CV disease were not consistently shown in three recent meta-analyses [218–220], whereas significant reduction in LDL cholesterol, and inflammatory and oxidants mediators were consistently reported with nuts consumption. It is important to note that the amount of walnuts consumed in previous trials was relatively large (30–108 g/day), representing 5–25% of total calories. This level of consumption appears to be difficult to maintain in a non-research setting. Recommended daily dose of nuts according to FDA is one ounce (28 g). The average nut consumption was 30 g/day in the nuts group in the PREDIMED study [6, 198]. For the first time, the PREDIMED study clearly showed that relatively small amount of nuts (30 g/day, about 180 kcal) is enough to reduce CV events.

6.4.4 Effects of olive oil in the US population and the PREDIMED-PLUS study

Although the results of the PREDIMED study have highlighted effects of olive oil and nuts, it is of note that CV benefits of olive oil and nuts were seen in conjunction with the other components of the Mediterranean diet. It still remains unclear what are the biological effects of EVOO and nuts that underlie the reduction of CV events. What is more important practically is whether similar effects on reduction in CV events is reproduced with supplements of EVOO and nuts on other types of diets, or whether lower amounts of EVOO and nuts have similar CV benefit as seen in the PREDIMED study.

All the previous studies in this area have been conducted in Mediterranean countries. The effects of olive oil on CV risk have not yet been evaluated in the U.S. population. As shown in **Figure 18**, the consumption of fish, fruit, and vegetables for the US population, important components in Mediterranean-style diet, is in the rage of 25–50% compared with that the participants in the PREDIMED study. Conversely, the consumption of meat for the US population is more than double. The critical question is whether olive oil or nuts can exhibit beneficial effects on CV risk on the background of the western style diet similarly as they have in previous observational, cohort, and RCTs of the Mediterranean diet. The recent pooled analysis from 61,181 women from the Nurses' Health Study and 31,797 men from the Health Professionals Follow-up Study has shown some answer for this important question [79]. Replacing about 1 teaspoon per day (5 g/day) of margarine, butter, or mayonnaise, or daily fat with an equivalent amount of olive oil was associated with a 5–7% lower risk for total CV disease. When olive oil was compared with other plant-derived oils, there were no significant associations. Mean intake in the group using the highest amount of olive oil was 12 g/day in this study, not as high as in the Spanish participants of the PREDIMED study at 50 g/day. This study has provided further support for the recommendation to replace saturated fat from animal fat with plant oils, such as olive oil, that contain more MUFA for the prevention of CV disease in the general population in the US.

The protocol of the PREDIMED study did not restrict total calorie intake and did not recommend any exercise therapy. Therefore, it was criticized as showing very small beneficial effects on body weight. Although the two Mediterranean diet groups consumed 200–270 kcal more, the incidence of new diabetes was reduced about 50% compared with the control group (10.1, 11 vs. 17.9%, EVOO, nuts vs. control) [221]. If the participants in the PREDIMED study could have received calorie-restricted diet with optimal exercise therapy, then this could have resulted in fewer incidence of new patients with diabetes.

Currently another study, the PREDIMED-PLUS study, a 6-year, multicenter, randomized clinical trial for the primary prevention of CVD is ongoing [222]. The objectives of this study is to compare an energy-restricted Mediterranean diet plus advice to increase physical activities with a control, energy-unrestricted Mediterranean diet without counseling on physical activities in 6874 older individuals (www.isrctn.com/ISRCTN 89898870). The energy-reduced Mediterranean diet features more restrictive limits for red and processed meats, butter, and carbonated sweetened drinks than an unrestricted Mediterranean diet. Although this is definitely the optimal treatment for overweight or obese individuals, the major challenge is participant adherence. However, initial results from a pilot study in 626 participants showed better adherence of the energy-reduced Mediterranean group [223]. This study is expected to result in more reduction in CV events with further fine-tuning of the Mediterranean diet in the future.

7. Final remarks

The two Mediterranean diet intervention studies, the Lyon Heart Diet and PREDIMED studies, have reduced CV events by 72 and 30%, respectively. The magnitude of efficacy of these results are more powerful compared with those in statin trials. CV specialists usually lack the nutrition education to effectively implement diet therapy. In the current era of a shift from disease treatment toward prevention, how can we maintain our knowledge for updated nutritional science to provide best diet therapy to patients? Characteristics of diet therapy should be simple, understandable, and long lasting for many subjects. For this purpose, physicians must keep studying nutritional science, and should be practicing healthy diet life by themselves. A recent study using an online survey has shown that only 20% of cardiologists eat 5 servings of vegetables and fruits per day [3]. Consuming healthy food by themselves will help to more confidently and comfortably recommend appropriate diet therapy to their patients. In contrast to evidence levels in pharmacological therapy, there have been few trustworthy RCTs in nutrition, which thus has created substantial inconsistent understanding of diet therapy at present. In the future, it is by far the most important task for related parties to be united to build up a foundation of high quality data of nutritional science.

Author details

Yasuhiro Nishikawa
Research and Development and Pharmacovigilance, Daiichi Sankyo, Co., Ltd., Tokyo, Japan

*Address all correspondence to: nishikawa.yasuhiro.cn@daiichisankyo.co.jp

References

[1] Collaborators TUBoD. The state of US health, 1990–2016: Burden of diseases, injuries, and risk factors among US States. JAMA. 2018;**319**:1444-1472. DOI: 10.1001/jama.2018.0158

[2] Devries S, Willett W, Bonow RO. Nutrition education in medical school, residency training, and practice. Journal of the American Medical Association. 2019;**321**:1351-1352. DOI: 10.1001/jama.2019.1581

[3] Devries S, Agatston A, Aggarwal M, Aspry KE, Esselstyn CB, Kris-Etherton P, et al. A deficiency of nutrition education and practice in cardiology. The American Journal of Medicine. 2017;**130**:1298-1305. DOI: 10.1016/j.amjmed. 2017.04.043

[4] Saitama Medical Center. The Department of Nutrition [Internet]. 2017. Available from: http://www.kawagoe.saitama-med.ac.jp/01consultation/centraldepartments/nutrition/ [Accessed: October 11, 2019]

[5] Kyorin University Hospital. Statistical Data in 2010 [Internet]. 2010. Available from: http://www.kyorin-u.ac. jp/hospital/introduction/pdf/22nenpou. pdf [Accessed: August 11, 2019]

[6] Estruch R, Ros E, Salas-Salvado J, Covas MI, Corella D, Aros F, et al. Primary prevention of cardiovascular disease with a Mediterranean diet supplemented with extra-virgin olive oil or nuts. The New England Journal of Medicine. 2018;**378**: e34. DOI: 10.1056/NEJMoa1800389

[7] Mair W, Dillin A. Aging and survival: The genetics of life span extension by dietary restriction. Annual Review of Biochemistry. 2008;**77**:727-754. DOI: 10.1146/annurev.biochem.77.061206.171059

[8] Wing RR, Bolin P, Brancati FL, Bray GA, Clark JM, Coday M, et al. Cardiovascular effects of intensive lifestyle intervention in type 2 diabetes. The New England Journal of Medicine. 2013;**369**:145-154. DOI: 10.1056/NEJMoa1212914

[9] Gregg EW, Chen H, Wagenknecht LE, Clark JM, Delahanty LM, Bantle J, et al. Association of an intensive lifestyle intervention with remission of type 2 diabetes. Journal of the American Medical Association. 2012;**308**:2489-2496. DOI: 10.1001/jama.2012.67929

[10] Phelan S, Kanaya AM, Subak LL, Hogan PE, Espeland MA, Wing RR, et al. Weight loss prevents urinary incontinence in women with type 2 diabetes: Results from the look AHEAD trial. Journal of Urology. 2012;**187**: 939-944. DOI: 10.1016/j.juro.2011.10.139

[11] Foster GD, Borradaile KE, Sanders MH, Millman R, Zammit G, Newman AB, et al. A randomized study on the effect of weight loss on obstructive sleep apnea among obese patients with type 2 diabetes: The sleep AHEAD study. Archives of Internal Medicine. 2009;**169**:1619-1626. DOI: 10.1001/archinternmed.2009.266

[12] Faulconbridge LF, Wadden TA, Rubin RR, Wing RR, Walkup MP, Fabricatore AN, et al. One-year changes in symptoms of depression and weight in overweight/obese individuals with type 2 diabetes in the look AHEAD study. Obesity. 2012;**20**:783-793. DOI: 10.1038/oby.2011.315

[13] Foy CG, Lewis CE, Hairston KG, Miller GD, Lang W, Jakicic JM, et al. Intensive lifestyle intervention improves physical function among obese adults with knee pain: Findings from the look AHEAD trial. Obesity. 2011;**19**:83-93. DOI: 10.1038/oby.2010.120

[14] Rejeski WJ, Ip EH, Bertoni AG, Bray GA, Evans G, Gregg EW, et al. Lifestyle change and mobility in obese adults with type 2 diabetes. The New England Journal of Medicine. 2012;**366**: 1209-1217. DOI: 10.1056/NEJMoa1110294

[15] Marsk R, Naslund E, Freedman J, Tynelius P, Rasmussen F. Bariatric surgery reduces mortality in Swedish men. British Journal of Surgery. 2010; **97**:877-883. DOI: 10.1002/bjs.6985

[16] Courcoulas AP, Christian NJ, Belle SH, Berk PD, Flum DR, Garcia L, et al. Weight change and health outcomes at 3 years after bariatric surgery among individuals with severe obesity. Journal of the American Medical Association. 2013;**310**: 2416-2425. DOI: 10.1001/jama.2013.280928

[17] Angrisani L, Santonicola A, Iovino P, Formisano G, Buchwald H, Scopinaro N. Bariatric surgery worldwide 2013. Obesity Surgery. 2015; **25**:1822-1832. DOI: 10.1007/s11695-015- 1657-z

[18] Sackner-Bernstein J, Kanter D, Kaul S. Dietary intervention for overweight and obese adults: Comparison of low-carbohydrate and low-fat diets. A meta-analysis. PLoS One. 2015;**10**:e0139817. DOI: 10.1371/journal.pone.0139817

[19] Tobias DK, Chen M, Manson JE, Ludwig DS, Willett W, Hu FB. Effect of low-fat diet interventions versus other diet interventions on long-term weight change in adults: A systematic review and meta-analysis. The Lancet Diabetes & Endocrinology. 2015;**3**:968-979. DOI: 10.1016/s2213-8587(15)00367-8

[20] Santos FL, Esteves SS, da Costa PA, Yancy WS Jr, Nunes JP. Systematic review and meta-analysis of clinical trials of the effects of low carbohydrate diets on cardiovascular risk factors. Obesity Reviews: An Official Journal of the International Association for the Study of Obesity. 2012;**13**:1048-1066. DOI: 10.1111/j.1467-789X.2012.01021.x

[21] Shimano H, Yahagi N, Amemiya-Kudo M, Hasty AH, Osuga J-I, Tamura Y, et al. Sterol regulatory element-binding Protein-1 as a key transcription factor for nutritional induction of lipogenic enzyme genes. The Journal of Biological Chemistry. 1999;**274**:35832-35839. DOI: 10.1074/jbc.274.50.35832

[22] Nordmann AJ, Nordmann A, Briel M, Keller U, Yancy WS Jr, Brehm BJ, et al. Effects of low-carbohydrate vs low-fat diets on weight loss and cardiovascular risk factors: A meta-analysis of randomized controlled trials. Archives of Internal Medicine. 2006;**166**:285-293. DOI: 10.1001/archinte.166.3.285

[23] Shai I, Schwarzfuchs D, Henkin Y, Shahar DR, Witkow S, Greenberg I, et al. Weight loss with a low-carbohydrate, Mediterranean, or low-fat diet. The New England Journal of Medicine. 2008;**359**:229-241. DOI: 10.1056/NEJMoa0708681

[24] Flegal KM, Carroll MD, Ogden CL, Johnson CL. Prevalence and trends in obesity among US adults, 1999–2000. Journal of the American Medical Association. 2002;**288**:1723-1727. DOI: 10.1001/jama.288.14.1723

[25] Cohen E, Cragg M, de Fonseka J, Hite A, Rosenberg M, Zhou B. Statistical review of US macronutrient consumption data, 1965–2011: Americans have been following dietary guidelines, coincident with the rise in obesity. Nutrition. 2015;**31**:727-732. DOI: 10.1016/j.nut.2015.02.007

[26] Appel LJ, Sacks FM, Carey VJ, Obarzanek E, Swain JF, Miller ER 3rd, et al. Effects of protein, monounsaturated fat, and carbohydrate

intake on blood pressure and serum lipids: Results of the OmniHeart randomized trial. Journal of the American Medical Association. 2005; **294**:2455-2464. DOI: 10.1001/jama.294.19.2455

[27] Stanhope KL, Schwarz JM, Keim NL, Griffen SC, Bremer AA, Graham JL, et al. Consuming fructose-sweetened, not glucose-sweetened, beverages increases visceral adiposity and lipids and decreases insulin sensitivity in overweight/obese humans. Journal of Clinical Investigation. 2009; **119**:1322-1334. DOI: 10.1172/jci37385

[28] Havel PJ. Dietary fructose: Implications for dysregulation of energy homeostasis and lipid/carbohydrate metabolism. Nutrition Reviews. 2005; **63**:133-157

[29] Hommes FA. Inborn errors of fructose metabolism. The American Journal of Clinical Nutrition. 1993;**58**: 788s-795s. DOI: 10.1093/ajcn/58.5.788S

[30] Seidelmann SB, Claggett B, Cheng S, Henglin M, Shah A, Steffen LM, et al. Dietary carbohydrate intake and mortality: A prospective cohort study and meta-analysis. The Lancet Public Health. 2018;**3**:e419-ee28. DOI: 10.1016/s2468-2667(18)30135-x

[31] Schwartz K, Chang HT, Nikolai M, Pernicone J, Rhee S, Olson K, et al. Treatment of glioma patients with ketogenic diets: Report of two cases treated with an IRB-approved energy-restricted ketogenic diet protocol and review of the literature. Cancer & Metabolism. 2015;**3**:3. DOI: 10.1186/s40170-015-0129-1

[32] Martuscello RT, Vedam-Mai V, McCarthy DJ, Schmoll ME, Jundi MA, Louviere CD, et al. A supplemented high-fat low-carbohydrate diet for the treatment of glioblastoma. Clinical Cancer Research: An Official Journal of the American Association for Cancer Research. 2016;**22**:2482-2495. DOI: 10.1158/1078-0432.Ccr-15-0916

[33] Welfare MoHLa. MHLW Overview of Dietary Reference Intakes for Japanese. 2015

[34] Japanse Diabetes Society. Practice Guideline in Diabetes. Tokyo, Japan: Nanko-do; 2016

[35] Kinoshita M, Yokote K, Arai H, Iida M, Ishigaki Y, Ishibashi S, et al. Japan atherosclerosis society (JAS) guidelines for prevention of atherosclerotic cardiovascular diseases 2017. Journal of Atherosclerosis and Thrombosis. 2018;**25**:846-984. DOI: 10.5551/jat.GL2017

[36] Evert AB, Boucher JL, Cypress M, Dunbar SA, Franz MJ, Mayer-Davis EJ, et al. Nutrition therapy recommendations for the management of adults with diabetes. Diabetes Care. 2014;**37**(Suppl 1):S120-S143. DOI: 10.2337/dc14-S120

[37] Egusa G, Yamane K. Lifestyle, serum lipids and coronary artery disease: Comparison of Japan with the United States. Journal of Atherosclerosis and Thrombosis. 2004;**11**:304-312. DOI: 10.5551/jat.11.304

[38] Eckel RH, Jakicic JM, Ard JD, Jesus JM, Miller NH, Hubbard VS, et al. AHA/ACC guideline on lifestyle management to reduce cardiovascular risk. Circulation. 2013, 2014;**129**:S76-S99. DOI: 10.1161/01.cir.0000437740.48606.d1

[39] Catapano AL, Graham I, De Backer G, Wiklund O, Chapman MJ, Drexel H, et al. 2016 ESC/EAS guidelines for the management of dyslipidaemias. European Heart Journal. 2016;**37**:2999-3058. DOI: 10.1093/eurheartj/ehw272

[40] USDA. USDA Scientific Report of the 2015 Dietary Guidelines Advisory

Committee [Internet]. 2015. Available from: https://health.gov/sites/default/files/2019-09/Scientific-Report-of-the-2015-Dietary-Guidelines-Advisory-Committee.pdf [Accessed: 15 July 2019]

[41] de Oliveira Otto MC, Mozaffarian D, Kromhout D, Bertoni AG, Sibley CT, Jacobs DR Jr, et al. Dietary intake of saturated fat by food source and incident cardiovascular disease: The multi-ethnic study of atherosclerosis. The American Journal of Clinical Nutrition. 2012;**96**:397-404. DOI: 10.3945/ajcn.112.037770

[42] Carlsen MH, Lillegaard IT, Karlsen A, Blomhoff R, Drevon CA, Andersen LF. Evaluation of energy and dietary intake estimates from a food frequency questionnaire using independent energy expenditure measurement and weighed food records. Nutrition Journal. 2010;**9**:37. DOI: 10.1186/1475-2891-9-37

[43] Praagman J, Beulens JW, Alssema M, Zock PL, Wanders AJ, Sluijs I, et al. The association between dietary saturated fatty acids and ischemic heart disease depends on the type and source of fatty acid in the European prospective investigation into cancer and nutrition-Netherlands cohort. The American Journal of Clinical Nutrition. 2016;**103**:356-365. DOI: 10.3945/ajcn.115.122671

[44] Temple NJ. How reliable are randomised controlled trials for studying the relationship between diet and disease? A narrative review. British Journal of Nutrition. 2016;**116**:381-389. DOI: 10.1017/s0007114516002129

[45] Ascherio A, Rimm EB, Giovannucci EL, Spiegelman D, Stampfer M, Willett WC. Dietary fat and risk of coronary heart disease in men: Cohort follow up study in the United States. British Medical Journal (Clinical Research Edition). 1996;**313**: 84-90. DOI: 10.1136/bmj.313.7049.84

[46] Kiage JN, Sampson UK, Lipworth L, Fazio S, Mensah GA, Yu Q, et al. Intake of polyunsaturated fat in relation to mortality among statin users and non-users in the southern community cohort study. Nutrition, Metabolism, and Cardiovascular Diseases: NMCD. 2015; **25**:1016-1024. DOI: 10.1016/j.numecd.2015.07.006

[47] Hu FB, Stampfer MJ, Manson JE, Rimm E, Colditz GA, Rosner BA, et al. Dietary fat intake and the risk of coronary heart disease in women. The New England Journal of Medicine. 1997; **337**:1491-1499. DOI: 10.1056/nejm199711203372102

[48] Ludwig DS, Willett WC, Volek JS, Neuhouser ML. Dietary fat: From foe to friend? Science. 2018;**362**:764-770. DOI: 10.1126/science.aau2096

[49] Guasch-Ferre M, Babio N, Martinez-Gonzalez MA, Corella D, Ros E, Martin-Pelaez S, et al. Dietary fat intake and risk of cardiovascular disease and all-cause mortality in a population at high risk of cardiovascular disease. The American Journal of Clinical Nutrition. 2015;**102**:1563-1573. DOI: 10.3945/ajcn.115.116046

[50] Holme I, Retterstol K, Norum KR, Hjermann I. Lifelong benefits on myocardial infarction mortality: 40-year follow-up of the randomized Oslo diet and antismoking study. Journal of Internal Medicine. 2016;**280**:221-227. DOI: 10.1111/joim.12485

[51] Wang DD, Li Y, Chiuve SE, Stampfer MJ, Manson JE, Rimm EB, et al. Association of specific dietary fats with total and cause-specific mortality. JAMA Internal Medicine. 2016;**176**: 1134-1145. DOI: 10.1001/jamainternmed.2016.2417

[52] Zong G, Li Y, Wanders AJ, Alssema M, Zock PL, Willett WC, et al. Intake of individual saturated fatty acids and risk of coronary heart disease in US men and

women: Two prospective longitudinal cohort studies. British Medical Journal (Clinical Research Edition). 2016;**355**: i5796. DOI: 10.1136/bmj.i5796

[53] Holme I. Long-term survival in pre-specified groups at risk in the Oslo study, 1972–1973. Scandinavian Journal of Public Health. 2015;**43**:117-122. DOI: 10.1177/1403494814558157

[54] Ford ES, Ajani UA, Croft JB, Critchley JA, Labarthe DR, Kottke TE, et al. Explaining the decrease in U.S. deaths from coronary disease, 1980–2000. The New England Journal of Medicine. 2007;**356**:2388-2398. DOI: 10.1056/NEJMsa053935

[55] Ramsden CE, Zamora D, Majchrzak-Hong S, Faurot KR, Broste SK, Frantz RP, et al. Re-evaluation of the traditional diet-heart hypothesis: Analysis of recovered data from Minnesota coronary experiment (1968–73). British Medical Journal (Clinical Research Edition). 2016;**353**:i1246. DOI: 10.1136/bmj.i1246

[56] Chowdhury R, Warnakula S, Kunutsor S, Crowe F, Ward HA, Johnson L, et al. Association of dietary, circulating, and supplement fatty acids with coronary risk: A systematic review and meta-analysis. Annals of Internal Medicine. 2014;**160**:398-406. DOI: 10.7326/m13-1788

[57] Svendsen K, Arnesen E, Retterstol K. Saturated fat -a never ending story? Food & Nutrition Research. 2017;**61**:1377572. DOI: 10.1080/16546628.2017.1377572

[58] Wang DD, Hu FB. Dietary fat and risk of cardiovascular disease: Recent controversies and advances. Annual Review of Nutrition. 2017;**37**:423-446. DOI: 10.1146/annurev-nutr-071816-064614

[59] Johnston BC, Zeraatkar D, Han MA, Vernooij RWM, Valli C, El Dib R, et al. Unprocessed red meat and processed meat consumption: Dietary guideline recommendations from the nutritional recommendations (NutriRECS) consortium. Annals of Internal Medicine. 2019;**171**:756-764. DOI: 10.7326/m19-1621

[60] Sacks FM, Lichtenstein AH, Wu JHY, Appel LJ, Creager MA, Kris-Etherton PM, et al. Dietary fats and cardiovascular disease: A presidential advisory from the American Heart Association. Circulation. 2017;**136**: e1-e23. DOI: 10.1161/cir.0000000000000510

[61] Dayton S, Pearce ML, Goldman H, Harnish A, Plotkin D, Shickman M, et al. Controlled trial of a diet high in unsaturated fat for prevention of atherosclerotic complications. Lancet (London, England). 1968;**2**:1060-1062

[62] Morris JN, Ball KP, Brigden WW, Burns-cox CJ, Hall CJL, Mcallen PM, et al. Controlled trial of soya-bean oil in myocardial infarction. Lancet (London, England). 1968;**2**:693-699

[63] Turpeinen O, Karvonen MJ, Pekkarinen M, Miettinen M, Elosuo R, Paavilainen E. Dietary prevention of coronary heart disease: The Finnish mental hospital study. International Journal of Epidemiology. 1979;**8**:99-118

[64] Leren P. The Oslo diet-heart study. Eleven-year report. Circulation. 1970; **42**:935-942

[65] Mihaylova B, Emberson J, Blackwell L, Keech A, Simes J, Barnes EH, et al. The effects of lowering LDL cholesterol with statin therapy in people at low risk of vascular disease: Meta-analysis of individual data from 27 randomised trials. Lancet (London, England). 2012;**380**:581-590. DOI: 10.1016/s0140-6736(12)60367-5

[66] Hamley S. The effect of replacing saturated fat with mostly n-6

polyunsaturated fat on coronary heart disease: A meta-analysis of randomised controlled trials. Nutrition Journal. 2017;**16**:30. DOI: 10.1186/s12937-017-0254-5

[67] Harcombe Z. US dietary guidelines: Is saturated fat a nutrient of concern? British Journal of Sports Medicine. 2019; **53**:1393-1396. DOI: 10.1136/bjsports- 2018-099420

[68] Temple NJ. Fat, sugar, whole grains and heart disease: 50 years of confusion. Nutrients. 2018;**10**:39-47. DOI: 10.3390/nu10010039

[69] Hooper L, Martin N, Abdelhamid A, Davey SG. Reduction in saturated fat intake for cardiovascular disease. The Cochrane Database of Systematic Reviews. 2015;**6**:CD011737. DOI: 10.1002/14651858.cd011737

[70] Mensink RP, Katan MB. Effect of dietary fatty acids on serum lipids and lipoproteins. A meta-analysis of 27 trials. Arteriosclerosis and Thrombosis: A Journal of Vascular Biology. 1992;**12**: 911-919

[71] Farvid MS, Ding M, Pan A, Sun Q, Chiuve SE, Steffen LM, et al. Dietary linoleic acid and risk of coronary heart disease: A systematic review and meta-analysis of prospective cohort studies. Circulation. 2014;**130**:1568-1578. DOI: 10.1161/circulationaha.114.010236

[72] Jacobs DR Jr, Meyer KA, Kushi LH, Folsom AR. Whole-grain intake may reduce the risk of ischemic heart disease death in postmenopausal women: The Iowa Women's health study. The American Journal of Clinical Nutrition. 1998;**68**:248-257. DOI: 10.1093/ajcn/68.2.248

[73] Li Y, Hruby A, Bernstein AM, Ley SH, Wang DD, Chiuve SE, et al. Saturated fats compared with unsaturated fats and sources of carbohydrates in relation to risk of coronary heart disease: A prospective cohort study. Journal of the American College of Cardiology. 2015;**66**:1538-1548. DOI: 10.1016/j.jacc.2015.07.055

[74] Schwingshackl L, Hoffmann G. Monounsaturated fatty acids, olive oil and health status: A systematic review and meta-analysis of cohort studies. Lipids in Health and Disease. 2014;**13**: 154. DOI: 10.1186/1476-511x-13-154

[75] Linseisen J, Welch AA, Ocke M, Amiano P, Agnoli C, Ferrari P, et al. Dietary fat intake in the European prospective investigation into cancer and nutrition: Results from the 24-h dietary recalls. European Journal of Clinical Nutrition. 2009;**63**(Suppl 4): S61-S80. DOI: 10.1038/ejcn.2009.75

[76] Misirli G, Benetou V, Lagiou P, Bamia C, Trichopoulos D, Trichopoulou A. Relation of the traditional Mediterranean diet to cerebrovascular disease in a Mediterranean population. American Journal of Epidemiology. 2012;**176**: 1185-1192. DOI: 10.1093/aje/kws205

[77] Fernandez-Jarne E, Martinez-Losa E, Prado-Santamaria M, Brugarolas-Brufau C, Serrano-Martinez M, Martinez-Gonzalez MA. Risk of first non-fatal myocardial infarction negatively associated with olive oil consumption: A case-control study in Spain. International Journal of Epidemiology. 2002;**31**:474-480. DOI: 10.1093/intjepid/31.2.474

[78] Guasch-Ferre M, Hu FB, Martinez-Gonzalez MA, Fito M, Bullo M, Estruch R, et al. Olive oil intake and risk of cardiovascular disease and mortality in the PREDIMED study. BMC Medicine. 2014;**12**:78. DOI: 10.1186/1741-7015-12-78

[79] Guasch-Ferré M, Liu G, Li Y, Sampson L, Manson JE, Salas-Salvadó J, et al. Olive oil consumption and cardiovascular risk in U.S. adults. Journal of the American College of

Cardiology. 2020;**75**:1729-1739. DOI: 10.1016/j. jacc.2020.02.036

[80] Soriguer F, Rojo-Martinez G, Goday A, Bosch-Comas A, Bordiu E, Caballero-Diaz F, et al. Olive oil has a beneficial effect on impaired glucose regulation and other cardiometabolic risk factors. Di@bet.es study. European Journal of Clinical Nutrition. 2013;**67**: 911-916. DOI: 10.1038/ejcn.2013.130

[81] Soriguer F, Almaraz MC, Garcia-Almeida JM, Cardona I, Linares F, Morcillo S, et al. Intake and home use of olive oil or mixed oils in relation to healthy lifestyles in a Mediterranean population. Findings from the prospective Pizarra study. British Journal of Nutrition. 2010;**103**:114-122. DOI: 10.1017/s0007114509991498

[82] de Lorgeril M, Renaud S, Salen P, Monjaud I, Mamelle N, Martin JL, et al. Mediterranean alpha-linolenic acid-rich diet in secondary prevention of coronary heart disease. The Lancet. 1994;**343**:1454-1459. DOI: 10.1016/ S0140-6736(94)92580-1

[83] de Lorgeril M, Salen P. Mediterranean diet in secondary prevention of CHD. Public Health Nutrition. 2011;**14**:2333-2337. DOI: 10.1017/s136898001100259x

[84] Statement from FDA Commissioner Scott Gottlieb, M.D., on a New Qualified Health Claim for Consuming Oils with High Levels of Oleic Acid to Reduce Coronary Heart Disease Risk [Internet]. 2018. Available from: https://www.fda.gov/news-events/press-announceme nts/statement-fda-commissioner-scott-gottlieb-md-new-qualified-health-claim-consuming-oils-high-levels?utm_campaign=111918_PR_FDA%20acknowledges%20new%20cardiovascular%20health%20c laim% 20for%20oleic%20acid&utm_medium=email&utm_ source =Eloqua [Accessed: 11 August 2019]

[85] Howard BV, Van Horn L, Hsia J, Manson JE, Stefanick ML, Wassertheil-Smoller S, et al. Low-fat dietary pattern and risk of cardiovascular disease: The Women's Health Initiative randomized controlled dietary modification trial. Journal of the American Medical Association. 2006;**295**:655-666. DOI: 10.1001/jama.295.6.655

[86] Siri-Tarino PW, Sun Q, Hu FB, Krauss RM. Saturated fat, carbohydrate, and cardiovascular disease. The American Journal of Clinical Nutrition. 2010;**91**:502-509. DOI: 10.3945/ ajcn.2008.26285

[87] Brennan CS. Dietary fibre, glycaemic response, and diabetes. Molecular Nutrition & Food Research. 2005;**49**:560-570. DOI: 10.1002/ mnfr.200500025

[88] Barclay AW, Petocz P, McMillan-Price J, Flood VM, Prvan T, Mitchell P, et al. Glycemic index, glycemic load, and chronic disease risk–a meta-analysis of observational studies. The American Journal of Clinical Nutrition. 2008;**87**: 627-637. DOI: 10.1093/ajcn/87.3.627

[89] Liu S. Intake of refined carbohydrates and whole grain foods in relation to risk of type 2 diabetes mellitus and coronary heart disease. Journal of the American College of Nutrition. 2002;**21**:298-306

[90] Yu D, Shu XO, Li H, Xiang YB, Yang G, Gao YT, et al. Dietary carbohydrates, refined grains, glycemic load, and risk of coronary heart disease in Chinese adults. American Journal of Epidemiology. 2013;**178**:1542-1549. DOI: 10.1093/aje/kwt178

[91] Eshak ES, Iso H, Date C, Yamagishi K, Kikuchi S, Watanabe Y, et al. Rice intake is associated with reduced risk of mortality from cardiovascular disease in Japanese men but not women. Journal of Nutrition. 2011;**141**:595-602. DOI: 10.3945/ jn.110.132167

[92] Gogebakan O, Kohl A, Osterhoff MA, van Baak MA, Jebb SA, Papadaki A, et al. Effects of weight loss and long-term weight maintenance with diets varying in protein and glycemic index on cardiovascular risk factors: The diet, obesity, and genes (DiOGenes) study: A randomized, controlled trial. Circulation. 2011;**124**:2829-2838. DOI: 10.1161/circulationaha.111.033274

[93] Pereira MA, Swain J, Goldfine AB, Rifai N, Ludwig DS. Effects of a low-glycemic load diet on resting energy expenditure and heart disease risk factors during weight loss. Journal of the American Medical Association. 2004; **292**:2482-2490. DOI: 10.1001/jama.292.20.2482

[94] Mozaffarian D, Ludwig DS. The 2015 US dietary guidelines: Lifting the ban on total dietary fat. Journal of the American Medical Association. 2015; **313**:2421-2422. DOI: 10.1001/jama.2015.5941

[95] Popkin BM, Hawkes C. Sweetening of the global diet, particularly beverages: Patterns, trends, and policy responses. The Lancet Diabetes & Endocrinology. 2016;**4**:174-186. DOI: 10.1016/S2213-8587(15)00419-2

[96] World Health Organization. Sugar Intake for Adults and Children [Internet]. 2015. Available from: https://apps.who.int/iris/bitstream/handle/10665/149782/9789241549028 eng.pdf ?sequence =1 [Accessed: 03 November 2019]

[97] Malik VS, Pan A, Willett WC, Hu FB. Sugar-sweetened beverages and weight gain in children and adults: A systematic review and meta-analysis. The American Journal of Clinical Nutrition. 2013;**98**:1084-1102. DOI: 10.3945/ajcn.113.058362

[98] Malik VS, Popkin BM, Bray GA, Després JP, Willett WC, Hu FB. Sugar-sweetened beverages and risk of metabolic syndrome and type 2 diabetes: A meta-analysis. Diabetes Care. 2010;**33**: 2477-2483. DOI: 10.2337/dc10-1079

[99] Fung TT, Malik V, Rexrode KM, Manson JE, Willett WC, Hu FB. Sweetened beverage consumption and risk of coronary heart disease in women. The American Journal of Clinical Nutrition. 2009;**89**:1037-1042. DOI: 10.3945/ajcn.2008.27140

[100] Narain A, Kwok CS, Mamas MA. Soft drinks and sweetened beverages and the risk of cardiovascular disease and mortality: A systematic review and meta-analysis. International Journal of Clinical Practice. 2016;**70**:791-805. DOI: 10.1111/ijcp.12841

[101] Ld K, Malik VS, Kellogg MD, Rimm EB, Willett WC, Hu FB. Sweetened beverage consumption, incident coronary heart disease, and biomarkers of risk in men. Circulation. 2012;**125**:1735-1741. DOI: 10.1161/CIRCULATIONAHA.111.067017

[102] World Health Organization. World Health Statistics Annual [Internet]. 1997–1999. Available from: http://www.who.int/whosis/whsa [Accessed: 07 August 2019]

[103] Mensink RP, Zock PL, Kester AD, Katan MB. Effects of dietary fatty acids and carbohydrates on the ratio of serum total to HDL cholesterol and on serum lipids and apolipoproteins: A meta-analysis of 60 controlled trials. The American Journal of Clinical Nutrition. 2003;**77**:1146-1155. DOI: 10.1093/ajcn/77.5.1146

[104] Siri-Tarino PW, Chiu S, Bergeron N, Krauss RM. Saturated fats versus polyunsaturated fats versus carbohydrates for cardiovascular disease prevention and treatment. Annual Review of Nutrition. 2015;**35**:517-543. DOI: 10.1146/annurev-nutr-071714-034449

[105] Jimenez-Gomez Y, Lopez-Miranda J, Blanco-Colio LM, Marin C,

Perez-Martinez P, Ruano J, et al. Olive oil and walnut breakfasts reduce the postprandial inflammatory response in mononuclear cells compared with a butter breakfast in healthy men. Atherosclerosis. 2009;**204**:e70-e76. DOI: 10.1016/j.atherosclerosis.2008.09.011

[106] Mata P, Alonso R, Lopez-Farre A, Ordovas JM, Lahoz C, Garces C, et al. Effect of dietary fat saturation on LDL oxidation and monocyte adhesion to human endothelial cells in vitro. Arteriosclerosis, Thrombosis, and Vascular Biology. 1996;**16**:1347-1355. DOI: 10.1161/01.atv.16.11.1347

[107] Bermúdez B, López S, Pacheco YM, Villar J, Muriana FJ, Hoheisel JD, et al. Influence of postprandial triglyceride-rich lipoproteins on lipid-mediated gene expression in smooth muscle cells of the human coronary artery. Cardiovascular Research. 2008;**79**:294-303. DOI: 10.1093/cvr/cvn082

[108] Bellido C, López-Miranda J, Blanco-Colio LM, Pérez-Martínez P, Muriana FJ, Martín-Ventura JL, et al. Butter and walnuts, but not olive oil, elicit postprandial activation of nuclear transcription factor kappaB in peripheral blood mononuclear cells from healthy men. The American Journal of Clinical Nutrition. 2004;**80**: 1487-1491. DOI: 10.1093/ajcn/80.6.1487

[109] McGuire S. Scientific report of the 2015 dietary guidelines advisory committee. Washington, DC: US Departments of agriculture and health and human services, 2015. Advances in Nutrition. 2016;**7**:202-204. DOI: 10.3945/an.115.011684

[110] Wheeler ML, Dunbar SA, Jaacks LM, Karmally W, Mayer-Davis EJ, Wylie-Rosett J, et al. Macronutrients, food groups, and eating patterns in the management of diabetes: A systematic review of the literature, 2010. Diabetes Care. 2012;**35**:434-445. DOI: 10.2337/dc11-2216

[111] Dinu M, Pagliai G, Casini A, Sofi F. Mediterranean diet and multiple health outcomes: An umbrella review of meta-analyses of observational studies and randomised trials. European Journal of Clinical Nutrition. 2018;**72**:30-43. DOI: 10.1038/ejcn.2017.58

[112] Esposito K, Giugliano D. Mediterranean diet and type 2 diabetes. Diabetes/Metabolism Research and Reviews. 2014;**30**(Suppl 1):34-40. DOI: 10.1002/dmrr.2516

[113] Georgoulis M, Kontogianni MD, Yiannakouris N. Mediterranean diet and diabetes: Prevention and treatment. Nutrients. 2014;**6**:1406-1423. DOI: 10.3390/nu6041406

[114] Guasch-Ferré M, Merino J, Sun Q, Fitó M, Salas-Salvadó J. Dietary polyphenols, Mediterranean diet, prediabetes, and type 2 diabetes: A narrative review of the evidence. Oxidative Medicine and Cellular Longevity. 2017;**2017**:6723931. DOI: 10.1155/2017/6723931

[115] Ley SH, Hamdy O, Mohan V, Hu FB. Prevention and management of type 2 diabetes: Dietary components and nutritional strategies. Lancet (London, England). 2014;**383**:1999-2007. DOI: 10.1016/s0140-6736(14)60613-9

[116] Takeya Y, Popper JS, Shimizu Y, Kato H, Rhoads GG, Kagan A. Epidemiologic studies of coronary heart disease and stroke in Japanese men living in Japan, Hawaii and California: Incidence of stroke in Japan and Hawaii. Stroke. 1984;**15**:15-23

[117] Yamagishi K, Iso H, Kokubo Y, Saito I, Yatsuya H, Ishihara J, et al. Dietary intake of saturated fatty acids and incident stroke and coronary heart disease in Japanese communities: The JPHC study. European Heart Journal. 2013;**34**:1225-1232. DOI: 10.1093/eurheartj/eht043

[118] Yamagishi K, Iso H, Yatsuya H, Tanabe N, Date C, Kikuchi S, et al. Dietary intake of saturated fatty acids and mortality from cardiovascular disease in Japanese: The Japan collaborative cohort study for evaluation of cancer risk (JACC) study. The American Journal of Clinical Nutrition. 2010;**92**:759-765. DOI: 10.3945/ajcn.2009.29146

[119] Ministry of Health Law. Surveys of Public Health and Nutrition [Internet]. 2010–2011. Available from: http://wwwmhlwgojp/bunya/kenkou/dl/kenkou_eiyou_chousa_tokubetsushuukei_h22pdf. [Accessed: 03 January 2020]

[120] Rehm CD, Penalvo JL, Afshin A, Mozaffarian D. Dietary intake among US adults, 1999–2012. Journal of the American Medical Association. 2016; **315**:2542-2553. DOI: 10.1001/jama.2016.7491

[121] Anderson TJ, Gregoire J, Pearson GJ, Barry AR, Couture P, Dawes M, et al. 2016 Canadian cardiovascular society guidelines for the Management of Dyslipidemia for the prevention of cardiovascular disease in the adult. The Canadian Journal of Cardiology. 2016;**32**:1263-1282. DOI: 10.1016/j.cjca.2016.07.510

[122] Mozaffarian D. Dietary and policy priorities for cardiovascular disease, diabetes, and obesity: A comprehensive review. Circulation. 2016;**133**:187-225. DOI: 10.1161/circulationaha.115.018585

[123] Wang Q, Afshin A, Yakoob MY, Singh GM, Rehm CD, Khatibzadeh S, et al. Impact of nonoptimal intakes of saturated, polyunsaturated, and trans fat on global burdens of coronary heart disease. Journal of the American Heart Association. 2016;**5**:1-23. DOI: 10.1161/jaha.115.002891

[124] Weggemans RM, Zock PL, Katan MB. Dietary cholesterol from eggs increases the ratio of total cholesterol to high-density lipoprotein cholesterol in humans: A meta-analysis. The American Journal of Clinical Nutrition. 2001;**73**: 885-891. DOI: 10.1093/ajcn/73.5.885

[125] Lecerf JM, de Lorgeril M. Dietary cholesterol: From physiology to cardiovascular risk. British Journal of Nutrition. 2011;**106**:6-14. DOI: 10.1017/s0007114511000237

[126] Herron KL, Vega-Lopez S, Conde K, Ramjiganesh T, Shachter NS, Fernandez ML. Men classified as hypo- or hyperresponders to dietary cholesterol feeding exhibit differences in lipoprotein metabolism. Journal of Nutrition. 2003;**133**:1036-1042. DOI: 10.1093/jn/133.4.1036

[127] Herron KL, Vega-Lopez S, Conde K, Ramjiganesh T, Roy S, Shachter NS, et al. Pre-menopausal women, classified as hypo- or hyperresponders, do not alter their LDL/HDL ratio following a high dietary cholesterol challenge. Journal of the American College of Nutrition. 2002;**21**: 250-258

[128] Yoshida A, Naito M, Miyazaki K. Japanese sisters associated with pseudohomozygous familial hypercholesterolemia and sitosterolemia. Journal of Atherosclerosis and Thrombosis. 2000; **7**:33-38

[129] Kritchevsky SB, Kritchevsky D. Egg consumption and coronary heart disease: An epidemiologic overview. Journal of the American College of Nutrition. 2000;**19**:549s-555s

[130] Jellinger PS, Handelsman Y, Rosenblit PD, Bloomgarden ZT, Fonseca VA, Garber AJ, et al. American Association of Clinical Endocrinologists and American College of Endocrinology Guidelines for Management of Dyslipidemia and Prevention of Cardiovascular Disease. Endocrine

Practice. 2017;**23**:1-87. DOI: 10.4158/ep171764.appgl

[131] Simopoulos AP, Leaf A, Salem N Jr. Workshop statement on the essentiality of and recommended dietary intakes for Omega-6 and Omega-3 fatty acids. Prostaglandins, Leukotrienes, and Essential Fatty Acids. 2000;**63**:119-121. DOI: 10.1054/plef.2000.0176

[132] Gabbs M, Leng S, Devassy JG, Monirujjaman M, Aukema HM. Advances in our understanding of oxylipins derived from dietary PUFAs. Advances in Nutrition. 2015;**6**:513-540. DOI: 10.3945/an.114.007732

[133] Simopoulos AP. The importance of the omega-6/omega-3 fatty acid ratio in cardiovascular disease and other chronic diseases. Experimental Biology and Medicine (Maywood, NJ). 2008;**233**: 674-688. DOI: 10.3181/0711-mr-311

[134] Stanley JC, Elsom RL, Calder PC, Griffin BA, Harris WS, Jebb SA, et al. UK Food Standards Agency workshop report: The effects of the dietary n-6:n-3 fatty acid ratio on cardiovascular health. British Journal of Nutrition. 2007;**98**: 1305-1310. DOI: 10.1017/s000711450784284x

[135] Harris WS, Davidson MH. RE: Plasma phospholipid fatty acids and prostate cancer risk in the SELECT trial. Journal of the National Cancer Institute. 2014;**106**:dju019. DOI: 10.1093/jnci/dju019

[136] Fritsche KL. Too much linoleic acid promotes inflammation-doesn't it? Prostaglandins, Leukotrienes, and Essential Fatty Acids. 2008;**79**:173-175. DOI: 10.1016/j.plefa.2008.09.019

[137] Harris WS, Von Schacky C. The Omega-3 index: A new risk factor for death from coronary heart disease? Preventive Medicine. 2004;**39**:212-220. DOI: 10.1016/j.ypmed.2004.02.030

[138] Metcalf RG, Cleland LG, Gibson RA, Roberts-Thomson KC, Edwards JR, Sanders P, et al. Relation between blood and atrial fatty acids in patients undergoing cardiac bypass surgery. The American Journal of Clinical Nutrition. 2010;**91**:528-534. DOI: 10.3945/ajcn.2009.28302

[139] Harris WS. Omega-3 fatty acids. In: Coates PM, Betz JM, Blackman MR, et al, eds. Encyclopedia of Dietary Supplements. 2nd ed. London and New York: Informa Healthcare; 2010. pp. 577-586

[140] MHLW (Ministry of Health Law). Surveys of Public Health and Nutrition [Internet]. 2015. Available from: https://wwwmhlwgojp/file/04-Houdouha ppyou-10904750-Kenkoukyoku-Ganta isakukenkouzoushinka/kekkagaiyoupdf. 2015. [Accessed: 21 January 2020]

[141] Board FaN. Dietary Reference Intakes, for Energy, Carbohydrate, Fiber, Fat, Fatty Acids, Cholesterol, Protein, and Amino Acids. Washington, DC: National Academies Press; 2005

[142] Kromann N, Green A. Epidemiological studies in the Upernavik district, Greenland. Incidence of some chronic diseases 1950–1974. Acta Medica Scandinavica. 1980;**208**:401-406

[143] Zhang J, Sasaki S, Amano K, Kesteloot H. Fish consumption and mortality from all causes, ischemic heart disease, and stroke: An ecological study. Preventive Medicine. 1999;**28**:520-529. DOI: 10.1006/pmed.1998.0472

[144] GISSI-Prevenzione Investigators. Dietary supplementation with n-3 polyunsaturated fatty acids and vitamin E after myocardial infarction: Results of the GISSI-Prevenzione trial. Gruppo Italiano per lo studio della Sopravvivenza nell'Infarto miocardico. Lancet (London, England). 1999;**354**: 447-455

[145] Kris-Etherton PM, Harris WS, Appel LJ. Fish consumption, fish oil, omega-3 fatty acids, and cardiovascular disease. Circulation. 2002;**106**: 2747-2757. DOI: 10.1161/01. cir.0000038493.65177.94

[146] de Goede J, Geleijnse JM, Boer JM, Kromhout D, Verschuren WM. Marine (n-3) fatty acids, fish consumption, and the 10-year risk of fatal and nonfatal coronary heart disease in a large population of Dutch adults with low fish intake. Journal of Nutrition. 2010;**140**: 1023-1028. DOI: 10.3945/ jn.109.119271

[147] Folsom AR, Demissie Z. Fish intake, marine omega-3 fatty acids, and mortality in a cohort of postmenopausal women. American Journal of Epidemiology. 2004;**160**:1005-1010. DOI: 10.1093/aje/kwh307

[148] Gillum RF, Mussolino ME, Madans JH. The relationship between fish consumption and stroke incidence. The NHANES I epidemiologic follow-up study (National Health and Nutrition Examination Survey). Archives of Internal Medicine. 1996;**156**:537-542

[149] Jarvinen R, Knekt P, Rissanen H, Reunanen A. Intake of fish and long-chain n-3 fatty acids and the risk of coronary heart mortality in men and women. British Journal of Nutrition. 2006;**95**:824-829

[150] Manger MS, Strand E, Ebbing M, Seifert R, Refsum H, Nordrehaug JE, et al. Dietary intake of n-3 long-chain polyunsaturated fatty acids and coronary events in Norwegian patients with coronary artery disease. The American Journal of Clinical Nutrition. 2010;**92**:244-251. DOI: 10.3945/ ajcn.2010.29175

[151] Morris MC, Manson JE, Rosner B, Buring JE, Willett WC, Hennekens CH. Fish consumption and cardiovascular disease in the physicians' health study: A prospective study. American Journal of Epidemiology. 1995;**142**:166-175

[152] Nakamura Y, Ueshima H, Okamura T, Kadowaki T, Hayakawa T, Kita Y, et al. Association between fish consumption and all-cause and cause-specific mortality in Japan: NIPPON DATA80, 1980–99. The American Journal of Medicine. 2005; **118**:239-245. DOI: 10.1016/j. amjmed.2004.12.016

[153] Orencia AJ, Daviglus ML, Dyer AR, Shekelle RB, Stamler J. Fish consumption and stroke in men. 30-year findings of the Chicago Western electric study. Stroke. 1996;**27**:204-209

[154] Streppel MT, Ocke MC, Boshuizen HC, Kok FJ, Kromhout D. Long-term fish consumption and n-3 fatty acid intake in relation to (sudden) coronary heart disease death: The Zutphen study. European Heart Journal. 2008;**29**:2024-2030. DOI: 10.1093/ eurheartj/ehn294

[155] Hooper L, Thompson RL, Harrison RA, Summerbell CD, Moore H, Worthington HV, et al. Omega 3 fatty acids for prevention and treatment of cardiovascular disease. The Cochrane Database of Systematic Reviews. 2004; **4**:CD003177. DOI: 10.1002/14651858. CD003177.pub2

[156] Bhatt DL, Steg PG, Miller M, Brinton EA, Jacobson TA, Ketchum SB, et al. Cardiovascular risk reduction with icosapent ethyl for hypertriglyceridemia. The New England Journal of Medicine. 2019;**380**:11-22. DOI: 10.1056/NEJMoa1812792

[157] Rauch B, Schiele R, Schneider S, Diller F, Victor N, Gohlke H, et al. OMEGA, a randomized, placebo-controlled trial to test the effect of highly purified omega-3 fatty acids on top of modern guideline-adjusted therapy after myocardial infarction.

Circulation. 2010;**122**:2152-2159. DOI: 10.1161/circulationaha.110.948562

[158] Kromhout D, Giltay EJ, Geleijnse JM. n-3 fatty acids and cardiovascular events after myocardial infarction. The New England Journal of Medicine. 2010;**363**:2015-2026. DOI: 10.1056/NEJMoa1003603

[159] Galan P, Kesse-Guyot E, Czernichow S, Briancon S, Blacher J, Hercberg S. Effects of B vitamins and omega 3 fatty acids on cardiovascular diseases: A randomised placebo controlled trial. British Medical Journal (Clinical Research Edition). 2010;**341**: c6273. DOI: 10.1136/bmj.c6273

[160] Bosch J, Gerstein HC, Dagenais GR, Diaz R, Dyal L, Jung H, et al. n-3 fatty acids and cardiovascular outcomes in patients with dysglycemia. The New England Journal of Medicine. 2012;**367**:309-318. DOI: 10.1056/NEJMoa1203859

[161] Roncaglioni MC, Tombesi M, Avanzini F, Barlera S, Caimi V, Longoni P, et al. n-3 fatty acids in patients with multiple cardiovascular risk factors. The New England Journal of Medicine. 2013;**368**:1800-1808. DOI: 10.1056/NEJMoa1205409

[162] Bowman L, Mafham M, Wallendszus K, Stevens W, Buck G, Barton J, et al. Effects of n-3 fatty acid supplements in diabetes mellitus. The New England Journal of Medicine. 2018; **379**:1540-1550. DOI: 10.1056/NEJMoa1804989

[163] Yokoyama M, Origasa H, Matsuzaki M, Matsuzawa Y, Saito Y, Ishikawa Y, et al. Effects of eicosapentaenoic acid on major coronary events in hypercholesterolaemic patients (JELIS): A randomised open-label, blinded endpoint analysis. Lancet (London, England). 2007;**369**:1090-1098. DOI: 10.1016/s0140-6736(07)60527-3

[164] EMA. Omega-3 Acid Ethyl Esters - Containing Medicinal Products for Oral in use in Secondary Prevention after Myocardial Infarction [Internet]. 2018. Available from: https://www.ema.europa.eu/en/medicines/human/referrals/omega-3-fatty-acid-medicines [Accessed: 13 February 2020]

[165] Siscovick DS, Barringer TA, Fretts AM, Wu JH, Lichtenstein AH, Costello RB, et al. Omega-3 polyunsaturated fatty acid (fish oil) supplementation and the prevention of clinical cardiovascular disease: A science advisory from the American Heart Association. Circulation. 2017;**135**:e867-ee84. DOI: 10.1161/cir.0000000000000482

[166] Abdelhamid AS, Brown TJ, Brainard JS, Biswas P, Thorpe GC, Moore HJ, et al. Omega-3 fatty acids for the primary and secondary prevention of cardiovascular disease. The Cochrane Database of Systematic Reviews. 2018;7: CD003177. DOI: 10.1002/14651858.CD003177.pub3

[167] Chiesa G, Busnelli M, Manzini S, Parolini C. Nutraceuticals and bioactive components from fish for dyslipidemia and cardiovascular risk reduction. Marine Drugs. 2016;**14**:113-127. DOI: 10.3390/ 70md14060113

[168] Clarke TC, Black LI, Stussman BJ, Barnes PM, Nahin RL. Trends in the use of complementary health approaches among adults: United States, 2002–2012. National Health Statistics Reports. 2015: 1-16

[169] Tavazzi L, Maggioni AP, Marchioli R, Barlera S, Franzosi MG, Latini R, et al. Effect of n-3 polyunsaturated fatty acids in patients with chronic heart failure (the GISSI-HF trial): A randomised, double-blind, placebo-controlled trial. Lancet (London, England). 2008;**372**: 1223-1230. DOI: 10.1016/s0140-6736(08)61239-8

[170] Eussen SR, Geleijnse JM, Giltay EJ, Rompelberg CJ, Klungel OH, Kromhout D. Effects of n-3 fatty acids on major cardiovascular events in statin users and non-users with a history of myocardial infarction. European Heart Journal. 2012;**33**:1582-1588. DOI: 10.1093/eurheartj/ehr499

[171] Iso H, Kobayashi M, Ishihara J, Sasaki S, Okada K, Kita Y, et al. Intake of fish and n3 fatty acids and risk of coronary heart disease among Japanese: The Japan public health center-based (JPHC) study cohort I. Circulation. 2006;**113**:195-202. DOI: 10.1161/circulationaha.105.581355

[172] Saito Y, Yokoyama M, Origasa H, Matsuzaki M, Matsuzawa Y, Ishikawa Y, et al. Effects of EPA on coronary artery disease in hypercholesterolemic patients with multiple risk factors: Sub-analysis of primary prevention cases from the Japan EPA lipid intervention study (JELIS). Atherosclerosis. 2008;**200**: 135-140. DOI: 10.1016/j.atherosclerosis.2008.06.003

[173] The BIP Study Group. Secondary prevention by raising HDL cholesterol and reducing triglycerides in patients with coronary artery disease. Circulation. 2000;**102**:21-27. DOI: 10.1161/01.cir.102.1.21

[174] Ginsberg HN, Elam MB, Lovato LC, Crouse JR 3rd, Leiter LA, Linz P, et al. Effects of combination lipid therapy in type 2 diabetes mellitus. The New England Journal of Medicine. 2010;**362**:1563-1574. DOI: 10.1056/NEJMoa1001282

[175] Kastelein JJP, Stroes ESG. FISHing for the miracle of eicosapentaenoic acid. The New England Journal of Medicine. 2019;**380**:89-90. DOI: 10.1056/NEJMe1814004

[176] Gao LG, Cao J, Mao QX, Lu XC, Zhou XL, Fan L. Influence of omega-3 polyunsaturated fatty acid-supplementation on platelet aggregation in humans: A meta-analysis of randomized controlled trials. Atherosclerosis. 2013;**226**:328-334. DOI: 10.1016/j.atherosclerosis.2012.10.056

[177] Mackay I, Ford I, Thies F, Fielding S, Bachoo P, Brittenden J. Effect of Omega-3 fatty acid supplementation on markers of platelet and endothelial function in patients with peripheral arterial disease. Atherosclerosis. 2012;**221**:514-520. DOI: 10.1016/j.atherosclerosis.2011.12.041

[178] Franzese CJ, Bliden KP, Gesheff MG, Pandya S, Guyer KE, Singla A, et al. Relation of fish oil supplementation to markers of atherothrombotic risk in patients with cardiovascular disease not receiving lipid-lowering therapy. The American Journal of Cardiology. 2015;**115**: 1204-1211. DOI: 10.1016/j.amjcard.2015.02.002

[179] Finnegan YE, Howarth D, Minihane AM, Kew S, Miller GJ, Calder PC, et al. Plant and marine derived (n-3) polyunsaturated fatty acids do not affect blood coagulation and fibrinolytic factors in moderately hyperlipidemic humans. Journal of Nutrition. 2003;**133**:2210-2213. DOI: 10.1093/jn/133.7.2210

[180] Cannon CP, Blazing MA, Giugliano RP, McCagg A, White JA, Theroux P, et al. Ezetimibe added to statin therapy after acute coronary syndromes. The New England Journal of Medicine. 2015;**372**:2387-2397. DOI: 10.1056/NEJMoa1410489

[181] Sabatine MS, Giugliano RP, Keech AC, Honarpour N, Wiviott SD, Murphy SA, et al. Evolocumab and clinical outcomes in patients with cardiovascular disease. The New England Journal of Medicine. 2017;**376**: 1713-1722. DOI: 10.1056/NEJMoa1615664

[182] Schwartz GG, Steg PG, Szarek M, Bhatt DL, Bittner VA, Diaz R, et al. Alirocumab and cardiovascular outcomes after acute coronary syndrome. The New England Journal of Medicine. 2018;**379**:2097-2107. DOI: 10.1056/NEJMoa1801174

[183] FDA. Summary of Qualified Health Claims Subject to Enforcement Discretion [Internet]. 2014. Available from:. https://wwwfdagov/Food/ResourcesForYou/Consumers/ucm393070htm [Accessed: 03 February 2020]

[184] AstraZeneca. Update on Phase III STRENGTH Trial for Epanova in Mixed Dyslipidaemia [Internet]. 2020. Available from: https://www.astrazeneca.com/media-centre/press-releases/2020/update-on-phase-iii-strength-trial-for-epanova-in-mixed-dyslipidaemia-13012020.html [Accessed: 03 February 2020]

[185] Preston MR. New insights into mechanisms of action for Omega-3 fatty acids in atherothrombotic cardiovascular disease. Current Atherosclerosis Reports. 2019;**21**:2. DOI: 10.1007/s11883-019-0762-1

[186] Bhatt DL, Miller M, Brinton EA, Jacobson TA, Steg PG, Ketchum SB, et al. Reduce-IT USA: Results from the 3146 patients randomized in the United States. Circulation. 2020;**141**:367-375. DOI: 10.1161/circulationaha.119.044440

[187] Weintraub WB. Cost-Effectiveness of Icosapent Ethyl in REDUCE-IT. AHA Meeting [Internet]. 2019. Available from: https://www.abstractsonline.com/pp8/#!/7891/presentation/35097 [Accessed: 24 February 2020]

[188] FDA. FDA Approves use of Drug to Reduce Risk of Cardiovascular Events in Certain Adult Patient Groups [Internet]. 2019. Available from: https://wwwfdagov/news-events/press-announceme nts/fda -approves- use- drug- reduce-risk-cardiovascular-events-certain-adult-patient-groups [Accessed: 24 February 2020]

[189] Deepak L. Bhatt. EPA Levels and Cardiovascular Outcomes in the Reduction of Cardiovascular Events with Icosapent Ethyl Intervention Trial [Internet]. ACC 2020 in Chicago. 2020. Available from: https://virtual.acc. org/on-demand [Accessed: 24 February 2020]

[190] Mente A, de Koning L, Shannon HS, Anand SS. A systematic review of the evidence supporting a causal link between dietary factors and coronary heart disease. Archives of Internal Medicine. 2009;**169**:659-669. DOI: 10.1001/archinternmed.2009.38

[191] Skeaff CM, Miller J. Dietary fat and coronary heart disease: Summary of evidence from prospective cohort and randomised controlled trials. Annals of Nutrition & Metabolism. 2009;**55**: 173-201. DOI: 10.1159/000229002

[192] Serra-Majem L, Roman B, Estruch R. Scientific evidence of interventions using the Mediterranean diet: A systematic review. Nutrition Reviews. 2006;**64**:S27-S47

[193] Sofi F, Abbate R, Gensini GF, Casini A. Accruing evidence on benefits of adherence to the Mediterranean diet on health: An updated systematic review and meta-analysis. The American Journal of Clinical Nutrition. 2010;**92**:1189-1196. DOI: 10.3945/ajcn.2010.29673

[194] Bloomfield HE, Koeller E, Greer N, MacDonald R, Kane R, Wilt TJ. Effects on health outcomes of a Mediterranean diet with No restriction on fat intake: A systematic review and meta-analysis. Annals of Internal Medicine. 2016;**165**: 491-500. DOI: 10.7326/m16-0361

[195] de Lorgeril M, Salen P, Martin JL, Monjaud I, Delaye J, Mamelle N.

Mediterranean diet, traditional risk factors, and the rate of cardiovascular complications after myocardial infarction: Final report of the Lyon diet heart study. Circulation. 1999;**99**: 779-785. DOI: 10.1161/01.cir.99.6.779

[196] Kris-Etherton P, Eckel RH, Howard BV, St Jeor S, Bazzarre TL. AHA science advisory: Lyon diet heart study. Benefits of a Mediterranean-style, National Cholesterol Education Program/American Heart Association step I dietary pattern on cardiovascular disease. Circulation. 2001;**103**: 1823-1825. DOI: 10.1161/01.cir.103.13.1823

[197] Pan A, Sun Q, Bernstein AM, Schulze MB, Manson JE, Stampfer MJ, et al. Red meat consumption and mortality: Results from 2 prospective cohort studies. Archives of Internal Medicine. 2012;**172**:555-563. DOI: 10.1001/archinternmed.2011.2287

[198] Estruch R, Ros E, Salas-Salvado J, Covas MI, Corella D, Aros F, et al. Primary prevention of cardiovascular disease with a Mediterranean diet. The New England Journal of Medicine. 2013; **368**:1279-1290. DOI: 10.1056/NEJMoa1200303

[199] Buckland G, Travier N, Barricarte A, Ardanaz E, Moreno-Iribas C, Sanchez MJ, et al. Olive oil intake and CHD in the European prospective investigation into cancer and nutrition Spanish cohort. British Journal of Nutrition. 2012;**108**:2075-2082. DOI: 10.1017/s000711451200298x

[200] Nielsen SJ, Kit BK, Ogden CL. Nut consumption among U.S. adults, 2009–2010. NCHS Data Brief. 2014;**176**:1-8

[201] Neal B, Perkovic V, Mahaffey KW, de Zeeuw D, Fulcher G, Erondu N, et al. Canagliflozin and cardiovascular and renal events in type 2 diabetes. The New England Journal of Medicine. 2017;**377**: 644-657. DOI: 10.1056/NEJMoa1611925

[202] Wiviott SD, Raz I, Bonaca MP, Mosenzon O, Kato ET, Cahn A, et al. Dapagliflozin and cardiovascular outcomes in type 2 diabetes. The New England Journal of Medicine. 2019;**380**: 347-357. DOI: 10.1056/NEJMoa1812389

[203] Marso SP, Daniels GH, Brown-Frandsen K, Kristensen P, Mann JF, Nauck MA, et al. Liraglutide and cardiovascular outcomes in type 2 diabetes. The New England Journal of Medicine. 2016;**375**:311-322. DOI: 10.1056/NEJMoa1603827

[204] Baigent C, Blackwell L, Collins R, Emberson J, Godwin J, Peto R, et al. Aspirin in the primary and secondary prevention of vascular disease: Collaborative meta-analysis of individual participant data from randomised trials. Lancet (London, England). 2009;**373**:1849-1860. DOI: 10.1016/s0140-6736(09)60503-1

[205] Sacks FM, Pfeffer MA, Moye LA, Rouleau JL, Rutherford JD, Cole TG, et al. The effect of pravastatin on coronary events after myocardial infarction in patients with average cholesterol levels. Cholesterol and recurrent events trial investigators. The New England Journal of Medicine. 1996; **335**:1001-1009. DOI: 10.1056/nejm199610033351401

[206] Patel A, MacMahon S, Chalmers J, Neal B, Woodward M, Billot L, et al. Effects of a fixed combination of perindopril and indapamide on macrovascular and microvascular outcomes in patients with type 2 diabetes mellitus (the ADVANCE trial): A randomised controlled trial. Lancet (London, England). 2007;**370**:829-840. DOI: 10.1016/s0140-6736(07)61303-8

[207] Wright JT Jr, Williamson JD, Whelton PK, Snyder JK, Sink KM, Rocco MV, et al. A randomized trial of intensive versus standard blood-pressure control. The New England Journal of Medicine. 2015;**373**:

2103-2116. DOI: 10.1056/NEJMoa1511939

[208] Cuspidi C, Negri F, Giudici V, Capra A, Sala C. Effects of antihypertensive drugs on carotid intima-media thickness: Focus on angiotensin II receptor blockers. A review of randomized, controlled trials. Integrated Blood Pressure Control. 2009;**2**:1-8. DOI: 10.2147/ibpc.s5174

[209] Nissen SE, Tuzcu EM, Schoenhagen P, Brown BG, Ganz P, Vogel RA, et al. Effect of intensive compared with moderate lipid-lowering therapy on progression of coronary atherosclerosis: A randomized controlled trial. Journal of the American Medical Association. 2004;**291**: 1071-1080. DOI: 10.1001/jama.291.9.1071

[210] Gerstein HC, Ratner RE, Cannon CP, Serruys PW, Garcia-Garcia HM, van Es GA, et al. Effect of rosiglitazone on progression of coronary atherosclerosis in patients with type 2 diabetes mellitus and coronary artery disease: The assessment on the prevention of progression by rosiglitazone on atherosclerosis in diabetes patients with cardiovascular history trial. Circulation. 2010;**121**: 1176-1187. DOI: 10.1161/circulationaha.109.881003

[211] Widmer RJ, Flammer AJ, Lerman LO, Lerman A. The Mediterranean diet, its components, and cardiovascular disease. The American Journal of Medicine. 2015;**128**: 229-238. DOI: 10.1016/j.amjmed.2014.10.014

[212] Jacobs DR Jr, Gross MD, Tapsell LC. Food synergy: An operational concept for understanding nutrition. The American Journal of Clinical Nutrition. 2009;**89**:1543s-1548s. DOI: 10.3945/ajcn.2009.26736B

[213] Sofi F, Macchi C, Abbate R, Gensini GF, Casini A. Mediterranean diet and health status: An updated meta-analysis and a proposal for a literature-based adherence score. Public Health Nutrition. 2014;**17**:2769-2782. DOI: 10.1017/s1368980013003169

[214] Sofi F, Cesari F, Abbate R, Gensini GF, Casini A. Adherence to Mediterranean diet and health status: Meta-analysis. British Medical Journal (Clinical Research Edition). 2008;**337**: a1344, 10.1136/bmj.a1344

[215] Cannon CP, Braunwald E, McCabe CH, Rader DJ, Rouleau JL, Belder R, et al. Intensive versus moderate lipid lowering with statins after acute coronary syndromes. The New England Journal of Medicine. 2004;**350**:1495-1504. DOI: 10.1056/NEJMoa040583

[216] Jain AK, Mehra NK, Swarnakar NK. Role of antioxidants for the treatment of cardiovascular diseases: Challenges and opportunities. Current Pharmaceutical Design. 2015;**21**: 4441-4455

[217] Buckland G, Mayen AL, Agudo A, Travier N, Navarro C, Huerta JM, et al. Olive oil intake and mortality within the Spanish population (EPIC-Spain). The American Journal of Clinical Nutrition. 2012;**96**:142-149. DOI: 10.3945/ajcn.111.024216

[218] Banel DK, Hu FB. Effects of walnut consumption on blood lipids and other cardiovascular risk factors: A meta-analysis and systematic review. The American Journal of Clinical Nutrition. 2009;**90**:56-63. DOI: 10.3945/ajcn.2009.27457

[219] Mozaffarian D, Hao T, Rimm EB, Willett WC, Hu FB. Changes in diet and lifestyle and long-term weight gain in women and men. The New England Journal of Medicine. 2011;**364**: 2392-2404. DOI: 10.1056/NEJMoa1014296

[220] Kelly RB. Diet and exercise in the management of hyperlipidemia. American Family Physician. 2010;**81**: 1097-1102

[221] Salas-Salvadó J, Bulló M, Babio N, Martínez-González M, Ibarrola-Jurado N, Basora J, et al. Reduction in the incidence of type 2 diabetes with the Mediterranean diet: Results of the PREDIMED-Reus nutrition intervention randomized trial. Diabetes Care. 2011; **34**:14-19. DOI: 10.2337/dc10-1288

[222] Salas-Salvadó J, Díaz-López A, Ruiz-Canela M, Basora J, Fitó M, Corella D, et al. Effect of a lifestyle intervention program with energy-restricted Mediterranean diet and exercise on weight loss and cardiovascular risk factors: One-year results of the PREDIMED-plus trial. Diabetes Care. 2019;**42**:777-788. DOI: 10.2337/dc18-0836

[223] Sayón-Orea C, Razquin C, Bulló M, Corella D, Fitó M, Romaguera D, et al. Effect of a nutritional and behavioral intervention on energy-reduced Mediterranean diet adherence among patients with metabolic syndrome: Interim analysis of the PREDIMED-plus randomized clinical trial. Journal of the American Medical Association. 2019; **322**:1486-1499. DOI: 10.1001/ jama.2019.14630

10

Regulatory Functions of α-Amylase in the Small Intestine Other than Starch Digestion: α-Glucosidase Activity, Glucose Absorption, Cell Proliferation, and Differentiation

Kimie Date

Abstract

Pancreatic α-amylase binds to the *N*-glycan of glycoproteins. Here, I will show that pancreatic α-amylase has regulatory functions in the small intestine other than starch digestion. These new functions were revealed by identification of α-amylase-binding proteins in the intestinal brush border membrane (BBM). This topic will include the following four parts: 1) identification of glycoproteins that bind pancreatic α-amylase in the small intestinal BBM; 2) interactions between pancreatic α-amylase and the binding glycoproteins, sucrose-isomaltase (α-glucosidase), and sodium/glucose co-transporter 1 (SGLT1), in which pancreatic α-amylase enhanced maltose degradation of sucrose-isomaltase under conditions including calcium and sodium, and inhibited glucose uptake of SGLT1; 3) localization of pancreatic α-amylase in the small intestine by binding to the BBM and being internalized into lysosomes through the endocytic pathway; and 4) expression of endogenous α-amylase in the duodenum: *AMY2B*, a pancreatic type α-amylase, is highly expressed in the human duodenum next to the pancreas. The α-amylase expression in the duodenum is required for proliferation and differentiation of human small intestinal epithelial cells.

Keywords: pancreatic α-amylase, small intestine, sucrase-isomaltase, SGLT1, cell proliferation, cell differentiation, endocytosis

1. Introduction

α-Amylase has been found in many organisms, including bacteria, mainly Bacilli, seeds of cereals and legumes, and digestive glands of animals such as humans and pigs. These α-amylases can be obtained as homogeneous preparations and utilized in various situations. For example, mammalian α-amylase is used as a gastrointestinal medicine and digestive agent. Microbial α-amylase is used in sugar production, food processing, clothing production, and detergents because it can be produced on an industrial scale. The uses of these amylases all focus on the ability of the amylase to degrade polysaccharides. The α-amylase in pancreatic juice and saliva clearly functions as a digestive enzyme. It is an endo-type enzyme that randomly cleaves α-1,4 glycosidic bonds such as starch and glycogen to produce maltose and oligosaccharides [1]. Therefore, α-amylase in digestive juices is an essential enzyme for animals consuming a starch diet. α-Amylase has been found in liver [2], brain [3], blood, urine, and cancer cells [4] in humans, but its physiological significance has not been completely elucidated yet.

It has been reported that porcine pancreatic α-amylase binds to an *N*-linked glycan of glycoproteins [5]. It has been shown that the binding of porcine pancre-atic α-amylase to *N*-linked glycans is different from that of the polysaccharide as a substrate. It shows that the carbohydrate-binding activities of pancreatic α-amylase are not common to all types of α-amylase. α-Amylases from barley, *Bacillus subtilis*, and mammalian saliva do not have this activity. Porcine pancreatic α-amylase binds mainly to transferrin having complex-type biantennary *N*-glycans, fetuin having complex-type triantennary *N*-glycans, and ribonuclease B having high-mannose *N*-glycans. However, it does not bind to bovine submandibular gland mucin having *O*-glycans or bovine serum albumin having no sugar chains. The carbohydrate-binding activities of porcine pancreatic α-amylase are affected by pH. Porcine pancreatic α-amylase has a high affinity for both complex type and high-mannose *N*-glycans under pH 5.5. On the other hand, the binding activity is seen with only the high-mannose *N*-glycans, and the binding to the complex *N*-glycans is reduced under neutral pH. Thus, pancreatic α-amylase selectively recognizes the structure of *N*-glycans of glycoproteins depending on pH.

The biological significance of the *N*-glycan binding found in pancreatic α-amylase in vivo is unknown. Pancreatic α-amylase is synthesized in pancreatic acinar cells, packed into acidic zymogen granules (pH 5.5), and secreted into alkaline pancreatic juice (pH 8.0) [6]. Pancreatic juice flows into the duodenum and mixes with gastric acid where it is neutralized, and pancreatic α-amylase exerts its enzymatic activity. The pH in the middle of the duodenum falls from pH 6.5 to 4.5 in a 3-hour period after a meal [7]. There are glycoproteins with *N*-glycans in pancreatic zymogen granules, its membrane, and the lumen of the small intestine [8–11]. These suggest that the *N*-glycan-binding activity of pancreatic α-amylase may be play a role in the packing of pancreatic zymogen granules, its exocytosis in the pancreas, and digestion and absorption of carbohydrates in the small intestine.

In this study, we elucidated the roles of the *N*-glycan-binding activity of pan-creatic α-amylase in the small intestine by identifying the glycoproteins to which the α-amylase binds on the small intestinal brush border membrane (BBM), the luminal surface of the small intestine where many glycoproteins are located. The functions and localizations of the identified α-amylase-binding-glycoproteins and analyses of interactions between α-amylase and the glycoproteins revealed that pan-creatic α-amylase has the following regulatory functions other than as a digestive enzyme: (1) enhancement of α-glucosidase, sucrase-isomaltase, (2) regulation of sodium-dependent glucose uptake, and (3) localization of pancreatic α-amylase in the small intestine. Furthermore, the new discoveries show that duodenal epithelial cells express α-amylase, which is essential for proliferation and differentiation of small intestinal epithelial cells.

2. Identification of glycoproteins that bind pancreatic α-amylase in the small intestinal BBM

In the small intestine, epithelial cells in the luminal villi have a brush border on the surface, and alkaline phosphatase and other membrane-type digestive enzymes are localized on the BBM. The BBM is covered with a glycocalyx composed of glycoproteins and proteoglycans [10, 12]. Lectin staining of rat small intestine tissue revealed that rat small intestinal BBM expresses glycoproteins having complex, high-mannose *N*-glycans, and core 1 *O*-glycans including NeuAcα2-6Gal/GalNAc, and Galβ1-3Gal [9]. It is reported that *N*-glycans of glycoproteins on the surface of porcine intestine have more complex types than those on the rats [13].

Previous reports have shown that pancreatic α-amylase binds to the *N*-glycans of purified glycoproteins [5], but it has not been confirmed whether or not pancreatic α-amylase binds to glycoproteins on small intestinal BBM. Furthermore, which glycoproteins bind to the pancreatic α-amylase and what role they play in interactions with the α-amylase were unknown. This study demonstrated the binding of α-amylase to pig small intestinal BBM by immunostaining, and identified the glycoproteins that bind α-amylase in the pig small intestinal BBM [14].

2.1 Binding of pancreatic α-amylase to small intestinal BBM

Tissue sections of pig duodenum were immunostained with an anti-pancreatic α-amylase antibody. Entire duodenal tissue sections were stained with the pancre-atic α-amylase antibody when there was a large amount of food in the stomach (dur-ing non-fasting), but hardly stained when there was little in the stomach (during fasting) [14]. The localization of exogenous pancreatic α-amylase was examined by staining a 1-cm section of the duodenum of a fasted pig with the pancreatic α-amylase antibody. Tissue sections fixed in formalin and embedded in paraffin were immunostained to detect pancreatic α-amylase. The duodenal sections were agitated in pancreatic α-amylase solution at 4°C. As a result, pancreatic α-amylase bound to the BBM, which is the upper end of the duodenal epithelium (**Figure 1**), and α-amylase staining increased in a time-dependent manner with agitation. Mannan inhibited the binding of pancreatic α-amylase to BBM duodenum sections incubated in α-amylase solution for 30 min. On the other hand, galactan and colominic acid inhibited binding of α-amylase to BBM after 10 min of agitation, but did not inhibit binding of α-amylase to BBM agitated for 30 min (data not shown) [14]. Pancreatic α-amylase bound to duodenum BBM, and its binding was inhibited by

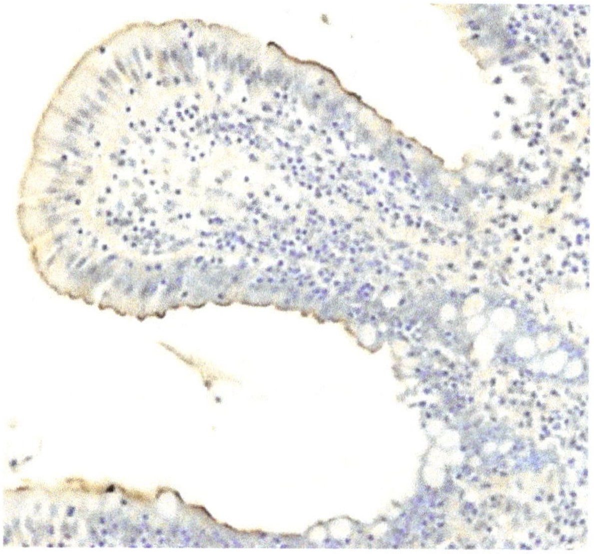

Figure 1.
Binding of pancreatic α-amylase to pig duodenum BBM.

mannan, indicating that α-amylase binds to duodenal BBM in a mannose-specific manner, even at the tissue level.

One-centimeter duodenum sections from fasted pigs were incubated with pancreatic α-amylase (10 μM) in PBS (pH 7.2) including phenylmethylsulfonyl fluoride (final concentratation 1 mM) at 4°C for 30 min, then fixed and paraffin-embedded. The paraffin sections were immunostained with rabbit anti-α-amylase IgGs-HRP. The color was developed with DAB/H_2O_2 and then counterstained with hematoxylin.

2.2 Separation and identification of glycoproteins from the small intestinal BBM that bind pancreatic α-amylase

It was shown that pig duodenal BBM contains glycoproteins that bind to pancreatic α-amylase having high mannose-type and complex-type *N*-glycans. Therefore, we separated and identified the glycoproteins binding α-amylase from fasted pig duodenal BBM [14]. The binding glycoproteins were separated from BBM solubilized with 1% TritonX-100 by using affinity chromatography with an α-amylase-Sepharose 6B column. The α-amylase-binding fractions were eluted by methyl-D-mannopyranoside and separated by molecular weight using SDS-PAGE. Seven main bands stained by SYPRO Ruby protein staining were cut out, treated with pepsin, and analyzed by LC–MS/MS for identification of the proteins in the bands. The major α-amylase-binding glycoproteins identified are shown in **Table 1**. The binding glycoproteins were grouped by functions and localizations. Group 1 consisted of membrane glycoproteins involved in α-glucosidase and sugar absorption, which function in glucose assimilation after starch digestion by α-amylase in the small intestine. Groups 2 and 3 consisted of membrane glycoproteins involved in transcytosis and proteolysis, respectively.

All seven bands were stained by lectins with ConA, GNA, and L-PHA, indicating the presence of *N*-glycans. ConA (concanavalin A), GNA (snowdrop lectin), and L-PHA (*Phaseolus vulgaris* lectin type L) bind specifically to *N*-glycans, high-mannose structures, and complex-type *N*-glycans, respectively. The identification of these α-amylase-binding proteins indicates that the *N*-glycan-binding activity

Identified proteins			
MW (kDa)	**Group 1**	**Group 2**	**Group 3**
202	SGLT1, SI		
144–156		VLA-2	Aminopeptidases, Enterokinase
110–122	SGLT1	DPP-IV, Integrin β1, ACE2	DPP-IV
99			Aminopeptidases
78	SGLT1	Transferrin, Transferrin receptor	
50–57	SGLT1	Na^+/K^+-ATPase β1-subunit	Enterokinase Amine oxidase B
46	Epoxide hydrase	CD Man-6-P receptor, Aminopeptidase N	Aminopeptidase N

SGLT1, sodium glucose co-transporter 1; SI, sucrose-isomaltase; VLA-2, integrin very late antigen-2; DPP-IV, dipeptidylpeptidase IV; ACE 2, angiotensin-converting enzyme 2.

Table 1.
Identification of α-amylase-binding proteins in intestinal BBM.

of pancreatic α-amylase in the duodenum may play a regulatory role involved in α-glucosidase/sugar absorption, transcytosis, and proteolysis.

3. Interaction between pancreatic α-amylase and binding glycoproteins in small intestinal BBM

First, effects of pancreatic α-amylase on the activities of glycoproteins in Group 1 were investigated. Group 1 consists of SI and SGLT1. SI, a membrane glycoprotein, digests sucrose, isomaltose, and maltose on the membrane as α-glucosidases. SGLT1 is also a membrane glycoprotein and plays an essential role in glucose absorption in the small intestine.

3.1 Effects of pancreatic α-amylase on α-glucosidase activity

SI plays an important role in the end digestion of starch because SI breaks down the maltose produced by α-amylase from starch into glucose as an α-glucosidase on the small intestinal membrane. SI is essential for the end digestion of starch, and its

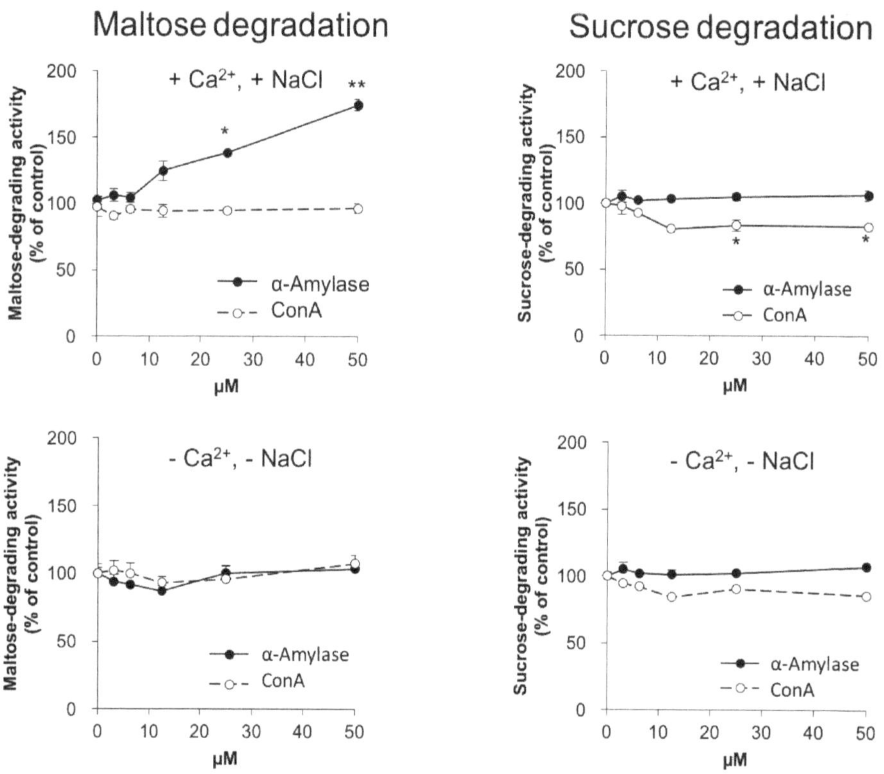

Figure 2.
*Effects of pancreatic α-amylase and ConA on maltose- and sucrose-degrading activity of pig duodenum BBM vesicles. A BBM vesicle suspension (50 μl) was pre-incubated with various concentrations of pancreatic α-amylase or ConA (0–50 μM) for 15 min at 37°C, and incubated with 0.056 M maltose (left) or 0.056 M sucrose (right) as substrate (50 μl) for 30 min (left) or 60 min (right) at 37°C. The maltose or sucrose hydrolysis was measured in the presence of 5 mM $CaCl_2$ and 0.15 M NaCl (upper) or in the absence of $CaCl_2$ and NaCl (lower). Phlorizin (0.5 mM), a glucose transporter inhibitor, was included in the substrate solution. The degrading activity by the production of glucose was measured using a glucose C-II test Wako (Wako, FUJIFILM). ●: α-amylase, ○: ConA. Results are given as means±SE; n = 6. *p < 0.05; **p < 0.01 compared with the absence of α-amylase or ConA by Student's* t-test *[14].*

deficiency and remarkable fluctuations in enzymatic activity are thought to have a significant effect on starch digestion and glucose absorption. In this study, a method was established for measuring SI activity using BBM that evaluates the effects of pancreatic α-amylase on SI activity as an α-glucosidase [14].

The effect of pancreatic α-amylase on SI activity was investigated with and without $CaCl_2$ and NaCl. As a comparison with α-amylase, the effects of concanavalin A (ConA), a lectin that recognizes α-mannose and α-glucose, were also measured because α-amylase shows a high affinity to α-mannose. In maltose degradation activity by SI, the α-amylase showed enhanced activity only in the presence of 5 mM $CaCl_2$ and 0.15 M NaCl, while no effect of α-amylase was shown in the absence of $CaCl_2$ and NaCl (**Figure 2**, left). ConA had no effect on the maltose degradation activity by SI. On the other hand, α-amylase did not affect the sucrose degradation activity, and ConA inhibited it by about 20% in the presence and absence of 5 mM $CaCl_2$ and 0.15 M NaCl, respectively (**Figure 2**, right).

3.2 Effects of pancreatic α-amylase on SGLT1 activity

SGLT1 is a glycoprotein having a complex-type *N*-glycan and a sodium-dependent glucose transporter indispensable for glucose absorption in the small intestine. The effect on the SGLT1 activity means that it directly affects the blood glucose concentration. This study shows the results of examining whether pancreatic α-amylase affects SGLT1 activity.

First, the timing of the addition of pancreatic α-amylase, where the effect of the α-amylase on SGLT1 activity is most frequently observed, was examined.

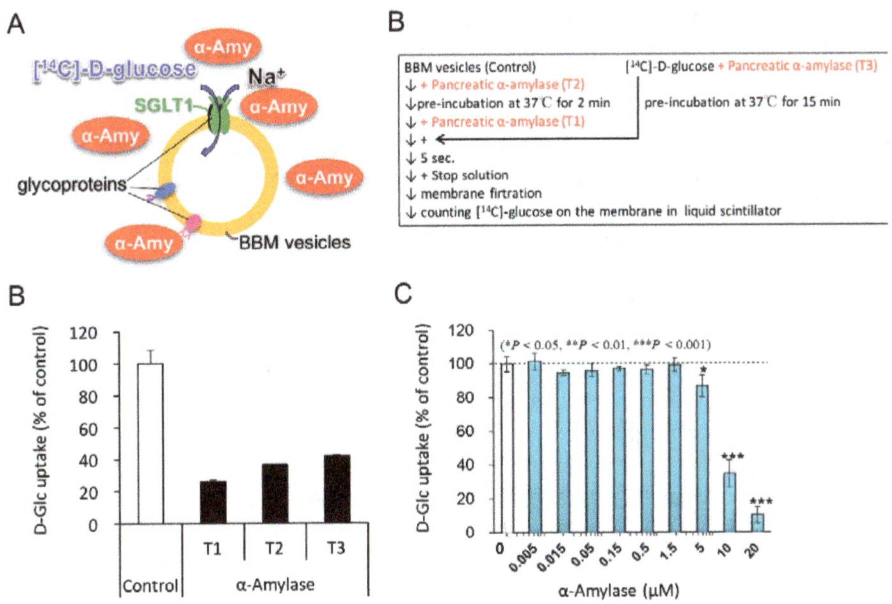

Figure 3.
*Effects of pancreaitc α-amylase on Na+-dependent glucose uptake. SGLT1 activity was assayed as Na+-dependent [14C]-D-glucose uptake (0.2 mM) in BBM vesicles prepared from pig duodenum. (A) Schematic illustration of the SGLT1 activity measurement system using BBM vesicles. (B) Timing of the α-amylase addition to the SGLT1 activity measurement system. T1: α-amylase was added to BBM vesicles prior to [14C]-D-glucose; T2: α-amylase was pre-incubated with BBM vesicles 2 min before addition of [14C]-D-glucose; T3: α-amylase was pre-incubated for 15 min with [14C]-D-glucose. □: Without pancreatic α-amylase (control), ■: With pancreatic α-amylase (10 μM). (C) Effects of pancreatic α-amylase on SGLT1 acrtivity under the three conditions. (D) Dose dependency of D-glucose (D-Glc) uptake on final concentrations of added α-amylase (μM). Pancreatic α-amylase was added at T1. Results are given as means ±SE; n = 6. *p < 0.05, ***p < 0.001 compared with the absence of polysaccharide by Student's* t-test *[14].*

T1: Pancreatic α-amylase was added just before the [^{14}C]-D-glucose substrate solution without preincubation. T2: The α-amylase was pre-incubated with BBM vesicle solution at 37°C for 2 min. T3: The α-amylase was pre-incubated with [^{14}C]-D-glucose substrate solution at 37°C for 15 min (**Figure 3A** and **B**). Inhibition of SGLT1 acitivity by pancreatic α-amylase was shown at all tested additions of the α-amylase, and T1 was the most efficient for SGLT1 inhibition (**Figure 3C**). The concentration-dependent effects of α-amylase on SGLT1 activity were examined under the T1 condition. SGLT1 activity was reduced from 5 μM of α-amylase, and inhibited to 34% at 10 μM and 10% at 20 μM (**Figure 3D**). The 50% inhibitory concentration (IC50) value was 8.1 μM.

Pancreatic α-amylase concentrations in pancreatic juice have been reported to be 4.2 mg/ml in pigs and 5–16 mg/ml in cows [15, 16]. Humans secrete 1–3 L of pancre-atic juice containing several to several tens of grams of protein per day. Therefore, pancreatic α-amylase is probably present in the order of mg/ml because the total concentration of α-amylase in pancreatic juice protein is 26.5% [17]. In this study, it was found that SGLT1 activity was inhibited by pancreatic α-amylase at more than 10 μM (≒ 0.56 mg/ml).

4. Localization of pancreatic α-amylase in the small intestine

α-Amylase synthesized in the pancreas and salivary glands is mostly secreted into the gastrointestinal tract where it digests starch. Part of the α-amylase enters the blood, one-quarter of which is excreted from the kidneys into the urine, and the remaining α-amylase is degraded (inactivated) by an unknown pathway. The α-amylase in the blood is maintained at a constant level by supply from the pancreas and salivary glands, excretion outside the body, and decomposition in the body. Therefore, the blood α-amylase activity is used for diagnosing pancreatitis and other diseases. The proportion of pancreatic α-amylase (unglycosylated 54 kDa) and saliva α-amylase (unglycosylated 54 kDa and glycosylated 57 kDa) is same when the concentration of α-amylase in human blood is examined by electropho-resis. When the pancrea is completely removed due to pancreatic cancer, the blood α-amylase activity temporarily decreases, but it returns to a normal level because the α-amylase in salivary glands increases. It is reported that fluorescently labeled α-amylase injected into rat small intestine was detected in intestinal epithelium and blood, indicating that the pancreatic α-amylase was transported into small intestine tissue (endocytosis) and blood (exocytosis) [18].

The pancreatic α-amylase-binding glycoproteins identified as Group 2 in Section 2.2 contain membrane glycoproteins that have an endocytic function. Transferrin receptor (TfR) binds to iron-bound transferrin and endocytoses iron-bound transferrin into enterocytes [19]. Similarly, aminopeptidase N, ACE2, and VLA- 2 bind to human coronavirus [20, 21], severe acute respiratory syndrome (SARS) virus [22], and matrix glycoproteins [23], respectively. Further, these ligands including viruses are able to endocytose into enterocytes. Mannose 6-phosphate receptor (Man-6-P-receptor) transports binding proteins to the lysosomal system [24]. DPP-IV does not stay in the BBM, and is transported into cells via the same pathway as aminopeptidase N and transferrin (51). This study demonstrated an endocytic pathway for α-amylase secreted into the duodenum from the pancreas [25].

4.1 Endocytosis of pancreatic α-amylase into the small intestine

Two kinds of experiments were performed using pig duodenum tissues and Caco-2 human intestinal epithelial cells that had differentiated into small intestine-like cells by culture in Transwells for 3 weeks. In the experiment using pig duodenum tissue, fasted duodenum with no stomach contents was cut into 1-cm pieces and agitated in a pig pancreatic α-amylase solution at 37°C. After agitation for various periods of time, the tissues were fixed with formalin, and paraffin-embedded sections were prepared. The sections were immunofluorescently stained with an anti-pancreatic α-amylase antibody to clarify the localization of the α-amylase. No staining was detected in the tissue sections after incubation for 0 min. The green fluorescence with anti-pancreatic α-amylase antibody was detected at the upper end of the duodenum corresponding to the BBM in the sections incubated with α-amylase for 10 min, and α-amylase was detected in the entire duodenal tissue incubation for 30 min (**Figure 4A**). In the experiment using differentiated Caco-2 cells, AlexaFluor488-labeled human pancreatic α-amylase was added to the culture medium. After incubation for 30 min at 4°C, the α-amylase in the medium was washed out, and chased for 0–60 min at 37°C in fresh medium without α-amylase. The cells were fixed with formalin, and AlexaFluor488-labeled α-amylase was detected by confocal microscopy. Green fluorescence indicating the localization of α-amylase was detected on the cell membrane only after incuba-tion at 4°C for 30 min. In the subsequent 37°C chase, the α-amylase was detected as punctates in the cells and had decreased at 60 min (**Figure 4B**). These results

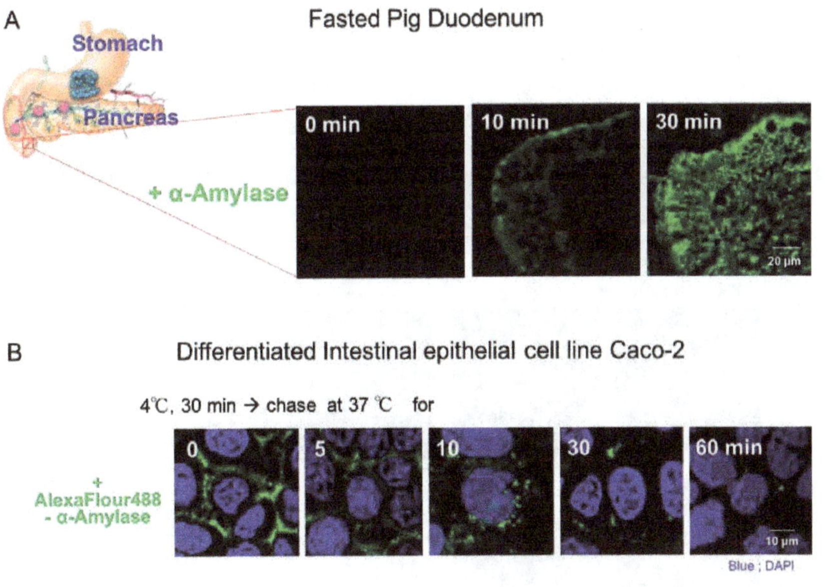

Figure4.
Incorporation of pancreatic α-amylase into pig duodenum tissue (A) and differentiated human epithelial cells Caco-2 (B). (A) One-centimeter duodenum sections from fasted pigs were incubated with pig pancreatic α-amylase (10 µM) in PBS (pH 7.2) including phenylmethylsulfonyl fluoride (final 0.1 mM) at 37°C for 0, 10, or 30 min. The duodenum sections were fixed and paraffin-embedded. The paraffin sections were immunostained with rabbit anti-pancreatic α-amylase antibody as a first antibody and Alexa Fluor 488-goat anti-rabbit antibody. The green fluorescence was detected by a microscope (Olympus FSX100). (B) Caco-2 cells were seeded at 2.6 × 10^5 cells/cm^2 on polyester Transwell permeable supports (0.4-µm pores, 12-mm diameter), and cultured for about 3 weeks in minimal essential medium (DMEM, Sigma) supplemented with 20% heat-inactivated (56°C, 30 min) fetal bovine serum (FBS, Gibco) and 0.1 mM non-essential amino acids (NEAA, Gibco) under a 95% air and 5% CO_2 atmosphere. The cells were starved in a DMEM-NEAA medium without FBS for 18 h. After being washed with Dulbecco's Phosphate-Buffered Saline (DPBS) with Ca^{2+} and Mg^{2+}, Alexa Fluor 488-human pancreatic α-amylase (20 µg/ml) in a DMEM-NEAA medium without FBS was added and incubated at 4°C for 30 min. The α-amylase was washed out, and cultured in DMEM including in 20% FBS and 1 mM NEAA at 37°C for 0–60 min. The cells were fixed, and Alexa Fluor 488-human pancreatic α-amylase was detected by confocal microscopy (ZEISS, LSM710). The nucleus was stained by 4',6-diamidino-2-phenylindole (DAPI) [25].

indicate that pancreatic α-amylase is incorporated into duodenal tissue and small intestinal epithelial cells in a time- and temperature-dependent manner.

4.2 Endocytosis pathway of pancreatic α-amylase to lysosomes

The results in **Figure 4B** showed that pancreatic α-amylase was internal-ized into the epithelial cells and disappeared. The cause of this disappearance is expected to be proteolysis. Among the α-amylase-binding proteins identified in Section 2.2, the membrane glycoprotein proteins classified into Group 3 are involved in protein degradation. In this study, co-localization with intracellular localization marker proteins was investigated to elucidate the endocytic pathway of the pancreatic α-amylase. Transferrin (Tf), early endosome antigen-1 (EEA1), and lysosomal-associated membrane protein 1 (LAMP1) were used as localization marker proteins of the cell membrane, early endosomes, and lysosomes, respectively, and were stained with an Alexa Fluor 594-labeled secondary antibody. Alexa Fluor 488-human pancreatic α-amylase (AF488-α-amylase) was mainly co-localized with Tf by chasing for 0–5 min at 37°C. Subsequently, the AF488- α-amylase was co-localized with EEA1 after chasing for 5–10 min, and then the α-amylase was finally co-localized with LAMP1 after a 30–60 min chase, followed by its disappearance (**Figure 5**). These results suggested that pancreatic α-amylase

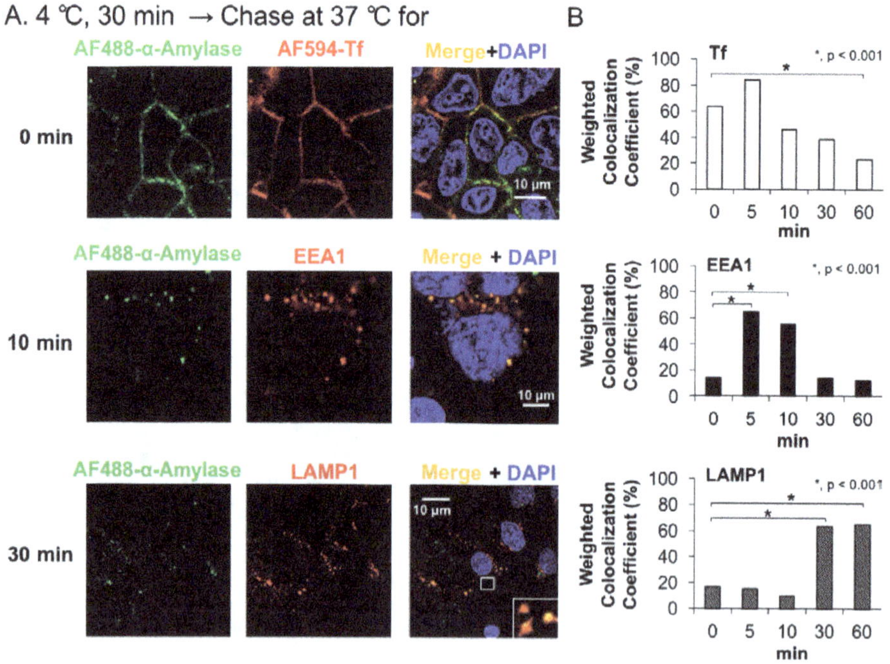

Figure 5.
Co-localization between human pancreatic α-amylase and localization marker proteins. Caco-2 cells were seeded at 2.6 × 10^5 cells/cm^2 on polyester Transwell permeable supports and cultured for about 3 weeks in DMEM supplemented with 20% heat-inactivated FBS and 0.1 mM NEAA under a 95% air and 5% CO_2 atmosphere. The cells were starved in a DMEM-NEAA medium without FBS for 18 h. After being washed with DPBS containing Ca^{2+} and Mg^{2+}, AF488-human pancreatic α-amylase (20 μg/ml) and/or Alexa Fluor 594 (AF594)-Tf in a DMEM-NEAA medium without FBS were added, and cells were incubated at 4°C for 30 min. The α-amylase was washed out, and cells were cultured in DMEM including 20% FBS and 1 mM NEAA at 37°C for 0–60 min. After the cells were fixed, they were stained with an anti-EEA1 antibody or anti-LAMP1 antibody as the first antibody, and followed by AF594-labeled secondary antibodies. The nucleus was stained by DAPI. The three kinds of fluorescence were detected by confocal microscopy (ZEISS, LSM710) (A) [25]. These weighted colocalizations were calculated as described previously [25] (B).

binds to the cell membrane and is transported into lysosomes though early endosomes and the α-amylase undergo degradation in the lysosome. The disappearance of AF488-amylases endocytosed into the cells was suppressed by chloroquine, which is an inhibitor of lysosome proteolysis (data not shown) [25]. In another experiment using pig duodenum tissue sections, α-amylase in the duodenum was well co-localized with LAMP1, and its degraded fragments were detected (data not shown) [25]. These results indicate that pancreatic α-amylase internalized by the endocytic pathway is undergoing proteolysis in the lysosome. Degraded α-amylase may be used as a source for rapid turnover in duodenal epithelial cells.

4.3 Biological significances of endocytosis of pancreatic α-amylase

Based on the SGLT1 inhibition of pancreatic α-amylase described in Section 3.2, the biological significance of endocytosis of the pancreatic α-amylase in Sections 4.1 and 4.2 is discussed as follows. **Figure 6** shows a hypothetical scheme of the biological function of α-amylase internalization [25]. (i) Within 30 min after food intake, pancreatic α-amylase has begun to be secreted from the pancreas into the duodenum, but its amount is not high. Therefore, the α-amylase on the surface of the duodenal BBM interacts with the SI on the BBM to promote starch digestion by both the α-amylase and SI. (ii) Approximately 30 min after food intake, the concentration of pancreatic α-amylase in the small intestinal lumen reaches a maximum, and the α-amylase binds to the glyco-proteins in the BBM. At this time, the glucose uptake of SGLT1 is inhibited by the α-amylase, whereby rapid glucose uptake is suppressed, and postprandial hyperglycemia is corrected. (iii) At 30–60 min after food intake, the α-amylase bound to the BBM is internalized into early endosomes in the epithelial cells.

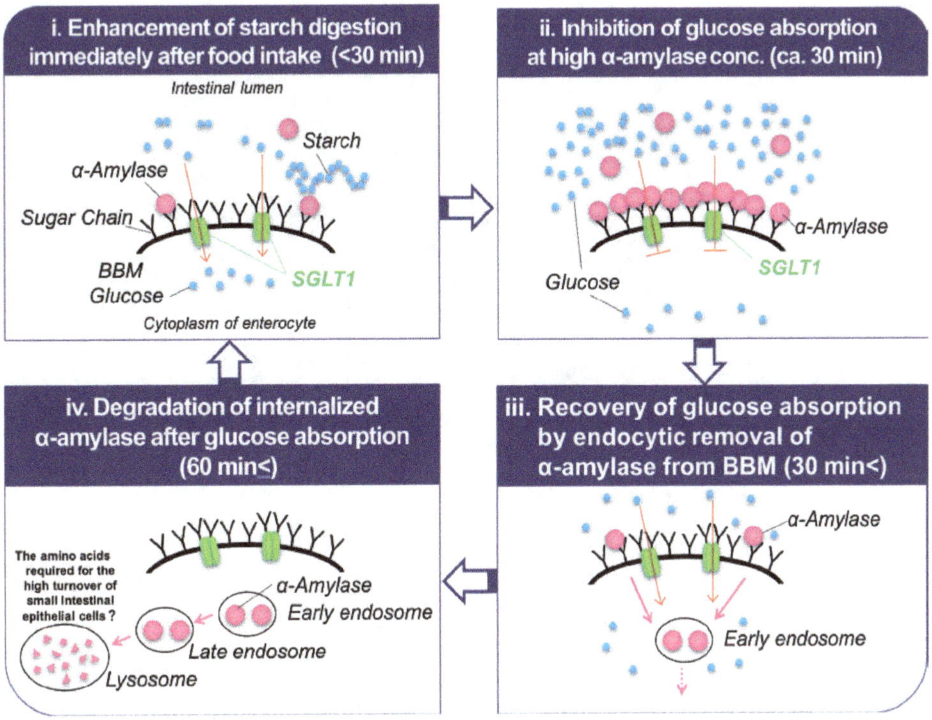

Figure 6.
A hypothetical schematic of the biological function of pancreatic α-amylase internalization.

That is, the inhibition of glucose uptake of SGLT1 in BBM by α-amylase is released, which means the blood glucose level can be maintained even when the blood glucose level drops during fasting. (iv) At 60 min or more after food ingestion, theα-amylase internalized into cells is transported to lysosomes and undergoes degradation.

5. Expression of endogenous α-amylase in the human duodenum

α-Amylase is abundantly expressed in the pancreas and salivary glands, and has been detected in liver [26], thyroid [27], parotid gland [28], white blood cells [29], lung carcinoma tissues [30], and brain [3] in humans. There are five isoforms of α-amylase including three salivary α-amylases (isoforms *AMY1A*, *AMY1B*, and *AMY1C*) and two pancreatic α-amylases (isoforms *AMY2A* and *AMY 2B*) [31]. The α-amylases in liver, white blood cells, and lung carcinoma tissues are encoded by *AMY2B* [2, 29, 30]. The brain amylases are encoded by *AMY1A* and *AMY2B* [3]. The parotid gland amylase is encoded by *AMY1C* [28]. It is reported that α-amylase activity is detected in small intestinal tissues [32]. It is not clear whether this α-amylase is an exogenous one that endocytoses pan-creatic α-amylase into small intestinal tissues or an endogenous α-amylase that is expressed in the small intestine itself. An endogenous α-amylase was stained in differentiated Caco-2 cells by immunostaining with an anti-α-amylase antibody during the experiments on internalization using fluorescence-labeled α-amylase in the cells described in Section 4. In this study, we demonstrated the expression of endogenous α-amylase in human duodenal epithelial cells and identified the isoform of the α-amylase expressed in the duodenal epithelial cells. Furthermore, the biological significances of α-amylase expression in the duodenum are shown [33].

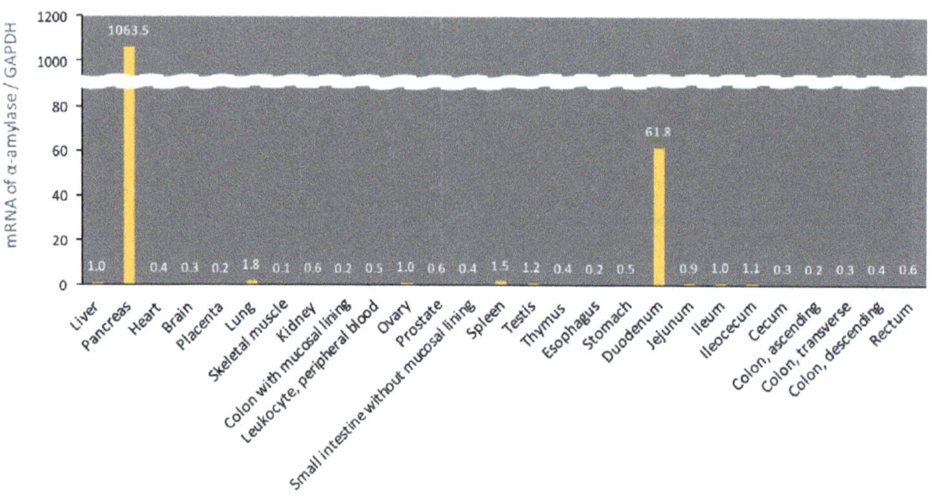

Figure 7.
Expression of α-amylase in human tissues. A reaction mixture was prepared by mixing Human MTC panel I, II or Digestive system MTC panel (Clontech) as a cDNA (5 μl), Power SYBER Green PCR Master mix (6.25 μl), 50 μM forward and reverse primers for AMY2B (0.2 μl each), and putting it in the 96-well reaction plate. Glyceraldehyde-3-phosphate dehydrogenase (GAPDH) was used as the internal standard. The sequences of primer sets for AMY2B and GAPDH were described previously [33]. Normalized data by GAPDH are shown with liver expression as 1.

5.1 Expression of *AMY2B* in human duodenum tissues

The mRNA expression of α-amylase in human tissues was measured by real-time PCR using human Multiple Tissue cDNA (MTC) Panels. The α-amylase was shown to be expressed most in the pancreas and then in the duodenum (**Figure 7**). The results mean that the α-amylase detected in the duodenum consists of both the endogenous α-amylase expressed in the duodenum and the exogenous α-amylase expressed by the pancreas and internalized into the duodenum. For further investigation, mRNA levels, protein levels, enzyme activities, and localization of the α-amylases were clarified using differentiated Caco-2 cells [33]. Caco-2 cells were originally human intestinal epithelial cells derived from the colon, but are known to gradually develop small intestine-like properties when differentiated by long-term culture for about 3 weeks. Therefore, we focused on the change in α-amylase expression in Caco-2 cells during differentiation into small intestine-like cells. The expression of α-amylase in Caco-2 cells increased with differentiation into small intestine-like cells in its mRNA level, protein level, enzyme activity, and immunostaining (**Figure 8**). Activity of α-amylase was detected in the cell extract but not in the culture medium, suggesting that the α-amylase was not secreted by the cells

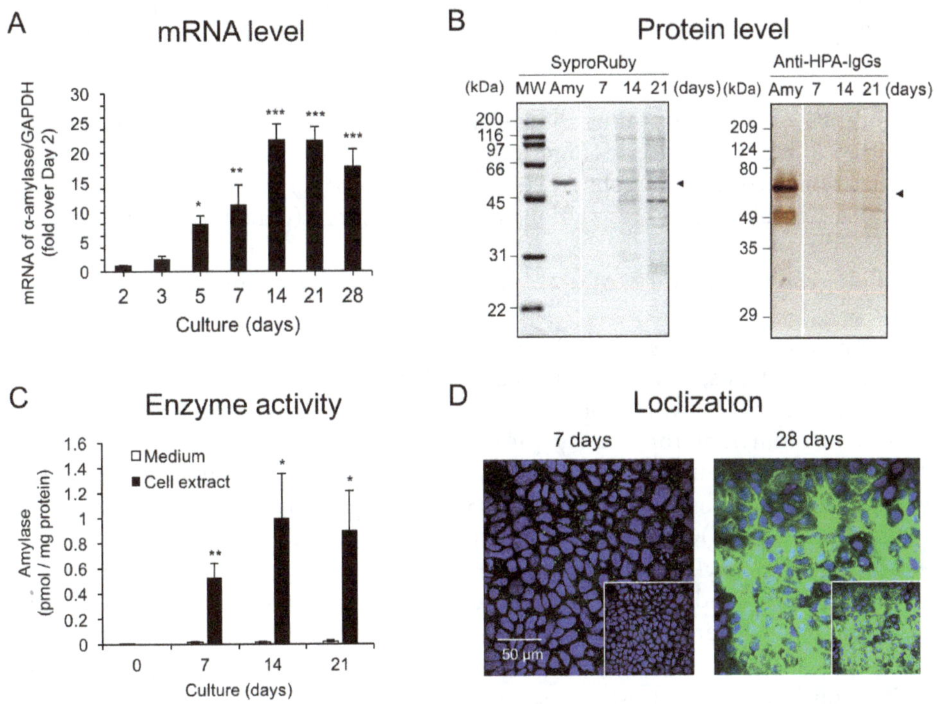

Figure 8.
*Expression of α-amylase in differentiated human epithelial cells. Caco-2 cells were seeded at 5 × 10⁴ cells/cm² in the wells and cultured for 3 weeks in DMEM supplemented with 20% heat-inactivated FBS and 0.1 mM NEAA under a 95% air and 5% CO_2 atmosphere. The cells were washed with DPBS and were prepared for each measurement as described previously [33]. (A) mRNA expression of α-amylase in the cells was measured by quantitative real-time PCR using a 7500 Real-Time PCR System (Applied Biosystems). *$p < 0.05$, **$p < 0.01$, ***$p < 0.001$ vs. Day 2 by one-way ANOVA with Dunnett's posthoc test. (B) Protein levels of α-amylase in the cell extract were detected by Western blotting using anti-human pancreatic α-amylase antibody (HPA IgGs) as a first antibody and HRP-labeled secondary antibodies. The staining was developed by 3,3'-diaminobenzidine (DAB) including H_2O_2. (C) Specific enzymatic activities of α-amylase in the culture medium and cell extract. *$p < 0.05$, **$p < 0.01$ vs. medium by paired* t*-test (D) Immunofluorescence staining of the permeabilized cells with anti-HPA IgGs as a first antibody and AF488-labeled secondary antibodies. The nucleus was stained by DAPI. The fluorescence was detected by confocal microscopy (ZEISS, LSM710). The lower right is an enlarged view [33].*

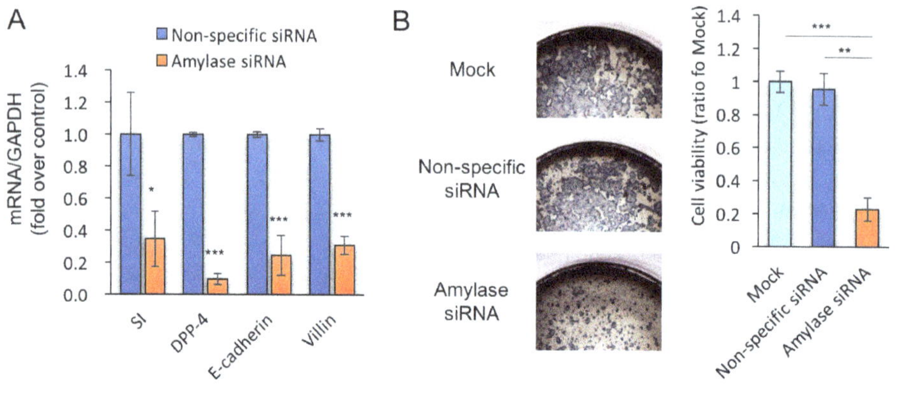

Figure 9.
*Effects of α-amylase suppression by siRNA on cell differentiation and proliferation. Nonspecific siRNA as a control or the siRNA targeting α-amylase was transfected to Caco-2 cells and these cells were seeded at 2 × 10⁵ cells/cm² (A) or 1 × 10⁵ cells/cm² (B) in the wells. The cells were cultured for 3 days in DMEM supplemented with 20% heat-inactivated FBS and 0.1 mM NEAA under a 95% air and 5% CO_2 atmosphere. (A) The cells were washed with DPBS and were prepared for mRNA expression as described previously [33]. mRNA expressions of α-amylase differentiation marker proteins (SI, DPP-4, E-cadherin, villin) in the cells were measured by quantitative real-time PCR using a 7500 Real-Time PCR System (Applied Biosystems). (B) The cells in the 96-well plates were stained with MTT, and the cell viability was measured by an MTT assay. Mock, the cells transfected with the transfection reagent only without siRNA. Data are shown as mean ± SE, *p < 0.05, **p < 0.01, ***p < 0.001, one-way ANOVA with Tukey's posthoc test [33].*

(**Figure 8C**). Immunostaining showed that the α-amylase in the cytoplasm was localized in a dotted pattern (**Figure 8D**). The isotype of the α-amylase expressed in differentiated Caco-2 cells was identified as pancreatic type *AMY2B* by a combina-tion of PCR and restriction enzyme treatment (data not shown) [33].

5.2 Biological significances of α-amylase expressed in the duodenum

α-Amylase has been shown to be expressed by tissues other than the pancreas and salivary glands, but the biological significance has not been elucidated. The increased α-amylase expression in obese mouse liver suggests that liver α-amylase may be a biomarker for obesity [34]. It has been hypothesized that α-amylase expressed in the brain may be an energy source in Alzheimer's disease [3]. Here, it was shown that the expression of α-amylase by Caco-2 cells was suppressed by RNA i nterference (RNAi), and affected cell proliferation and differentiation [33]. The expression of α-amylase was suppressed to about 30% by siRNA (small interfering RNA), and four kinds of cell differentiation markers were quantified by real-time PCR. All four differentiation markers were reduced in cells transfected with α-amylase siRNA compared to cells transfected with control siRNA (**Figure 9A**). This result indicates that α-amylase expression is required for cell differentiation. Furthermore, it was shown that the cell proliferation of cells transfected with α-amylase siRNA was dramatically reduced depending on the cell-seeding concen-tration (**Figure 9B**).

6. Conclusion

This study showed new functions of both exogenous and endogenous pan-creatic α-amylase other than starch digestion in the small intestine. Exogenous α-amylase synthesized by the pancreas and secreted into the small intestinal tract enhances α-glucosidase activity and inhibits glucose uptake by SGLT1 in the small intestine BBM. The exogenous α-amylase was internalized into lysosomes and degraded in intestinal epithelial cells. On the other hand, endogenous α-amylase is highly expressed in the duodenum, where it enhances cell proliferation and differentiation.

Acknowledgements

This work was supported in part by the Japan Society for the Promotion of Science Grants 22.10385, 26.40058 and 19K16072 (to K. D.), the Dr. Yoshifumi Jigami Memorial Fund, the Society of Yeast Scientists (to K. D.), and the Lotte Shigemitsu Prize (to K. D.).

Thanks

Special thanks to Dr. Haruko Ogawa from Ohcanomizu University for advices on identification of α-amylase-binding proteins and other experiments in this study. Thanks to Dr. Nana Kawasaki from National Institute of Health Sciences for LC–MS/MS analysis and database search. Thanks to Dr. Ayano Satoh from Okayama University for advices on Caco-2 cell culture. Thanks to Dr. Tomomi Yamazaki for advices on identification of α-amylase isoforms and measurement of mRNA expres-sion by real-time PCR. Thanks to Katherine Ono for editing the English.

Author details

Kimie Date
Institute for Human Life Innovation, Ochanomizu University, Tokyo, Japan

*Address all correspondence to: date.kimie@ocha.ac.jp

References

[1] Ishikawa K, Matsui I, Kobayashi S, Nakatani H, Honda K. Substrate recognition at the binding site in mammalian pancreatic alpha-amylases. Biochemistry. 1993;**32**:6259-6265

[2] Koyama I, Komine S, Iino N, Hokari S, Igarashi S, Alpers DH, et al. Alpha-Amylase expressed in human liver is encoded by the AMY-2B gene identified in tumorous tissues. Clinica Chimica Acta. 2001;**309**:73-83. DOI: 10.1016/s0009-8981(01)00501-0

[3] Byman E, Schultz N, Netherlands Brain B, Fex M, Wennstrom M. Brain alpha-amylase: A novel energy regulator important in Alzheimer disease? Brain Pathology. 2018;**28**:920-932. DOI: 10.1111/bpa.12597

[4] Tomita N, Matsuura N, Horii A, Emi M, Nishide T, Ogawa M, et al. Expression of alpha-amylase in human lung cancers. Cancer Research. 1988;**48**:3292-3296

[5] Matsushita H, Takenaka M, Ogawa H. Porcine pancreatic alpha-amylase shows binding activity toward N-linked oligosaccharides of glycoproteins. The Journal of Biological Chemistry. 2002;**277**:4680-4686. DOI: 10.1074/jbc.M105877200;M105877200

[6] Thorn P, Fogarty KE, Parker I. Zymogen granule exocytosis is characterized by long fusion pore openings and preservation of vesicle lipid identity. Proceedings of the National Academy of Sciences of the United States of America. 2004;**101**:6774-6779. DOI: 10.1073/pnas.0400336101

[7] Ovesen L, Bendtsen F, Tage- Jensen U, Pedersen NT, Gram BR, Rune SJ. Intraluminal pH in the stomach, duodenum, and proximal jejunum in normal subjects and patients with exocrine pancreatic insufficiency. Gastroenterology. 1986;**90**:958-962. DOI: 10.1016/0016-5085(86)90873-5

[8] Gupta R, Jaswal VM, Meenu MA. Intestinal epithelial cell surface glycosylation in mice. I. Effect of high-protein diet. Annals of Nutrition & Metabolism. 1992;**36**:288-295

[9] Pusztai A, Ewen SW, Grant G, Peumans WJ, Van Damme EJ, Coates ME, et al. Lectins and also bacteria modify the glycosylation of gut surface receptors in the rat. Glycoconjugate Journal. 1995;**12**:22-35

[10] Roth J. Cellular sialoglycoconjugates: A histochemical perspective. The Histochemical Journal. 1993;**25**:687-710

[11] Smits HL, Kramer MF. Human duodenal gland (Brunner's gland) mucus glycoprotein analysis. Archives of Biochemistry and Biophysics. 1984;**228**:64-70. DOI: 0003-9861(84)90047-X

[12] Van Halbeek H, Gerwig GJ, Vliegenthart JF, Smits HL, Van Kerkhof PJ, Kramer MF. Terminal alpha (1 leads to 4)-linked N-acetylglucosamine: A characteristic constituent of duodenal-gland mucous glycoproteins in rat and pig. A high-resolution 1H-NMR study. Biochimica et Biophysica Acta. 1983;**747**:107-116

[13] Hedemann MS, Hojsgaard S, Jensen BB. Lectin histochemical characterisation of the porcine small intestine around weaning. Research in Veterinary Science. 2007;**82**:257-262. DOI: 10.1016/j.rvsc.2006.06.007

[14] Asanuma-Date K, Hirano Y, Le N, Sano K, Kawasaki N, Hashii N, et al. Functional regulation of sugar assimilation by N-glycan-specific interaction of pancreatic alpha-amylase

with glycoproteins of duodenal brush border membrane. The Journal of Biological Chemistry. 2012;**287**:23104-23118. DOI: 10.1074/jbc.M111.314658

[15] Fiedorowicz M, Chaczatrian G. Effect of illumination with the visible polarized and nonpolarized light on alpha-amylolysis of starches of different botanical origin. Journal of Agricultural and Food Chemistry. 2003;**51**:7815-7819. DOI: 10.1021/jf026202r

[16] Uc A, Giriyappa R, Meyerholz DK, Griffin M, Ostedgaard LS, Tang XX, et al. Pancreatic and biliary secretion are both altered in cystic fibrosis pigs. American Journal of Physiology. Gastrointestinal and Liver Physiology. 2012;**303**:G961-G968. DOI: 10.1152/ajpgi.00030.2012

[17] Fukuoka S. Gene family of GPI linked proteins involved in intracellular sorting of secretory proteins. Tanpakushitsu Kakusan Koso. 1992;**37**:795-809

[18] Cloutier M, Gingras D, Bendayan M. Internalization and transcytosis of pancreatic enzymes by the intestinal mucosa. The Journal of Histochemistry and Cytochemistry. 2006;**54**:781-794. DOI: 10.1369/jhc.5A6877.2006

[19] Testa U, Kuhn L, Petrini M, Quaranta MT, Pelosi E, Peschle C. Differential regulation of iron regulatory element-binding protein(s) in cell extracts of activated lymphocytes versus monocytes-macrophages. The Journal of Biological Chemistry. 1991;**266**:13925-13930

[20] Renold A, Cescato R, Beuret N, Vogel LK, Wahlberg JM, Brown JL, et al. Basolateral sorting signals differ in their ability to redirect apical proteins to the basolateral cell surface. The Journal of Biological Chemistry. 2000;**275**:9290- 9295. DOI: 10.1074/jbc.275.13.9290

[21] Hansen GH, Delmas B, Besnardeau L, Vogel LK, Laude H, Sjostrom H, et al. The coronavirus transmissible gastroenteritis virus causes infection after receptor-mediated endocytosis and acid-dependent fusion with an intracellular compartment. Journal of Virology. 1998;**72**:527-534

[22] Crackower MA, Sarao R, Oudit GY, Yagil C, Kozieradzki I, Scanga SE, et al. Angiotensin-converting enzyme 2 is an essential regulator of heart function. Nature. 2002;**417**:822-828. DOI: 10.1038/nature00786

[23] Le Varlet B, Staquet MJ, Dezutter-Dambuyant C, Gaucherand M, Schmitt D. Expression and endocytosis of integrin VLA receptors for collagen, fibronectin and laminin by normal human keratinocytes. Journal of Dermatological Science. 1991;**2**:287-299. DOI: 10.1016/0923-1811(91)90053-z

[24] Russell MR, Nickerson DP, Odorizzi G. Molecular mechanisms of late endosome morphology, identity and sorting. Current Opinion in Cell Biology. 2006;**18**:422-428. DOI: 10.1016/j.ceb.2006.06.002

[25] Date K, Satoh A, Iida K, Ogawa H. Pancreatic alpha-amylase controls glucose assimilation by duodenal retrieval through N-glycan-specific binding, endocytosis, and degradation. The Journal of Biological Chemistry. 2015;**290**:17439-17450. DOI: 10.1074/jbc.M114.594937

[26] Samuelson LC, Wiebauer K, Gumucio DL, Meisler MH. Expression of the human amylase genes: Recent origin of a salivary amylase promoter from an actin pseudogene. Nucleic Acids Research. 1988;**16**:8261-8276. DOI: 10.1093/nar/16.17.8261

[27] Otsu N, Oami H, Okawa M, Aotsuka S, Yokohari R. Amylase in the thyroid gland. Histochemistry.

1982;**74**:21-26. DOI: 10.1007/bf00495048

[28] Ting CN, Rosenberg MP, Snow CM, Samuelson LC, Meisler MH. Endogenous retroviral sequences are required for tissue-specific expression of a human salivary amylase gene. Genes & Development. 1992;**6**:1457-1465. DOI: 10.1101/gad.6.8.1457

[29] Hokari S, Miura K, Koyama I, Kobayashi M, Komine S, Komoda T. A restriction endonuclease assay for expression of human alpha-amylase isozymes. Clinica Chimica Acta. 2002;**322**:113-116. DOI: 10.1016/s0009-8981(02)00161-4

[30] Yokouchi H, Horii A, Emi M, Tomita N, Doi S, Ogawa M, et al. Cloning and characterization of a third type of human alpha-amylase gene, AMY2B. Gene. 1990;**90**:281-286. DOI: 10.1016/0378-1119(90)90191-s

[31] Gumucio DL, Wiebauer K, Caldwell RM, Samuelson LC, Meisler MH. Concerted evolution of human amylase genes. Molecular and Cellular Biology. 1988;**8**:1197-1205. DOI: 10.1128/mcb.8.3.1197

[32] Whitten RO, Chandler WL, Thomas MG, Clayson KJ, Fine JS. Survey of alpha-amylase activity and isoamylases in autopsy tissue. Clinical Chemistry. 1988;**34**:1552-1555

[33] Date K, Yamazaki T, Toyoda Y, Hoshi K, Ogawa H. Alpha-amylase expressed in human small intestinal epithelial cells is essential for cell proliferation and differentiation. Journal of Cellular Biochemistry. 2020;**121**:1238-1249. DOI: 10.1002/jcb.29357

[34] Mojbafan M, Afsartala Z, Amoli MM, Mahmoudi M, Yaghmaei P, Larijani B, et al. Liver alpha-amylase gene expression as an early obesity biomarker. Pharmacological Reports. 2017;**69**:229-234. DOI: 10.1016/j.pharep.2016.11.001

11

Etiology of Cancer Associated Thromboembolism (CAT) and Diet, Lifestyle and Medicine to Reduce Cancer and Venous Thromboembolism

Kenji Yokoyama

Abstract

Cancer is one of the leading causes of death in developed countries, and cancer patients often develop venous thromboembolism (VTE). VTE is the second leading cause of death in cancer patients receiving chemotherapy. The incidence of VTE varies among cancers, and it is highest in pancreatic cancer patients. Increased white blood cells and thrombocytosis are risk factors for developing cancer-associated VTE. Some other proteins (tissue factor, podoplanin, P-selectin, and plasminogen activator inhibitor-1) may also play roles in thrombus formation in cancer patients. Certain diets and nutrition (e.g., enough fish, vegetables, and fruits) may reduce the risk of VTE. Certain diets and nutrition also may reduce the risk of cancer, and alcohol drinking and cigarette smoking definitely increase risk of cancer. Some studies suggest that aspirin, a widely used antiplatelet drug, may reduce cancer incidence and mortality, but other studies fail to show the beneficial effects of aspirin.

Keywords: cancer, venous thromboembolism, fish, vegetables, aspirin

1. Introduction

Cancer is one of the leading causes of death in developed countries gincludin Japan. According to the Japanese Cancer Institute registry data,nts 1,017,200 patie were estimated to be newly diagnosed with cancer, and 380,300 patients were estimated to die from cancer in 2019 [1]. Colonosed cancer is the most often diagn in Japanese people, followed by gastric andenlung cancer. Lung cancer most oft causes death related to cancer, followed tely by colon and gastric cancer. Approxima half of Japanese people sufferd die from cancer during their lifetime, and one-thir from cancer. Venous lica-thromboembolism (VTE) is common and serious comption in patientsher with cancer. The risk of VTE in cancer patients isseveralfold hig than that in useindividuals without cancer [2, 3], and VTE is the second leading ca of death in cancer patients undergoing chemotherapy after death directly related to cancer [4]. Therefore, it is important to prevent and treat cancer-associated VTE to improve prognosis of cancer.

2. History of cancer-associated thrombosis

French physician Armand Trousseau first described the relationship between cancer and thrombosis when he reported multiple cancer patients complicated with "phlegmasia alba dolens" caused by deep vein thrombosis in 1865 [5]. He speculated that excess of fibrin and hypercoagulable state of blood caused thrombosis in these patients. Two years later, he suffered from "phleg-masia alba dolens," and he died from gastric cancer. Since then, many studies have revealed the relationships between cancer and thrombosis. Presently, it is well known that thrombosis, i.e., venous thromboembolism (VTE), arterial thrombosis, disseminated intravascular coagulation, and thrombotic microan-giopathy, often occurs in cancer patients, and thrombosis occurring in cancer patients become to be recognized as cancer-associated thrombosis (CAT) (**Table 1**).

Venous thromboembolism
Arterial thrombosis
Disseminated intravascular coagulation
Thrombotic microangiopathy

Table 1.
Cancer-associated thrombosis.

3. Epidemiology and etiology of venous thromboembolism

Among CAT, VTE most often occurs in cancer patients. VTE is a disease that includes deep vein thrombosis (DVT), which usually occurs in the lower legs, and pulmonary embolisms (PE). Most isolated distal DVTs do not extend to the proximal veins and remain uneventful, whereas parts of clot may break off from proximal DVTs and they may cause potentially life-threatening PE. VTE is the third frequent cardiovascular diseases in Western countries next to myocardial infarction and stroke, and it is estimated that annual incidence of VTE is 1–2 per 1000 adults in the USA [6]. Racial differences may exist in the incidence of VTE, and it is reported that the incidence of VTE in whites is five times higher than that in Asians [7]. Previously, the incidence of VTE in Japanese population was supposed to be low, but more Japanese patients have been diagnosed with VTE, recently. The number of patients diagnosed with PE was 28 per 1,000,000 people in 1996, and it increased to 126 in 2011 [8].

There are several risk factors that induce VTE, and cancer is one of the main risk factors for VTE (**Table 2**). It has been reported that cancer is associated with 18% of all VTE, and the overall risk of VTE was increased sevenfold in patients with a malignancy (odds ratio [OR], 6.7; 95% confidence interval [CI], 5.2–8.6) vs. persons without malignancy [9].

Major surgery
Cancer
Pregnancy
Delivery
Acute medical illness
Paralysis
Prolonged bed rest
Oral contraceptive
Obesity
Elderly
Thrombophilia

Table 2.
Risk factors for venous thromboembolism.

4. Risk factors for cancer-associated venous thromboembolism

Incidence rates of VTE increase with age in the general population. Likewise, cancer-associated VTE occurs more often in the elderly population than younger population. Khorana et al. reported that age 65 or older is an independent risk factor for developing cancer-associated VTE. Cancer-associated VTE is more common in female sex and black race [3]. Obesity; complications such as respiratory disease, kidney disease, and infection; and poor performance status are also risk factors for cancer-associated VTE [10–12].

The risk of VTE varies by cancer site, and meta-analysis of several studies proves that the incidence of VTE is highest in the pancreatic cancer patients, followed by hematological malignancy and brain tumor patients [13]. VTE more often occurs in patients with advanced cancer than in patients with early cancer [14]. The incidence of VTE also varies by cancer histology, is higher in lung adenocarcinoma patients than in lung squamous cell carcinoma patients [15], and is higher in high-grade lymphoma patients than in low-grade lymphoma patients [16, 17].

Cancer treatment also affects VTE incidence. VTE is a common complication of surgery, regardless of whether it is cancer surgery or not, and adequate prophylaxis is recommended in guidelines including Japanese guideline [18]. However, among cancer patients who received adequate VTE prophylaxis after surgery, 2.1% of them developed massive VTE and 0.8% of them died [19]. Many types of anticancer drugs, such as cisplatin, l-asparaginase, and bevacizumab, also increase risk of thrombosis in cancer patients. Especially, the incidence of VTE is very high in multiple myeloma patients receiving immunomodulatory drugs (e.g., thalido-mide, lenalidomide, and pomalidomide), and these patients need primary preven-tion of VTE by using antithrombotic drugs. Cancer patients often need indwelling central venous catheter (CVC) for delivery of intravenous drugs, parenteral nutrition, and collecting blood samples. Indwelling CVC increases risk of develop-ing VTE, and it is estimated that the risk of symptomatic catheter thrombosis is 0.3–28% [20].

Considering these factors, several risk models to predict the occurrence of cancer-associated VTE have been published. Khorana score is the most widely used risk model among them [21]. Five predictive variables are identified in this score: site of cancer (2 points for very high-risk site, 1 point for high-risk site), platelet count of 350 × 10 ^{9} /L or more, hemoglobin less than 100 g/L (10 g/dL) and/or the use of erythropoiesis-stimulating agents, leukocyte count more than 11 × 10^9/L, and body mass index of 35 kg/m^2 or more (1 point each). Rates of VTE have been reported to be 0.3% in low-risk (score = 0), 2% in intermediate-risk (score = 1–2), and 6.7% in high-risk (score ≥ 3) category over a median of 2.5 months.

5. Pathogenesis of cancer-associated venous thromboembolism

Stasis of blood flow, hypercoagulability, and endothelial injury are known as Virchow's triad, and they are involved in thrombus formation. Stasis of blood flow caused by several factors, such as poor performance status, indwelling CVC, and venous compression by tumor, is thought to be involved in the pathogenesis of VTE in cancer patients.

Blood cells also play an important role in the occurrence of VTE in cancer patients. Leukocyte count 11 × 10^9/L or above is a risk factor of VTE in cancer patients [21]. Increased leukocyte is found in 20–30% of cancer patients, and it is common in colon and lung cancer patients. Increased expression of granulocyte colony stimulating factor, granulocyte-macrophage colony stimulating factor, and interleukin-6 causes leukocyte increase in cancer patients [22, 23]. Neutrophils may enhance thrombosis through formation of neutrophil extracellular traps (NETs), which take in erythrocytes and platelets, and bind to tissue factor (TF) resulting in activation of coagulation [24, 25]. Increased incidences of VTE are reported both in cancer patients with thrombocytosis prior to cancer diagnosis and thrombocy-tosis at cancer diagnosis [11, 26, 27]. Higher expression of platelet factor 4, which activates platelets, in cancer patients may be related to the development of VTE [28, 29]. Platelets also play a regulatory role in NETs formation. These may play an important role in the pathogenesis of cancer-associated VTE.

Some proteins also have been reported to be involved in the pathogenesis of cancer-associated VTE. TF plays an important role in hemostasis and activates factor IX and factor X to initiate extrinsic coagulation pathway by forming a complex with factor VII or activated factor VII. VTE most frequently occurs in pancreatic cancer patients, and pancreatic cancer expresses TF. Expression levels of TF correlate with histologic grades of cancer, and the incidence of VTE is higher in patients with pancreatic cancer with high TF expression level [30, 31]. Podoplanin is a protein which activates platelets by binding to platelet C-type lectin receptor 2 (CLEC-2) [32, 33]. The relationships between podoplanin and VTE are proven in patients with glioblastoma multiforme (GBM). Expression levels of podoplanin vary by GBM subtype. GBM with high podoplanin expression level has a high number of platelet aggregates in tumor vessels and is reported to have high incidence of VTE [34].

P-selectin is a protein that exists in platelets and endothelial cells, and soluble form of P-selectin exists in plasma. P-selectin induces leukocytes to damaged endothelium for thrombus formation. The incidence of VTE is reported to be higher in cancer patients with high levels of soluble P-selectin [35]. Inhibition of P-selectin reduces thrombus formation in animal models [36].

Plasminogen activator inhibitor-1 (PAI-1) inhibits plasmin, which is synthesized from plasminogen to dissolve thrombus. Increased level of PAI-1 causes thrombotic tendency. The incidence of VTE is high in pancreatic cancer patients with increased levels of PAI-1 [37]. It is reported that administration of bevacizumab to mice trans-planted with lung cancer cells increases PAI-1 expression and enlarges the size of thrombus. Administration of PAI-1 inhibitor to these mice decreases the thrombus size [38]. These findings suggest that increased PAI-1 may be related to the occur-rence of cancer-associated VTE (**Figure 1**).

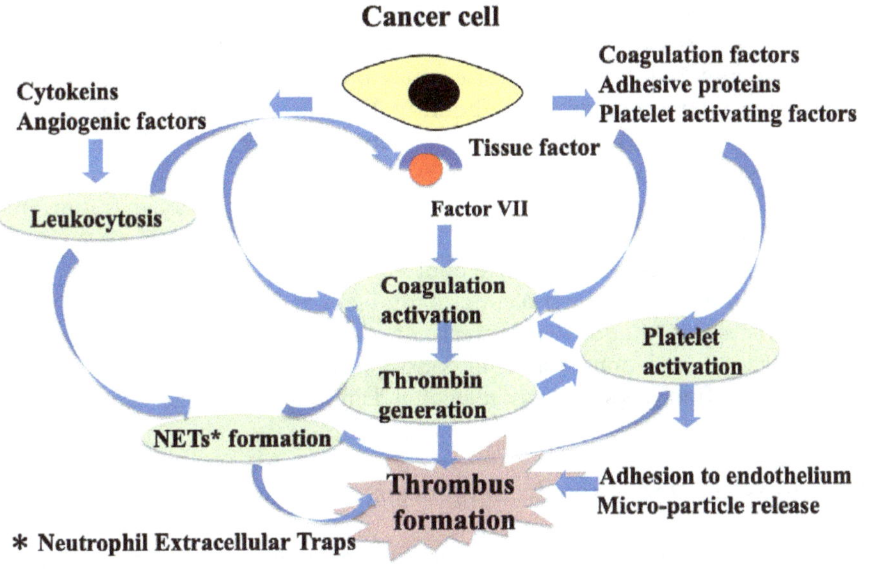

Figure 1.
Pathogenesis of cancer-associated venous thromboembolism. Cancer cells express and release various proteins. These induce leukocytosis and thrombocytosis and activate coagulation resulting in thrombus formation.

6. Diet, nutrition, and VTE

Considering the pathogenesis of cancer-associated VTE described in the previous section, it is unlikely that certain diets and nutrition can suppress the development of cancer-associated VTE specifically. Then, are there any diets and nutrition which may prevent the development of VTE in general, not just cancer-associated? The associa-tion between diet and nutrition and thrombosis has not necessarily been well ana-lyzed for VTE, but it has been well analyzed for arterial thrombosis such as ischemic heart disease or cerebral infarction. In 2010, the American College of Cardiology announced seven lifestyles to reduce deaths caused by cardiovascular and cerebral infarction by 20% by 2020: (1) nonsmoking, (2) body mass index <25 kg/m^2, (3) physical activity at goal levels, (4) pursuit of a diet consistent with the current guide-line recommendations, (5) untreated total cholesterol <200 mg/dL, (6) untreated blood pressure < 120/<80 mm Hg, and (7) fasting blood glucose <100 mg/dL [39]. Do these lifestyles also reduce the incidence of VTE? Hypertension, hypercholester-olemia, diabetes (these are related to diet and nutrition), and smoking are risk factors for atherosclerotic cardiovascular disease, and meta-analysis of nine clinical trials revealed that only smoking is a risk factor for VTE among them [40]. These results suggest that diets and nutrition to prevent arterial thrombosis are not necessarily effective for VTE prevention. On the other hand, obesity, one of the risk factors for arterial thrombosis, is also known to be one of the risk factors for the development of VTE. Analysis of the association between 95 BMI-related gene polymorphisms and VTE development proves that five of the polymorphisms are associated with VTE development [41]. Therefore, taking a diet without too much calories or carbohy-drates to maintain proper body weight is considered to be useful for VTE prevention.

Other reports examining the relationship between diet and nutrition and VTE are as follow. The incidence of VTE is 22% lower for those who eat fish three or more times a week than for those who eat twice or less a week [42] and is low for those who eat enough fish, vegetables, and fruits and eat less red meat and processed meat [43]. These reports suggest that diets to prevent arterial thrombosis might also be useful to prevent VTE. Furthermore, consumption of grape suppresses thrombin generation and enhances fibrinolysis [44]. Diets with 20, 30, and 50% of their calories on protein, lipids, and carbohydrates for 12 months result in reduction of abdominal circumference, increased HDL-C, decreased fibrinogen, and significantly increased interleukin-10 in those with metabolic syndrome [45]. These reports suggest that diet and nutrition might directly affect the blood coagulation and fibrinolysis which play an important role in the development of VTE.

Several reports related to the alcohol consumption and VTE have also been published. Women consuming alcohol daily were at 26% lower risk of VTE than non-consumers [46], and the analysis of three large US cohorts showed no evidence of an association of alcohol consumption amount or frequency with PE risk [47]. These findings suggest that alcohol drinking is not a risk factor for VTE.

7. Factors associated with carcinogenesis

The accumulation of various genetic abnormalities in normal cells causes carcinogenesis. Some cancers are caused by congenital genetic abnormalities, but most genetic abnormalities causing cancers are acquired abnormalities. It is estimated that smoking contributes to 20% of cancers and 23% of cancer deaths and infection with helicobacter pylori, hepatitis virus, etc. contributes to 21% of cancers and 22% of cancer deaths in Japanese population, and these are thought to be the main risk factors for cancer in Japanese population. Drinking alcohol contributes to 6% of both cancers and cancer deaths, and it is also a significant risk factor for cancer in Japanese population. Consumption of salt more than 6 g per day, deficiency of fruit intake, and deficiency of vegetable intake also contribute to 1.6, 0.7, and 0.6% of cancers and 1.4, 0.8, and 0.6% of cancer deaths, respectively [48]. Diet and nutrition seem to have some effects on the development of cancer and cancer mortality.

8. Diet, nutrition, and cancer

According to a report "Food, Nutrition, Physical Activity, and the Prevention of Cancer: A Global Perspective" published by World Cancer Research Fund and American Institute for Cancer Research, it is convincing that adult body fatness has increased risks of esophageal, pancreatic, liver, colorectal, postmenopausal breast, endometrial, and kidney cancer. As for diets and nutrition, there exist causal relationships between aflatoxin and liver cancer, lean and processed meat and colon cancer, arsenic in drinking water and lung cancer, and high-dose beta-carotene supplements and lung cancer. On the other hand, whole grains and food containing dietary fiber decrease colorectal cancer. Non-starchy vegetables and fruits decrease aerodigestive cancer and some other cancers [49]. It is not fully understood how each diet and nutrition has effects on carcinogenesis, a diet with enough vegetables and fruits, less lean and processed meat, reduced carbohydrate and fat to prevent obesity, and low in salt might be useful to reduce cancer incidence.

9. Alcohol, cigarette smoking, and cancer

In 2017, the American Society of Clinical Oncology announced that alcohol drinking had been established as a risk factor for cancer, and avoiding excessive

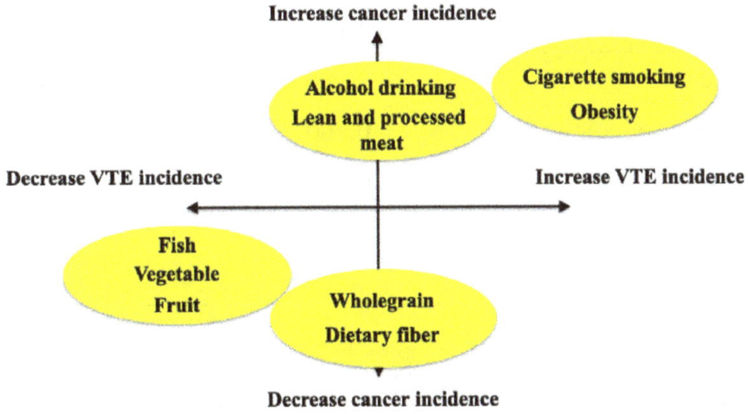

Figure 2.
Effects of diets and lifestyle on cancer and venous thromboembolism (VTE). Fish, vegetables, and fruits may decrease the incidences of both cancer and VTE. Cigarette smoking and obesity increase the incidences of both cancer and VTE. Drinking alcohol and consuming lean and processed meat increase the incidence of cancer. Whole grain and dietary fiber decrease the incidence of cancer.

drinking was important to prevent cancer [50]. The development of pharyngeal, laryngeal, esophageal, liver, breast, and colorectal cancer was obviously related to alcohol drinking. The incidence of esophageal cancer was 1.3 times higher for small drinkers, 2.2 times for moderate drinkers, and 5 times for heavy drinkers than non-drinkers. Ethanol itself is not carcinogenic, but acetaldehyde, its metabolite, binds to DNA and proteins to be carcinogenic and mutagenic. It is proven that administra-tion of large amount of ethanol or acetaldehyde causes cancer in animal experi-ments [51]. Acetaldehyde is metabolized by aldehyde dehydrogenase 2 (ALDH2). Higher percentage of Japanese people has inactive form of ALDH2 compared to the Western. It might result in adverse effects of alcohol drinking on carcinogenesis in Japanese population.

Smoking is a well-known risk factor for cancer. The International Agency for Research on Cancer (IRAC) assessed causal relationships in 2009 and stated that smoking is related to oral, pharyngeal, laryngeal, esophageal, lung, gastric, colon, liver, pancreatic, renal cell, renal pelvis, ureter, bladder, cervical, and ovarian cancer and chronic myelogenous leukemia. Passive smoking is a risk factor for lung cancer [52]. To prevent cancer of yourself, your family, and your colleagues, no smoking is mandatory (**Figure 2**).

10. Aspirin and cancer

Aspirin is a widely used antiplatelet drug that inhibits platelets' cyclooxygenase (COX), resulting in decreased platelet aggregation. Numerous studies have demonstrated the effects of aspirin on the secondary prevention of arterial thrombosis, and several studies have investigated the effects of aspirin use for the primary prevention of atherosclerotic diseases. Meta-analyses of these studies have shown that daily regular aspirin use reduce the incidence of colon colon cancancer, mortality cer, and mof etastasis of colon cancer. The incidenc e or mo rtality of other types of cancer might also be reduced [53–55]. Increased COX expression results in tumor growth and progression, and inhibition of COX reduces carcinogenesis in animal experiments. Platelets are known to play an important role in tumormetastasis [56]. These might be related to the inhibitory effects of aspirin on cancer

Representative reports of large-scale meta-analysis		
Outcome	HR	Reference
Incidnce of colon cancer	0.76(0.60 – 0.96)	[53]
Death due to colon cancer	0.65(0.48 – 0.88)	[53]
Death due to cancer	0.79(0.68 – 0.92)	[54]
Cancer with disant metastasis	0.64(0.48 – 0.84)	[55]
Recent publications		
Outcome	HR	Reference
Incidence of cacer	1.24(1.06 –1.46)	[57]
Death due to cancer	1.08(0.85 –1.38)	[57]
Death due to cancer	1.31(1.10 –1.56)	[58]
Incidence of cacer	1.01(0.92 –1.11)	[59]

HR: Hazard ratio (aspirin vs placebo or no-aspirin).

Table 3.
Effects of aspirin on cancer incidence and cancer mortality.

regular aspirin use does not decrease cancer incidence or cancer mortality [57–59] (**Table 3**). Further studies are needed to confirm the effects of aspirin on cancer incidence and cancer mortality.

11. Conclusion

Various factors are involved in carcinogenesis and occurrence of cancer-associated VTE. Certain diets and nutrition may reduce the risk of VTE. Some lifestyles may reduce cancer incidence, and other lifestyles increase the risk of cancer. Further studies are needed to create ideal diet, nutrition, and lifestyle to reduce the risk of cancer and cancer-associated VTE.

Author details

Kenji Yokoyama
Department of Hematology/Oncology, Tokai University Hachioji, Hachioji, Japan

*Address all correspondence to: yk092750@tsc.u-tokai.ac.jp

References

[1] Available from: https://ganjoho.jp/reg_stat/statistics/stat/short_pred.html

[2] Khorana AA, Francis CW, Culakova E, Lyman GH. Risk factors for chemotherapy-associated venous thromboembolism in a prospective observational study. Cancer. 2005;**104**:2822-2829

[3] Khorana AA, Francis CW, Culakova E, Kuderer NM, Lyman GH. Frequency, risk factors, and trends for venous thromboembolism among hospitalized cancer patients. Cancer. 2007;**110**:2339-2346

[4] Eichinger S. Cancer associated thrombosis: Risk factors and outcomes. Thrombosis Research. 2016;**140**:S12-S17

[5] Trousseau A. Phlegmasia alba dolens. In: Clinique Medicale de L'hotel-dieu de Paris. 2nd ed. Vol. 3. Paris, France: J.-B. Bailliere et fils; 1865. pp. 654-712

[6] Naess IA, Christiansen SC, et al. Incidence and mortality of venous thrombosis: A population-based study. Journal of Thrombosis and Haemostasis. 2007;**5**:692-699

[7] Stein PD, Kayali F, et al. Pulmonary thromboembolism in Asians/Pacific islanders in the United States: Analysis of data from the National Hospital Discharge Survey and the United States Bureau of the Census. The American Journal of Medicine. 2004;**116**:435-442

[8] Nakamura M, Yamada N, et al. Current management of venous thromboembolism in Japan: Current epidemiology and advances in anticoagulant therapy. Journal of Cardiology. 2015;**66**:451-459

[9] Blom JW, Doggen CJ, et al. Malignancies, prothrombotic mutations, and the risk of venous thrombosis. JAMA. 2005;**293**:715-722

[10] Khorana AA, Francis CW, et al. Thromboembolism in hospitalized neutropenic cancer patients. Journal of Clinical Oncology. 2006;**24**:484-490

[11] Khorana AA, Francis CW, et al. Risk factors for chemotherapy-associated venous thromboembolism in a prospective observational study. Cancer. 2005;**104**:2822-2829

[12] Al AD. Cancer-related venous thromboembolism: Insight into underestimated risk factors. Hematology Oncology and Stem Cell Therapy. 2010;**3**:191-195

[13] Horsted F, West J, et al. Risk of venous thromboembolism in patients with cancer: A systematic review and meta-analysis. PLoS Medicine. 2012;**9**:e1001275

[14] Dickmann B, Ahlbrecht J, et al. Regional lymph node metastases are a strong risk factor for venous thromboembolism: Results from the Vienna cancer and thrombosis study. Haematologica. 2013;**98**:1309-1314

[15] Blom JW, Osanto S, et al. The risk of a venous thrombotic event in lung cancer patients: Higher risk for adenocarcinoma than squamous cell carcinoma. Journal of Thrombosis and Haemostasis. 2004;**2**:1760-1765

[16] Mahajan A, Wun T, et al. Lymphoma and venous thromboembolism: Influence on mortality. Thrombosis Research. 2014;**133**(Suppl 2):S23-S28

[17] Caruso V, Di Castelnuvo A, et al. Thrombotic complications in adult patients with lymphoma: A meta-analysis of 29 independent cohorts including 18 018 patients and 1149 events. Blood. 2010;**115**:5322-5328

[18] Available from: http://j-circ. or.jp/guideline/pdf/JCS2017_ito_h.pdf#search=%27

[19] Agnelli G, Bolis G, et al. A clinical outcome-based prospective study on venous thromboembolism after cancer surgery. The @RISTOS project. Annals of Surgery. 2006;**243**:89-95

[20] Verso M, Agnelli G. Venous thromboembolism associated with long-term use of central venous catheters in cancer patients. Journal of Clinical Oncology. 2003;**21**:3665-3675

[21] Khorana AA, Kuderer MM, et al. Development and validation of a predictive model for chemotherapy-associated thrombosis. Blood. 2008;**111**:4902-4907

[22] Granger JM, Kontoyiannis DP. Etiology and outcome of extreme leukocytosis in 758 nonhematologic cancer patients: A retrospective, single-institution study. Cancer. 2009;**115**:3919-3923

[23] Kasuga I, Makino S, et al. Tumor-related leukocytosis is linked with poor prognosis in patients with lung carcinoma. Cancer. 2001;**92**:2399-2405

[24] Olsson AK, Cedervall J. NETosis in cancer - platelet-neutrophil crosstalk promotes tumor-associated pathology. Frontiers in Immunology. 2016;**21**:373

[25] Massberg S, Grahl L, et al. Reciprocal coupling of coagulation and innate immunity via neutrophil serine proteases. Nature Medicine. 2010;**16**:887-896

[26] Jensvoll H, Blix K, et al. Platelet count measured prior to cancer development is a risk factor for future symptomatic venous thromboembolism: The Tromsø study. PLoS One. 2014;**9**:e92011

[27] Simanek R, Vormittag R, et al. High platelet count associated with venous thromboembolism in cancer patients: Results from the Vienna cancer and thrombosis study (CATS). Journal of Thrombosis and Haemostasis. 2010;**8**:114-120

[28] Riedl J, Hell L. Association of platelet activation markers with cancer-associated venous thromboembolism. Platelets. 2016;**27**:80-85

[29] Poruk KE, Firpo MA, et al. Serum platelet factor 4 is an independent predictor of survival and venous thromboembolism in patients with pancreatic adenocarcinoma. Cancer Epidemiology, Biomarkers & Prevention. 2010;**19**:2605-2610

[30] Khorana AA, Adhrendt SA, et al. Tissue factor expression, angiogenesis, and thrombosis in pancreatic cancer. Clinical Cancer Research. 2007;**13**:2870-2875

[31] Khorana AA, Francis CW, et al. Plasma tissue factor may be predictive of venous thromboembolism in pancreatic cancer. Journal of Thrombosis and Haemostasis. 2008;**6**:1983-1985

[32] Suzuki-Inoue K, Inoue O, et al. Novel platelet activation receptor CLEC-2: From discovery to prospects. Journal of Thrombosis and Haemostasis. 2011;**9**(S1):44-55

[33] Watson SP, Herbert JM, et al. GPVI and CLEC-2 in hemostasis and vascular integrity. Journal of Thrombosis and Haemostasis. 2010;**8**:1456-1467

[34] Riedl J, Preusser M, et al. Podoplanin expression in primary brain tumors induces platelet aggregation and increases risk of venous thromboembolism. Blood. 2017;**129**:1831-1839

[35] Ay C, Simanek R, et al. High plasma levels of soluble P-selectin are predictive of venous thromboembolism in cancer

patients: Results from the Vienna cancer and thrombosis study (CATS). Blood. 2008;**112**:2703-2708

[36] Thomas GM, Panicot-Dubois L, et al. Cancer cell-derived microparticles bearing P-selectin glycoprotein ligand 1 accelerate thrombus formation in vivo. The Journal of Experimental Medicine. 2009;**206**:913-1927

[37] Andren-Sandberg A, Lecander I, et al. Peaks in plasma plasminogen activator inhibitor-1 concentration may explain thrombotic events in cases of pancreatic carcinoma. Cancer. 1992;**69**:2884-2887

[38] Chen N, Ren M, et al. Bevacizumab promotes venous thromboembolism through the induction of PAI-1 in a mouse xenograft model of human lung carcinoma. Molecular Cancer. 2015;**14**:1-7

[39] Lloyd-Jones DM, Hong Y, et al. Defining and setting national goals for cardiovascular health promotion and disease reduction: The American Heart Association's strategic impact goal through 2020 and beyond. Circulation. 2010;**121**:586-613

[40] Mahmoodi BK, Cushman M, et al. Association of traditional cardiovascular risk factors with venous thromboembolism: An individual participant data meta-analysis of prospective studies. Circulation. 2017;**135**:7-16

[41] Lindstrom S, Germain M, et al. Assessing the causal relationship between obesity and venous thromboembolism through a Mendelian randomization study. Human Genetics. 2017;**136**:897-902

[42] Hansen-Krone IJ, Enga KF, et al. High fish plus fish oil intake is associated with slightly reduced risk of venous thromboembolism: The Tromsø study. The Journal of Nutrition. 2014;**144**:861-867

[43] Steffen LM, Folsom AR, et al. Greater fish, fruit, and vegetable intakes are related to lower incidence of venous thromboembolism: The longitudinal investigation of thromboembolism etiology. Circulation. 2007;**115**:188-195

[44] Ammollo CT, Semeraro F, et al. Grape intake reduces thrombin generation and enhances plasma fibrinolysis. Potential role of circulating procoagulant microparticles. The Journal of Nutritional Biochemistry. 2017;**50**:66-73

[45] Rahamon SK, Fabian UA, et al. Changes in mediators of inflammation and pro-thrombosis after 12 months of dietary modification in adults with metabolic syndrome. African Health Sciences. 2017;**17**:453-462

[46] Lutsey PL, Steffen LM, et al. Diet and incident venous thromboembolism: The Iowa Women's health study. American Heart Journal. 2009;**157**:1081-1087

[47] Harrington LB, Hagan KA, et al. Alcohol consumption and the risk of incident pulmonary embolism in US women and men. Journal of Thrombosis and Haemostasis. 2018;**16**:1753-1762

[48] Inoue M, Sawada N, et al. Attributable causes of cancer in Japan in 2005--systematic assessment to estimate current burden of cancer attributable to known preventable risk factors in Japan. Annals of Oncology. 2012;**23**:1362-1369

[49] Available from: https://www.wcrf.org/dietandcancer/interactive-cancer-risk-matrix

[50] LoConte NK, Brewster AM, et al. Alcohol and cancer: A statement of the American Society of Clinical Oncology. Journal of Clinical Oncology. 2018;**36**:83-93

[51] Poschl G, Seitz HK. Alcohol and cancer. Alcohol and Alcoholism. 2004;**39**:155-165

[52] Available from: https://monographs.iarc.fr/wp-content/uploads/2018/06/mono100E-6.pdf#search=%27IRAC、2009%2C+smoking%27

[53] Rothwell PM, Wilson M, et al. Long-term effect of aspirin on colorectal cancer incidence and mortality: 20-year follow-up of five randomized trials. Lancet. 2010;**376**:1741-1750

[54] Rothwell PM, Fowkes FG, et al. Effect of daily aspirin on long-term risk of death due to cancer: Analysis of individual patient data from randomised trials. Lancet. 2011;**377**:31-41

[55] Rothwell PM, Wilson M, et al. Effect of daily aspirin on risk of cancer metastasis: A study of incident cancers during randomised controlled trials. Lancet. 2012;**379**:1591-1601

[56] Santilli F, Boccatonda A, et al. Aspirin, platelets, and cancer: The point of view of the internist. European Journal of Internal Medicine. 2016;**34**:11-20

[57] Yokoyama K, Ishizuka N, et al. Effects of daily aspirin on cancer incidence and mortality in the elderly Japanese. Research and Practice in Thrombosis and Haemostasis. 2018;**2**:274-281

[58] McNeil JJ, Nelson MR, et al. Effect of aspirin on all-cause mortality in the healthy elderly. The New England Journal of Medicine. 2018;**379**:1519-1528

[59] Bowman L, Mafham M, et al. Effects of aspirin for primary prevention in persons with diabetes mellitus. The New England Journal of Medicine. 2018;**379**:1529-1539

12

Lipid Peroxidation as a Link between Unhealthy Diets and the Metabolic Syndrome

Arnold N. Onyango

Abstract

Unhealthy diets, such as those high in saturated fat and sugar accelerate the development of non-communicable diseases. The metabolic syndrome is a conglomeration of disorders such as abdominal obesity, hypertension, impaired glucose regulation and dyslipidemia, which increases the risk for diabetes and cardiovascular disease. The prevalence of the metabolic syndrome is increasing globally, and dietary interventions may help to reverse this trend. A good understanding of its pathophysiological mechanisms is needed for the proper design of such interventions. This chapter discusses how lipid peroxidation is associated with the development of this syndrome, mainly through the formation of bioactive aldehydes, such as 4-hydroxy-2-nonenal, malondialdehyde, acrolein and glyoxal, which modify biomolecules to induce cellular dysfunction, including the enhancement of oxidative stress and inflammatory signaling. It gives a current understanding of the mechanisms of formation of these aldehydes and how dietary components such as saturated fatty acids promote oxidative stress, leading to lipid oxidation. It also outlines mechanisms, apart from free radical scavenging and singlet oxygen quenching, by which various dietary constituents prevent oxidative stress and lipid oxidation in vivo.

Keywords: Oxidative stress, lipid peroxidation, insulin resistance; metabolic syndrome

1. Introduction

The metabolic syndrome (MS) refers to the occurrence in an individual of multiple physiological disorders related to obesity, hypertension, dysregulated blood glucose and dysregulated blood lipids, and is a risk factor for diabetes and cardiovascular disease [1]. It has been defined more specifically, and in slightly different ways by the National Cholesterol Education Program (NCEP) Adult Treatment Panel III, and by the World Health Organization (WHO). According to the former, MS is characterized by at least three of the following five clinical or biochemical abnormalities: abdominal obesity, arterial hypertension, elevated fasting blood glucose, high plasma triglycerides, and reduced high density lipoprotein cholesterol (HDL-c) [2]. On the other hand, WHO defined it as the occurrence of impaired glu-cose tolerance or impaired fasting glucose or diabetes and any two of the following: hypertension; elevated trigycerides or low HDL-c; abdominal obesity or obesity as determined by BMI; or microalbuminaria [1].

A proper understanding of the etiology of MS is necessary for its prevention and treatment. This chapter focuses on the role of lipid peroxidation in this pathophysiological process. It begins with a current understanding of the mechanisms of lipid oxidation, with emphasis on the formation of highly reactive lipid oxidation products such as 4-hydroxy-2-nonenal, malondialdehyde, acrolein and glyoxal. This is followed by a discussion of how these aldehydes and other lipid oxidation products contribute to the different MS components. The role of major dietary components in the initiation of oxidative stress and lipid oxidation, as well as mechanisms by which specific dietary components inhibit such undesirable events are also discussed.

2. Mechanisms of lipid peroxidation (LPO) and the formation of bioactive lipid oxidation products

In cells, extensive lipid oxidation and the accumulation of lipid oxidation products occurs under conditions of oxidative stress, when the concentrations of reactive oxygen species (ROS) such as superoxide anions, hydrogen peroxide and singlet oxygen increase, and are not matched by an increase in the cellular antioxidant capacity [3]. Electron leakage from the mitochondrial electron transport chain, or the actions of enzymes such as NADPH oxidases and xanthine oxidase generate superoxide anions ($^{\cdot-}O_2$), which are converted by superoxide dismutase to hydrogen peroxide (H_2O_2), which may be converted by ferrous ions (Fe^{2+}) to hydroxyl radicals (·OH) according to the Fenton reaction Eq. (1). Superoxide anion also reacts with nitric oxide (NO), formed by nitric oxide synthases, to form the highly reactive peroxynitrite anion (-OONO), which reacts with H_2O_2 to form sin-glet oxygen according to Eq. (2), and this is only one of many possible mechanisms of formation of singlet oxygen in biological systems [4–6].

$$\mathrm{HOOH} + Fe^{2+} \rightarrow Fe^{3+} + {}^{-}\mathrm{OH} + HO^{\cdot} \tag{1}$$

$$\mathrm{ONOO}^{-} + \mathrm{HOOH} \rightarrow {}^{1}\mathrm{O}_2 + ONO^{-} + \mathrm{H_2O} \tag{2}$$

Lipid peroxidation involves a reaction between unsaturated lipids and oxygen. This may be enzyme-catalysed or non-enzymatic. Non-enzymatic lipid oxidation is either mediated by singlet oxygen, or it may involve free radical oxidation [7]. Singlet oxygen reacts by electrophilic addition to any of the double bonds in an unsaturated fatty acid such as linoleic acid (LA) to form hydroperoxide isomers such as the 10-, 12- and 13-LA hydroperoxides (10-LA-OOH, 12-LA-OOH and 13-LAOOH) as shown in **Figure 1**.

On the other hand, free radical oxidation begins by the abstraction of a hydrogen atom from a fatty acid, for example by the hydroxyl radical, to form a carbon centred radical, which rearranges to form a relatively stable conjugated radical (**Figure 2**). The latter reacts with oxygen to form a peroxyl radical, which abstracts a hydrogen from another fatty acid molecule to form a hydroperoxide and a new carbon centred radical, hence establishing a free radical chain reaction (**Figure 2**).

A fatty acid hydroperoxide can be converted to an alkoxyl radical by Fe^{2+} (**Figure 3**), in analogy to the conversion of H_2O_2 to the hydroxyl radical accord-ing to Eq. (1). The alkoxyl radical can be converted to a number of non-aldehydic products, including a hydroxy acid and a keto-acid, or it can cyclize to form an epoxy-allylic radical whose further oxygenation affords a hydroperoxy-epoxide

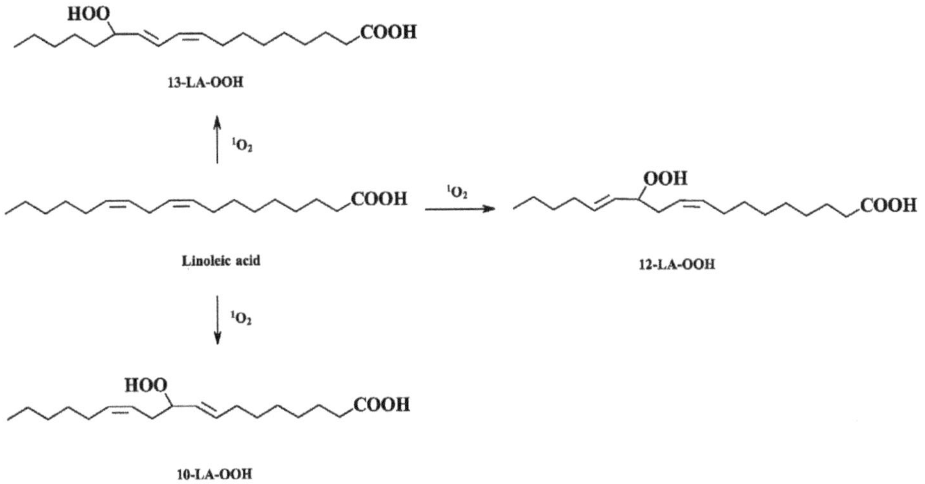

Figure 1.
Formation of different hydroperoxide isomers by the singlet oxygen-mediated oxidation of linoleic acid.

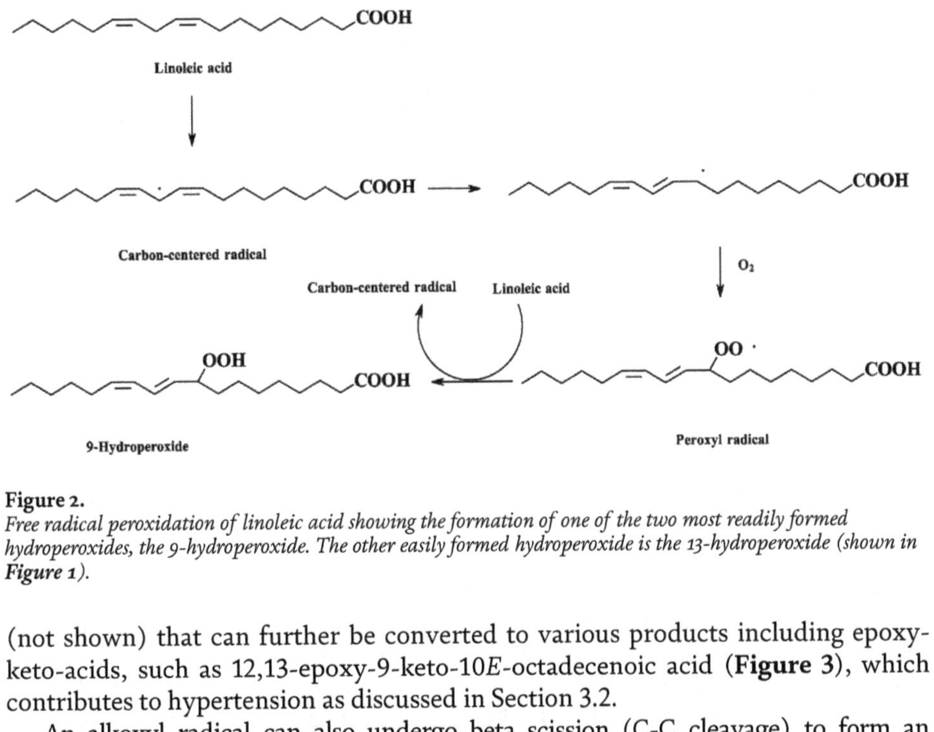

Figure 2.
*Free radical peroxidation of linoleic acid showing the formation of one of the two most readily formed hydroperoxides, the 9-hydroperoxide. The other easily formed hydroperoxide is the 13-hydroperoxide (shown in **Figure 1**).*

(not shown) that can further be converted to various products including epoxy-keto-acids, such as 12,13-epoxy-9-keto-10*E*-octadecenoic acid (**Figure 3**), which contributes to hypertension as discussed in Section 3.2.

An alkoxyl radical can also undergo beta scission (C-C cleavage) to form an aldehyde and a carbon centred radical, and this is only facile if the latter is a resonance stabilized allylic radical, such as would be formed from the 10-LA-OOH (**Figure 4**) or 12-LA-OOH but not 13-LA-OOH [8]. Beta scission is also facile if the carbon bearing the alkoxyl radical occurs next to another oxygen-bearing carbon [9]. Various pathways fulfilling these conditions have been proposed for the formation of the major bioactive lipid-derived aldehydes such as MDA, HNE, acrolein and glyoxal [9, 10].

Acrolein is mainly formed from PUFAS with more than two double bonds, such as arachidonic acid, eicosapentaenoic acid (EPA), docosapentaenoic acid (DPA) and docosahexaenoic acid (DHA) [9]. **Figure 5** shows examples of how MDA, HNE and glyoxal can all be formed from linoleic acid, the most abundant PUFA in most human tissues [3–6]. It starts with the 13-LA-OOH, formed by singlet

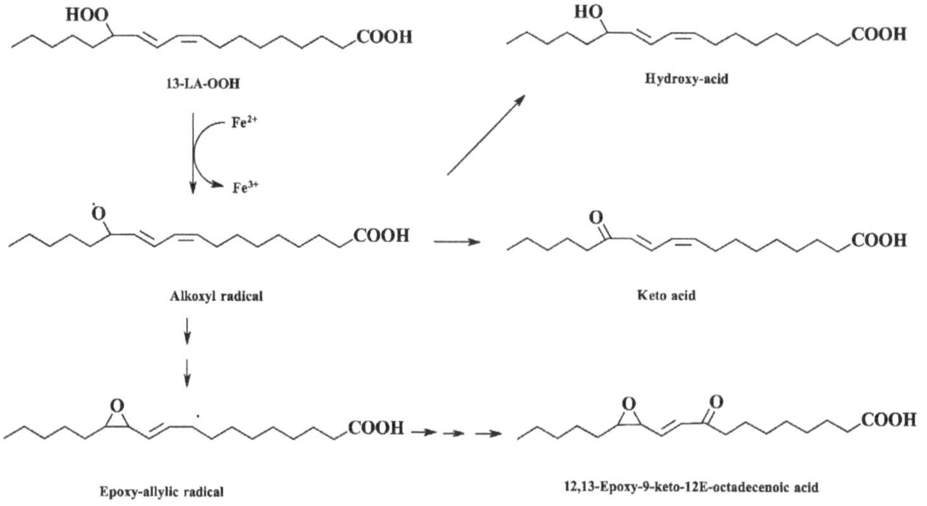

Figure 3.
Conversion of the 13-hydroperoxide of linoleic acid (13-LA-OOH) via the corresponding alkoxyl radical to different types of non-aldehydic products.

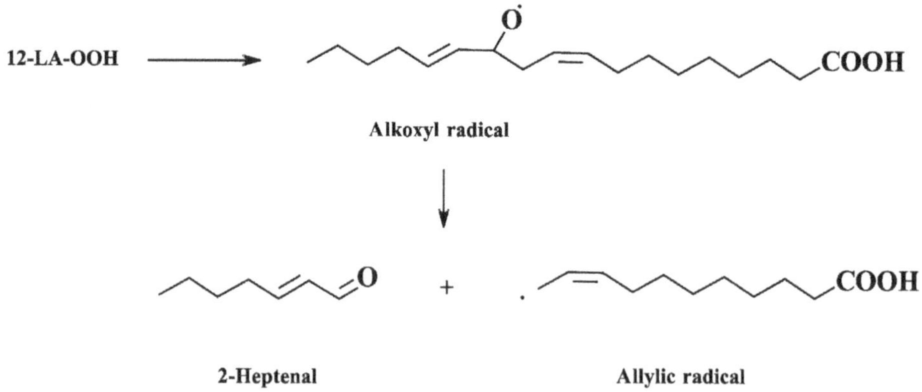

Figure 4.
b-Scission of an alkoxy radical to form an aldehyde (2-heptenal) and an allylic radical. Scission on the other side of the alkoxyl radical to form a vinyl radical and 12-oxo-9-dodecenoic acid is energetically unfavourable.

oxygen -mediated or free radical oxidation, which further reacts with singlet oxygen to form a hydroperoxy-dioxetane (addition of singlet oxygen to a conjugated double bond system forms dioxetanes rather than hydroperoxides). The dioxetane is unstable, and decomposes to form two aldehydes, namely 9-oxononanoic acid and 4-hydroperoxy-2-nonenal (4-HPNE). The former is one of the predominant products of linoleic acid oxidation, and contributes to hypertension through acti-vating phospholipase A2 (Section 3.2). A primary amine (RNH_2) such as lysine or phosphatidylethanolamine may catalyse the conversion of 4-HPNE via a dioxetanyl anion to a dioxetane whose cleavage affords MDA and hexanal (**Figure 5**). While it has long been known that linoleic acid is a precursor of MDA, albeit not as readily as from more highly unsaturated PUFAS, its mechanism of formation from linoleic acid remained elusive [11]. 4-HPNE can alternatively react with another singlet oxygen molecule to form a hydroperoxy-dioxetanyl aldehyde whose decomposi-tion affords glyoxal and 2-hydroperoxy-heptanal (not shown). 4-HPNE can also be converted to an alkoxyl radical, which can abstract a hydrogen to form 4-HNE, or to an epoxy-alkyl radical which can rearrange to an ether radical whose further

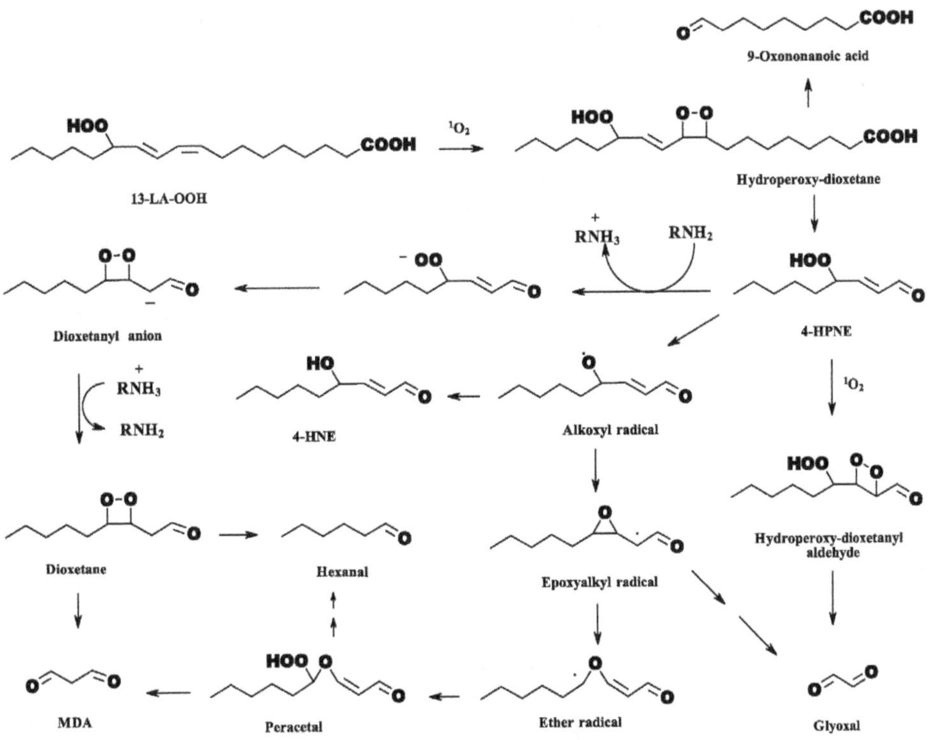

Figure 5.
Mechanisms of the conversion of the 13-hydroperoxide of linoleic acid (LA-OOH) to 4-HNE, MDA, glyoxal, hexanal and 9-oxo-nonanoic acid. Other pathways to these products exist but are not shown.

reaction with oxygen leads to formation of a per acetal that can decompose to MDA and hexane. The epoxy-alkyl radical can also directly react with oxygen to form a hydroperoxy-epoxide whose decomposition affords glyoxal. In the cell, glutathione peroxidase may contribute to the conversion of 4-HPNE to 4-HNE.

3. Lipid peroxidation products contribute to the development of the metabolic syndrome

Lipid oxidation products influence the pathogenesis of metabolic syndrome components such as obesity, hypertension, impaired fasting glucose/diabetes, and dyslipidemia, in various ways [12].

3.1 Obesity

Obesity occurs when adipocytes increase in number and/or size, coupled with increased fat storage and reduced fat oxidation. Adipose tissue (AT) is functionally classified as brown or white (BAT and WAT, respectively). BAT consists of adipocytes specialized for thermogenesis, and hence contribute to reduction of obesity; while WAT, the major type of adipose tissue in humans, has less capacity for fat oxidation, and may contribute to obesity [13]. White adipocytes can exist in or acquire a brown-like (beige or brite) phenotype with higher fat oxidation than ordinary white adipocytes, and a higher number of beige adipocytes reduces an individual's susceptibility to obesity [13]. Expansion of WAT by differentiation of preadipocytes (hyperplasia) into mature adipocytes with adequate lipid filling and fat oxidation capacity is beneficial for safe storage of fat; but mere expansion of mature adipocytes because of excessive lipid filling and reduced fat oxidation (hypertrophy) is associated with adverse health outcomes.

A certain amount of ROS is required for proper preadipocyte and mature adipocyte physiology. However, oxidative stress and excessive autophagy may inhibit preadipocyte differentiation and promote hypertrophy of mature adipocytes (**Figure 6**) [14]. Likewise, brown or beige adipocytes have many mitochondria for the enhanced fat oxidation, but mitochondrial oxidative stress causes loss of the mitochondria through mitophagy, thus leading to whitening, increased lipid storage and hypertrophy (**Figure 6**) [15]. Adenosine 5-monophosphate kinase (AMPK), sirtuins 1 and 3, protein kinase B (akt), peroxisome proliferator activated receptor gamma and alpha (PPARγ and PPARα, respectively), and PPARγ coactivator-1α (PGC-1α) are among the proteins that reduce oxidative stress and/or promote mitochondrial biogenesis in adipocytes [16, 17]. Both protein kinase A (PKA) and akt are required for PPARγ expression [18], which is required for differentiation of both brown and white adipocytes [19]. PPARγ promotes thermogenesis in mature brown adipocytes through activation of uncoupled protein 1 (UCP-1), and by upregulating glycerol kinase which catalyses glycerol-3-phosphate synthesis, which is required for TG synthesis [20]. While this looks paradoxical, TG synthesis may help reduce the lipotoxicity and oxidative stress induction by free fatty acids (discussed in Section 4), and allow targeted, β-adrenergic signaling-associated release of fatty acids for mitochondrial oxidation. AMPK activates autophagy and induces the transcription factor nrf2; and the latter upregulates antioxidant enzymes such as catalase, glutathione peroxidase, superoxide dismutase and heme oxygenase 1 [21]. Sirt1, which is mainly localized in the nucleus, increases the expression catalase and SOD as reviewed by Iside et al. [22]. In addition, it upregulates autophagy genes, and autophagy defect associated with its inhibition promotes release of exosomes which induce toll-like receptor 4 (TLR4) signaling, downstream activation of nuclear factor kappa B (NF-kB), and NF-kB-mediated upregulation of oxidative stress and inflammation-promoting genes [23].

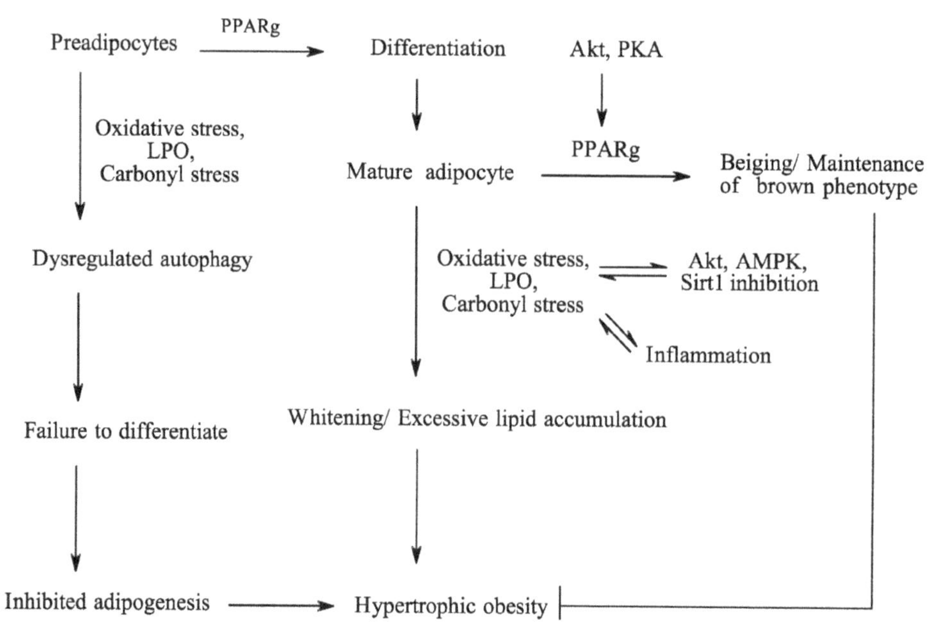

Figure 6.
Role of oxidative stress and lipid oxidation-induced carbonyl stress in the pathogenesis of hypertrophic obesity.

Conditions that promote adipose tissue oxidative stress, including inappropriate diets (Section 4), induce lipid oxidation, and the latter generates carbonyl stress due to formation of various aldehydes as explained in Section 2. These aldehydes, including HNE and acrolein modify and inhibit AMPK and sirt1, thus amplifying oxidative stress and their own formation (**Figure 6**) [24–26]. HNE also carbonylates insulin receptor substrate1/2 (IRS1), leading to degradation and inhibition of the latter, thus inducing insulin resistance and downstream akt inhibition [27]. Thus, insulin resistant obese individuals have lower akt, AMPK ad sirt1 activity, but higher reactive carbonyls and carbonylated proteins [28]. Acrolein and HNE additionally aggravate oxidative stress through readily reacting with, and depleting the antioxidant glutathione [29, 30]. They modify the endoplasmic reticulum calcium pump SERCA, leading to its inhibition and ER stress [3], which aggravates oxidative stress, insulin resistance, sirt1 inhibition, expression of the pro-inflammatory cytokines, TNFα and IL6, and adipocyte whitening [31, 32]. Glutathionylated HNE and other aldehydes released from adipocytes under conditions of oxidative stress promote macrophage infiltration into WAT, and their acquisition of a proinflammatory M1 phenotype [33]. Malondialdehyde reacts with albumin, and the MDA-albumin conjugates promote a proinflammatory phenotype in macrophages and T cells [34]. Cytokines such as interleukin1-β, released from inflammatory macrophages, in turn promote adipocyte oxidative stress and whitening [35].

3.2 Hypertension

Arterial hypertension occurs because of (i) increased renal retention of sodium and water (ii) dysregulation of vasodilators and vasoconstrictors and (iii) arte-rial stiffness. Obesity is a major risk factor for hypertension [36]. For example, adiponectin inhibits adrenal production of aldosterone, a potent inducer of hypertension [37], but obesity reduces adiponectin secretion and increases circulating aldosterone [38]. Thus, by promoting obesity, lipid peroxidation products indirectly promote hypertension. However, they also induce hypertension independently of obesity. For example, the non-aldehydic linoleic acid oxidation product, 12,13-epoxy-9-keto-10-*E*-octadecenoic acid (Shown in **Figure 3**) also promotes adrenal production of aldosterone to induce hypertension [39].

Aldosterone binds to the renal tubular epithelial cell mineralocorticoid receptor, which, as a transcription factor, upregulates the expression of the epithelial sodium channel, which promotes sodium retention [40]. Independently of gene transcription, aldosterone activates the non-receptor tyrosine kinase cSrc in these cells, probably through the angiotensin receptor type 1 (AT1R), and cSrc activates epidermal growth factor receptor (EGFR) signaling, leading to activation of the mitogen activated protein kinase Erk1/2 [40]. Erk1/2 activates Na^+/K^+ ATPase, which promotes sodium and water retention [41]. Aldosterone-cSrc signaling also induces oxidative stress [40], which induces formation of lipid oxidation products. 4-HNE, inhibits AMPK and sirt1, thus inhibiting eNOS, leading to reduced NO bioavailability, and this causes increased transactivation of EGFR and downstream Erk1/2 [42–44]. Thus, blood HNE levels are increased in hypertension [45], and the latter can be ameliorated by carbonyl quenching [46]. Oxidized low density lipoprotein, which contains oxidatively modified lipids such as HNE, induces oxidative stress in renal tubular endothelial cells, which activates the renal renin-angiotensin system (RAS); whose component, angiotensin 2, overstimulates sodium transporters and thus induces hypertension [47, 48]. Hypertension in turn promotes oxidative stress and LDL oxidation, thereby creating a vicious circle [49].

Inhibition of endothelial cell sirt1, sirt3 and AMPK, which can be mediated by LPO products, causes inhibition of endothelial nitric oxide synthase (eNOS) and decreases production of NO, the main arterial vasodilator [50–52]. HNE induces endothelial cell insulin resistance, and the associated akt inhibition both inhibits eNOS and upregulates the vasoconstrictor, endothelin [3, 53]. The dysfunctional endothelial cells further produce pro-inflammatory factors such as TNFα, IL-1β, IL-8 and MCP-1 which recruit circulating neutrophils, platelets and monocytes, and the latter differentiate into macrophages [53, 54]. Neutrophils, monocytes and macrophages secrete myeloperoxidase [55]. Myeloperoxidase oxidizes LDL [56]. It also promotes the activation of endothelial cyp4a12a, which catalyzes the formation of 20-hydroxy-eicosatetraenoic acid (20-HETE) from arachidonic acid [57]. 20-HETE upregulates endothelial RAS components including angiotensin 2, a potent vasoconstrictor, which also induces aldosterone secretion [58]. Both angio-tensin 2 and aldosterone aggravate endothelial oxidative stress and dysfunction. Androgens promote 20-HETE synthesis, and this may explain the higher occur-rence of hypertension in men than women [58].

Stiffness of the coronary artery and other major arteries inhibits their systolic dilatation, and thus promotes systolic hypertension [59]. Degradation of the elastic fiber, elastin, in the walls of the major arteries, and its replacement with collagen fibres is a hallmark of the pathogenesis of arterial stiffness [59]. The myeloper-oxidase product, 20-HETE, activates matrix metalloproteinase 12 (MMP-12, macrophage elastase), which degrades elastin [60]. Myeloperoxidase additionally inhibits the elastase inhibitor, α1, and this is antagonized by sulfur compounds such as glutathione [61]. Acrolein and HNE, on the other hand, deplete glutathione [62]. 20-HETE additionally sensitizes vascular smooth muscle cells to stimuli that promote their dedifferentiation and proliferation [58], which contributes to arterial stiffening especially of the muscular arteries [63]. One of the most readily formed aldehydic linoleic acid oxidation products, 9-oxononanoic acid (**Figure 3**) activates phospholipase A2 (PLA_2) leading to generation of eicosanoids and thromboxane A2 in blood [64]. Thromboxane A_2 causes vasoconstriction and the proliferation of smooth muscle cells [65].

Malondialdehyde forms collagen crosslinks that prevent collagen degradation, thus promoting arterial stiffness [66]. Thus, MDA-modified LDL independently predicts arterial stiffness [67]. Glyoxal contributes to arterial stiffness by reacting with collagen to form advanced glycation end products such as GOLA, GOLD, GODIC and carboxymethyl lysine (CML) [68]. CML induces endothelial oxidative stress through the RAGE receptor, which activates components of NF-kB signaling that promote expression of collagen 1 and 2 [69, 70].

3.3 Dyslipidemia

Dyslipidemia in metabolic syndrome is defined by elevated circulating triglycerides (hypertriglyceridemia) or low levels of high-density lipoprotein cholesterol (low HDLc); and hepatic steatosis, a component of non-alcoholic fatty liver disease (NAFLD) is its main risk factor [71]. This is because, in hepatic steatosis, there occurs greater production and secretion of triglyceride-rich very low-density lipoproteins (VLDL), leading to hypertriglyceridemia; as well as higher hepatic lipase activity, which increases the hepatic uptake and degradation of HDL [71]. Hepatocyte oxidative stress, ER stress and associated lipid peroxidation are involved in the development of hepatic steatosis [72, 73], and this makes lipid peroxidation an important factor in the development of dyslipidemia [74].

Low HDLc also occurs in obesity independently of elevated triglyc-erides, indicating that it occurs even independently of NAFLD [75]. Hypoadiponectinemia, which depends on obesity rather than NAFLD [76], may cause reduced HDLc through increased hepatic lipase activity; reduced hepatic expression of the HDL protein apo A; reduced expression of the cholesterol export protein ABCA1 which transfers cholesterol to HDL; and upregulated synthesis of LCAT which transfers cholesterol from HDLc to chylomicrons [77]. Obesity is also associated with increased plasma TNFα [78] which suppresses hepatocyte apo AI gene expression via ERK and JNK [79]. HNE contributes to JNK over-activation in hepatocytes [80].

3.4 Prediabetes and diabetes

Diabetes is a state of elevated postprandial and/or fasting blood glucose that, if not controlled, leads to the damage of various organs; while prediabetes refers to an intermediate level of fasting and/or postprandial blood glucose, higher than normal but less than diabetic blood glucose levels [1]. It is an earlier stage toward the development of diabetes, but which can revert to normoglycemia. The major causes of (pre)diabetes are pancreatic alpha and beta cell dysfunctions leading to glucagon over-secretion and insulin under-secretion, respectively; coupled with skeletal muscle, adipose and/or hepatic insulin resistance [81].

Both obesity and hypertension contribute to the pathogenesis of prediabetes, hence the lipid oxidation products that induce obesity and hypertension indirectly promote diabetes thereby. Nevertheless, lipid oxidation products also directly promote (pre)diabetes. For example, malondialdehyde was found to dose-dependently reduce the insulin content in the pancreas and to contribute to beta cell death [82]. HDL prevents beta cell apoptosis and diabetes by promoting cholesterol efflux from these cells, but acrolein- or MDA-modified HDL loses this protective property [83–85]. oxLDL impairs insulin gene expression and causes death of pancreatic beta cells, through induction of oxidative stress and ER stress [86]. As already discussed, lipid oxidation products induce endothelial dysfunction. Pancreatic endothelial cell dysfunction contributes to diabetes, being associated with leukocyte recruitment and increased production of proinflammatory cytokines [87]. Cytokines such as IL-1β and TNFα induce alpha and beta cell oxidative stress [88] and associated lipid peroxidation. Insulin resistance, which can be induced by HNE and acrolein, is part of the alpha cell and beta cell dysfunctions leading to diabetes [81].

4. Role of dietary constituents in inducing tissue oxidative stress, lipid peroxidation and the metabolic syndrome

Diets high in saturated fatty acids, cholesterol, sugar, salt, and red meat, contribute to higher lipid oxidation in the tissues and organs that have a central role in the metabolic syndrome, such as adipose tissue, endothelial tissue, muscle, liver and pancreas.

Although saturated fatty acids do not undergo peroxidation, they contribute to the induction of oxidative stress in cells, which then leads to peroxidation of unsaturated fatty acids. For example, the most abundant saturated fatty acid in the diet, palmitic acid, is a key substrate for the first reaction in ceramide biosynthesis [89]. Ceramides induce oxidative stress, for example by inhibiting components of the electron transport chain [90].

Palmitate also induces oxidative stress and ER stress independently of ceramide. For example, it increases diacylglycerol levels, which is associated with activation of protein kinase C (PKC), which inhibits the Kreb's cycle enzymes aconitase and isocitrate dehydrogenase [91]. Thus, the acetyl COA generated from peroxisomal and mitochondrial fatty acid beta oxidation accumulates in the cell, promoting acetylation of mammalian target of rapamycin complex (MTORC-1) and high mobility group box-1 (HMGB-1), as has been demonstrated in hepatocytes [92]. Acetylation activates MTORC-1, which inhibits akt and further promotes oxidative stress by upregulating the expression of TLR4, thus upregulating the NF-kB-NADPH oxidase/iNOS axis [92]. Acetylation of HMGB-1 causes its translocation out of the cell, enabling it to induce oxidative stress by interacting with the receptor for advanced glycation end products (RAGE) as well as TLR4, which both induce NF-kB activation [93]. Obesity is associated with increased circulating HMGB-1, which accelerates the pathogenesis of obesity, hypertension and diabetes [72, 73, 94, 95]. TLR2/4 signaling also activates RAS components including angiotensin 2, whose signaling via its receptor AT1R induces NFkB and oxidative stress [3, 96].

PUFAS undergo peroxidation during cooking as well as in the digestive tract [97]. This is more pronounced when they are part of a meal containing meat, especially red meat, which has higher myoglobin content; since iron from the latter promotes lipid oxidation [98]. This leads to a postprandial increase in circulating carbonyls such as malondialdehyde and HNE, which promote oxidative stress, HDL modification and postprandial inflammation [98, 99]. On the other hand, absorbed, unoxidized unsaturated fatty acids including MUFAs and PUFAs reduce palmitate-induced oxidative stress and lipotoxicity in many cell types by promoting the incorporation of palmitate into TGs for safe storage [100–102]. Nevertheless, high concentrations of arachidonic acid also induce deleterious effects. Thus, supplementation of arachidonic acid to a high fat diet led to enhanced obesity in mice [103], which is attributable to the fact that this n-6 fatty acid promotes adipogenesis from preadipocytes, but its cyclooxygenase-mediated oxidation products, prostaglandins E2 and F2a (PGE2 and PGF2a) inhibit browning via ERK activation and associated decrease in UCP-1 expression [104, 105]. These prostaglandins activate NF-kB, diminish adiponectin production, upregulate pro-inflammatory mediators such as TNFα and MCP-1, and thus promote macrophage activation [106]. They promote oxidative stress and lipid oxidation, and the lipid oxidation product HNE in turn induces cyclooxygenase 2 [107]. Adipose inflammation has systemic effects, hence adipose tissue arachidonic acid was found to be independently associated with abdominal obesity, dyslipidemia, hypertension and fasting glucose [108]. Its myeloperoxidase products, 20-HETE is associated with insulin resistance and hyperglycemia [109]. Since humans synthesize arachidonic acid from linoleic acid, the arachidonic acid content in human adipose tissues does not necessarily reflect its dietary intake [110].

Although linoleic acid is a precursor of arachidonic acid, studies of its effects on the metabolic syndrome have given mixed results, with both harmful and protective roles reported [111–113]. The differences are partly due to genetic factors. For example, there are individual and ethnic differences in the expression of fatty acid desaturase 1 and 2 (FADS 1/2); with genotypes favouring greater FADS1/2 activ-ity and arachidonic acid synthesis being associated with greater susceptibility to metabolic dysregulation [114, 115]. Black people and Indians significantly generate arachidonic acid from dietary linoleic acid, unlike people of European origin [114, 116]. A high adipose tissue linoleic: arachidonic acid is inversely associated with cardiovascular mortality and hypertension [112]. Likewise, a low linoleic: arachidonic acid ratio in plasma phospholipids is associated with hypertension [117]. Polymorphisms in the receptor for oxLDL, Lox-1, might also determine differences in the response to increased dietary linoleic acid; since this PUFA increases Lox-1 expression in aortic endothelial cells [118]. The effects of linoleic acid may also be dependent on the overall diet. If the diet is high in other factors that induce oxidative stress such as dietary sugar and salt, the pro-oxidative environment thus created may abrogate potential linoleic acid benefits through its increased oxidation. This is in analogy to the fact that high glycemic index foods abrogate the anti-obesity effects of fish oil [119]. A high linoleic acid diet may also be unfavourable for people who have already developed some component of the metabolic syndrome and thus have a more pro-inflammatory status.

Oleic acid is the major dietary fatty acid in the Mediterranean diet, which is generally associated with health benefits. This fatty acid is relatively resistant to peroxidation. Besides promoting the safe storage of palmitate in TGs, it induces thermogenesis by upregulating adipose triglyceride lipase and hormone sensitive lipase, which induce lipolysis coupled with fatty acid oxidation [120]. It promotes M2 macrophage phenotype in visceral adipose [121].

The dietary n-3 fatty acids are generally highly susceptible to oxidation because they all contain at least 3 double bonds. Although they are not 4-HNE precursors, decomposition of their hydroperoxides very readily produces acrolein, MDA, glyoxal and methylglyoxal. Despite this, they are largely beneficial, suppressing development of the metabolic syndrome [122]. In adipocytes, their binding to the GPR120/Ffar4 receptor inhibits TLR2 and TLR4 signaling and associated NFkB activation, oxidative stress and inflammation [123]. This receptor also upregulates miR-30b and 378, and induces FGF21 secretion, whose signaling activates AMPK, promotes browning and induces adiponectin [123–126]. The n-3 PUFAs are metabolized by cyclooxygenase to resolvins, protectins, maresins and isoprostanes which help in resolving inflammation [127].

A high dietary n-3: n-6 PUFA ratio has been found to be protective against the metabolic syndrome in some studies but not others [128, 129]. This might be partly due to inter-individual differences in the metabolism of n-6 fatty acids.

High carbohydrate diets promote obesity because excess sugars are stored as lipids. High sucrose or high fructose diets are particularly obesogenic [130]. Fructose metabolism robustly increases palmitate synthesis in adipocytes [131]. Moreover, fructose metabolism is associated with decreased cellular ATP, purine degradation and activation of xanthine oxidase which generates reactive oxygen species and associated lipid peroxidation [132], which is involved in adipocyte whitening and less thermogenesis. Uric acid, a product of purine degradation also induces oxidative stress through increased NADPH oxidase activity and RAS activation [131–134].

High salt (sodium chloride) diets promote obesity, by salt-induced activation of adipocyte Na/K+ ATPase, which is coupled to activation of src, which generates ROS, and transactivates PI3-K-Akt–MTOR and EGFR-ERK/MAPK pathways [135, 136]. This is associated with increased expression of proinflammatory mediators such as TNFα, MCP-1, COX-2, IL-17A, IL-6, leptin, and leptin [136, 137]. Sodium chloride also activates Na+/K+ ATPase and induces oxidative stress in endothelial cells and renal tubular epithelial cells, thereby promoting hypertension [132], and this is also subject to genetic susceptibility [138].

High dietary cholesterol is associated with a high risk of dyslipidemia [139]. Cholesterol-rich chylomicron remnants mainly deliver their cholesterol to the liver, and cholesterol accumulation in hepatocytes strongly induces oxidative stress, by modification of the mitochondrial membrane and limiting import of glutathione into the mitochondria, as well by inducing ER stress and proinflammatory cytokines [140].

The lipopolysaccharide (LPS) component of the walls of gram-negative bacteria is a pro-inflammatory molecule that contributes to metabolic low-grade inflamma-tion (endotoxemia), by signaling through TLR2 and 4 in various cell types, leading to NFkB activation and release of pro-inflammatory cytokines. High sucrose and high saturated fat diets promote the growth of gram-negative bacteria, and thus increase the entry of LPS into the circulation [141].

5. Mechanisms of the antioxidant and metabolic syndrome-suppressing effects of dietary factors

While some food components promote a pro-oxidative and pro-inflammatory state as discussed in the previous section, other dietary factors inhibit oxidative stress and inflammation. They do this through various mechanisms, but the most widely considered mechanisms are those associated with lipid oxidation, including scavenging of free radicals such as peroxyl radicals and alkoxyl radicals, chelation of metal ions that participate in formation of such radicals, and singlet oxygen quenching.

5.1 Free radical scavenging and singlet oxygen quenching

Carotenoids, phenolic substances, tocopherols and ascorbic acid are well known for their antioxidant activities targeting the neutralization of reactive radicals and/or singlet oxygen quenching. Thus, carotenoids reduce oxidative stress and lipid oxidation, resulting in adipocyte beiging and obesity prevention [142]. There is decreased adipose beta carotene in obese subjects, and this was suggested to at least partly be due to their depletion under the high ROS environment [142]. Likewise, tocopherols and tocotrienols have been shown to be protective against all components of the metabolic syndrome [143]. Thus, the high tocotrienol content of palm oil may reduce its potential harm from the high palmitate content [144]. Unfortunately, radical scavenging antioxidants also exhibit pro-oxidant activity, depending on their concentrations and the level of prooxidative factors [145]. Hence, there is need to consider a broad range of dietary factors that prevent oxidative by alternative mechanisms, such as those outlined hereafter. A single molecule can act by multiple mechanisms, and the more mechanisms involved, the greater might be the benefit.

5.2 Insulin-mimicking

Insulin signaling activates akt, which reduces oxidative stress by promoting mitophagy and by activating nrf2 to induce antioxidant enzymes [81, 146]. Moreover, nrf2, via heme oxygenase 1 (HO-1), inhibits NFkB and associated upregulation of NADPH oxidase and iNOS [147]. Quercetin and ferulic acid are examples of molecules that have demonstrated oxidative stress and metabolic syndrome amelioration at least partly through PI3K-akt signaling in various cell types [148–150]. Resveratrol and ferulic acid inhibit LPS- and oxidative stress-induced intestinal barrier injury through this signaling pathway [151, 152].

5.3 AMPK and SIRT1 activation

AMPK and/or sirt1 reduce mitochondrial oxidative stress in adipocytes, pancre-atic beta cells, hepatocytes, endothelial cells, and thus are useful in preventing all aspects of the metabolic syndrome. In addition to insulin mimicking, quercetin and ferulic acid, also activate these proteins [153–155].

5.4 Adiponectin and adiponectin receptor enhancement

Compounds that activate AMPK, sirt1 and/or PI3K-akt in adipose tissues limit adipocyte hypertrophy and inflammation, and enhance adiponectin production. Adiponectin has systemic effects in reducing insulin resistance and oxidative stress, because it activates both PI3K-akt and AMPK in insulin target tissues, and also promotes anti-inflammatory polarization of macrophages [156]. Dietary compounds than ameliorate metabolic syndrome through enhanced adiponectin secretion and/or upregulating adiponectin receptor include n3-fatty acids, sesamin, the citrus derived polymethoxyflavonoids nobiletin and tangeretin, quercetin and resveratrol [157–160].

5.5 Ceramide reduction

Adiponectin signaling increases ceramidase activity, thus reducing ceramide levels [161]. Hence, the adiponectin and adiponectin receptor enhancers should contribute to reducing ceramide-induced oxidative stress. Not much research has been done along this line, but it has been reported that DHA inhibits ceramide biosynthesis [162]. In mice, dietary inulin reduces ceramide synthesis by suppressing neutral sphingomyelinase expression and activity [163].

5.6 Vasodilation

Vasodilation reduces blood pressure, and thus reduces pressure-dependent oxidative stress as well as LDL oxidation and Lox-1 dependent oxidative stress [164]. Thus, for people with prehypertension or hypertension, vasodilation may be a major strategy for reducing oxidative stress and lipid oxidation. Cinnamaldehyde has vasodilatory and antihypertensive activity through effects on smooth muscle contractility [165]. Dietary nitrate achieves vasodilation through NO release, and this is associated not only with pressure regulation, but also other components of the metabolic syndrome including blood glucose and lipid improvement [166]. Adiponectin induces AMPK dependent eNOS activation in endothelial cells, hence adiponectin enhancers such as imperatorin also promote NO synthesis and vasodilatation [167].

5.7 Reactive carbonyl, ALEs and AGEs scavenging

Scavengers of reactive carbonyls such as HNE, acrolein and MDA have been demonstrated to ameliorate oxidative stress, lipid peroxidation and the metabolic syndrome. Examples of compounds with such effects include carnosine, carnosinol, epigallocatechin-3-gallate and the mulberry anthocyanins cyanidin 3-glucoside (C3G) and cyanidin 3-rutinoside (C3R) [46, 168–170]. Aminoguanidine attenuates hypertension by scavenging AGES [171].

5.8 Gut microbiota modulation

Probiotic microorganisms suppress the growth of pathogenic microorganisms. They also produce metabolites such as short chain fatty acids with beneficial effects on the metabolic syndrome. For example, butyrate promotes PI3K-akt signaling to prevent oxidative stress and maintain intestinal barrier integrity [172, 173]. Quercetin, resveratrol and n-3 fatty acids have been demonstrated to positively influence gut microbiota and decrease intestinal barrier permeability in animal studies [153, 174].

6. Conclusions

Lipid peroxidation is a major contributor to the pathogenesis of the metabolic syndrome, especially through highly reactive and bioactive aldehydes such as acrolein, 4-hydroxy-2-nonenal, malondialdehyde and glyoxal. Mechanisms of formation of these products are now well-understood. For example, this article has highlighted that formation of MDA from linoleic acid may be easier than previously thought. The mentioned aldehydes propagate oxidative stress and inflammation by inducing insulin resistance, inhibiting sirt1 and AMPK, reducing adiponectin secretion, as well as forming AGEs and ALEs that activate the RAGE receptor. Inhibiting LPO and the LPO product-associated oxidative stress and inflammation is necessary for preventing and/or ameliorating progression of the metabolic syndrome. This may not be effectively accomplished by dietary agents that merely scavenge free radicals and/or quench singlet oxygen, but also by those that inhibit the signaling pathways that generate non-lipid ROS, or scavenge the reactive carbonyls, ALEs and AGEs. In addition, saturated fat, sugar, meat, and salt, that fuel the signaling pathways that initiate LPO should be reduced. The metabolic influence of some dietary compo-nents such as salt and n-6 PUFAs is particularly influenced by genetics, and this should be duly considered when making dietary recommendations.

Author details

Arnold N. Onyango
School of Food and Nutrition Sciences, Jomo Kenyatta University of Agriculture and Technology, Nairobi, Kenya

*Address all correspondence to: arnold.onyango@jkuat.ac.ke

References

[1] Alberti, K. G. M.M, Zimmet, P.Z. for the WHO Consultation (1998). Definition, diagnosis and classification of diabetes mellitus and its complications. Part 1: diagnosis and classification of diabetes mellitus. Provisional report of a WHO Consultation. Diabetic Medicine 1998; 15: 539-553

[2] National Cholesterol Education Program (NCEP): Expert Panel on Detection and Treatment of High Blood Cholesterol in Adults (2002). Third Report of the National Cholesterol Education Program (NCEP) Expert Panel on Detection, Evaluation, and Treatment of High Blood Cholesterol in Adults (Adult Treatment Panel III) final report. Circulation 106, 3143-3421

[3] Onyango, A. N. (2018). Cellular stresses and stress responses in the pathogenesis of insulin resistance. *Oxidative Medicine and Cellular Longevity*, Article ID 4321714.

[4] Onyango, A. N. (2016). Endogenous generation of singlet oxygen and ozone in human and animal tissues: mechanisms, biological significance, and influence of dietary components. Oxidative Medicine and Cellular Longevity, *2016*.

[5] Onyango, A. N. (2016). Formation of aldehydic phosphatidylcholines during the anaerobic decomposition of a phosphatidylcholine bearing the 9-hydroperoxide of linoleic acid. *BioMed Research International*, Article ID 8218439.

[6] Onyango, A. N. (2017). The contribution of singlet oxygen to insulin resistance. *Oxidative Medicine and Cellular Longevity*, Article ID 8765972.

[7] Girotti, A. W. (1985). Mechanisms of lipid peroxidation. Journal of Free Radicals in Biology & Medicine, *1*(2), 87-95.

[8] Onyango, A. N., Inoue, T., Nakajima, S., Baba, N., Kaneko, T., Matsuo, M., & Shimizu, S. (2001). Synthesis and stability of phosphatidylcholines bearing polyenoic acid hydroperoxides at the sn-2 position. Angewandte Chemie International Edition, *40*(9), 1755-1757.

[9] Onyango, A. N. (2012). Small reactive carbonyl compounds as tissue lipid oxidation products; and the mechanisms of their formation thereby. Chemistry and physics of lipids, *165*(7), 777-786.

[10] Schneider, C., Porter, N. A., & Brash, A. R. (2008). Routes to 4-hydroxynonenal: fundamental issues in the mechanisms of lipid peroxidation. Journal of Biological Chemistry, *283*(23), 15539-15543.

[11] Onyango, A. N., & Baba, N. (2010). New hypotheses on the pathways of formation of malondialdehyde and isofurans. Free Radical Biology and Medicine, *49*(10), 1594-1600.

[12] Pillon, N. J., & Soulage, C. O. (2012). Lipid peroxidation by-products and the metabolic syndrome. Lipid peroxidation, 409-436.

[13] Zoico, E., Rubele, S., De Caro, A., Nori, N., Mazzali, G., Fantin, F., ... & Zamboni, M. (2019). Brown and beige adipose tissue and aging. Frontiers in endocrinology, *10*, 368.

[14] Castro, J. P., Grune, T., & Speckmann, B. (2016). The two faces of reactive oxygen species (ROS) in adipocyte function and dysfunction. Biological Chemistry, *397*(8), 709-724.

[15] Cedikova, M., Kripnerová, M., Dvorakova, J., Pitule, P., Grundmanova, M., Babuska, V., ... & Kuncova, J. (2016). Mitochondria in white, brown, and beige adipocytes. *Stem cells international*, *2016*.

[16] Andrade, J. M. O., Barcala-Jorge, A. S., Batista-Jorge, G. C., Paraíso, A. F., de Freitas, K. M., de Farias Lelis, D., ... & Santos, S. H. S. (2019). Effect of resveratrol on expression of genes involved thermogenesis in mice and humans. Biomedicine & Pharmacotherapy, *112*, 108634.

[17] Bargut, T. C. L., Souza-Mello, V., Aguila, M. B., & Mandarim-de-Lacerda, C. A. (2017). Browning of white adipose tissue: lessons from experimental models. Hormone molecular biology and clinical investigation, *31*(1).

[18] Kim, S. P., Ha, J. M., Yun, S. J., Kim, E. K., Chung, S. W., Hong, K. W., ... & Bae, S. S. (2010). Transcriptional activation of peroxisome proliferator-activated receptor-γ requires activation of both protein kinase A and Akt during adipocyte differentiation. Biochemical and Biophysical Research Communications, *399*(1), 55-59.

[19] Sanchez-Gurmaches, J., Calejman, C. M., Jung, S. M., Li, H., & Guertin, D. A. (2019). Brown fat organogenesis and maintenance requires AKT1 and AKT2. Molecular Metabolism, *23*, 60-74.

[20] Lasar, D., Rosenwald, M., Kiehlmann, E., Balaz, M., Tall, B., Opitz, L., ... & Wolfrum, C. (2018). Peroxisome proliferator activated receptor gamma controls mature brown adipocyte inducibility through glycerol kinase. Cell Reports, *22*(3), 760-773.

[21] Xu, Q., Fan, Y., Loor, J. J., Liang, Y., Sun, X., Jia, H., ... & Xu, C. (2021). Adenosine 5′-monophosphate-activated protein kinase ameliorates bovine adipocyte oxidative stress by inducing antioxidant responses and autophagy. Journal of Dairy Science.

[22] Iside, C., Scafuro, M., Nebbioso, A., & Altucci, L. (2020). SIRT1 activation by natural phytochemicals: an overview. Frontiers in Pharmacology, *11*, 1225.

[23] Li, F., Li, H., Jin, X., Zhang, Y., Kang, X., Zhang, Z., ... & Sun, H. (2019). Adipose-specific knockdown of Sirt1 results in obesity and insulin resistance by promoting exosomes release. Cell Cycle, *18*(17), 2067-2082.

[24] Lu, Q., Mundy, M., Chambers, E., Lange, T., Newton, J., Borgas, D., ... & Rounds, S. (2017). Alda-1 protects against acrolein-induced acute lung injury and endothelial barrier dysfunction. American Journal of Respiratory Cell and Molecular Biology, 57(6), 662-673.

[25] Shearn, C. T., Backos, D. S., Orlicky, D. J., Smathers-McCullough, R. L., & Petersen, D. R. (2014). Identification of 5′ AMP-activated kinase as a target of reactive aldehydes during chronic ingestion of high concentrations of ethanol. Journal of Biological Chemistry, *289*(22), 15449-15462.

[26] Zhang, X., Wang, Z., Li, J., Gu, D., Li, S., Shen, C., & Song, Z. (2013). Increased 4-hydroxynonenal formation contributes to obesity-related lipolytic activation in adipocytes. PLoS One, *8*(8), e70663.

[27] D. Demozay, J. C. Mas, S. Rocchi, E. Van Obberghen, FALDH reverses the deleterious action of oxidative stress induced by lipid peroxidation product 4-hydroxynonenal on insulin signaling in 3T3-L1 adipocytes. Diabetes 57, 1216-1226 (2008).

[28] Xu, X. J., Gauthier, M. S., Hess, D. T., Apovian, C. M., Cacicedo, J. M., Gokce, N., ... & Ruderman, N. B. (2012). Insulin sensitive and resistant obesity in humans: AMPK activity, oxidative stress, and depot-specific changes in gene expression in adipose tissue. Journal of lipid research, *53*(4), 792-801.

[29] Kehrer, J. P., & Biswal, S. S. (2000). The molecular effects of acrolein. Toxicological Sciences, *57*(1), 6-15.

[30] Pillon, N. J., Croze, M. L., Vella, R. E., Soulère, L., Lagarde, M., & Soulage, C. O. (2012). The lipid peroxidation by-product 4-hydroxy-2-nonenal (4-HNE) induces insulin resistance in skeletal muscle through both carbonyl and oxidative stress. Endocrinology, *153*(5), 2099-2111.

[31] Kawasaki, N., Asada, R., Saito, A., Kanemoto, S., & Imaizumi, K. (2012). Obesity-induced endoplasmic reticulum stress causes chronic inflammation in adipose tissue. Scientific reports, 2(1), 1-7.

[32] Lee, J. M., Park, S., Lee, D., Ginting, R. P., Lee, M. R., Lee, M. W., & Han, J. (2021). Reduction in endoplasmic reticulum stress activates beige adipocytes differentiation and alleviates high fat diet-induced metabolic phenotypes. *Biochimica et Biophysica Acta (BBA)-Molecular Basis of Disease*, *1867*(5), 166099.

[33] Frohnert, B. I., Long, E. K., Hahn, W. S., & Bernlohr, D. A. (2014). Glutathionylated lipid aldehydes are products of adipocyte oxidative stress and activators of macrophage inflammation. Diabetes, *63*(1), 89-100.

[34] Rahman, M., Steuer, J., Gillgren, P., Végvári, Á., Liu, A., & Frostegård, J. (2019). Malondialdehyde conjugated with albumin induces pro-Inflammatory activation of T cells isolated from human atherosclerotic plaques both directly and via dendritic cell–mediated mechanism. JACC: Basic to Translational Science, *4*(4), 480-494.

[35] Keuper, M. (2019). On the role of macrophages in the control of adipocyte energy metabolism. Endocrine Connections, *8*(6), R105-R121.

[36] Jiang, S. Z., Lu, W., Zong, X. F., Ruan, H. Y., & Liu, Y. (2016). Obesity and hypertension. Experimental and therapeutic medicine, *12*(4), 2395-2399.

[37] Kargi, A. Y., & Iacobellis, G. (2014). Adipose tissue and adrenal glands: novel pathophysiological mechanisms and clinical applications. *International Journal of Endocrinology*, *2014*.

[38] Sarzani, R., Guerra, F., Mancinelli, L., Buglioni, A., Franchi, E., & Dessì-Fulgheri, P. (2012). Plasma aldosterone is increased in class 2 and 3 obese essential hypertensive patients despite drug treatment. American Journal of Hypertension, 25, 818-826

[39] Goodfriend, T. L., Ball, D. L., Egan, B. M., Campbell, W. B., & Nithipatikom, K. (2004). Epoxy-keto derivative of linoleic acid stimulates aldosterone secretion. Hypertension, *43*(2), 358-363.

[40] Cannavo, A., Bencivenga, L., Liccardo, D., Elia, A., Marzano, F., Gambino, G., ... & Paolocci, N. (2018). Aldosterone and mineralocorticoid receptor system in cardiovascular physiology and pathophysiology. *Oxidative medicine and cellular longevity*, Article ID 1204598.

[41] Zhong, Z., Kotova, O., Davidescu, A., Ehren, I., Ekberg, K., Jörnvall, H., ... & Chibalin, A. V. (2004). C-peptide stimulates Na+, K+-ATPase via activation of ERK1/2 MAP kinases in human renal tubular cells. Cellular and Molecular Life Sciences CMLS, *61*(21), 2782-2790.

[42] Beltowski, J., Wójcicka, G., Jamroz-Wiśniewska, A., Borkowska, E., & Marciniak, A. (2005). Antioxidant treatment normalizes nitric oxide production, renal sodium handling and blood pressure in experimental hyperleptinemia. Life sciences, *77*(15), 1855-1868.

[43] Beltowski, J. (2010). Leptin and the regulation of renal sodium handling and renal Na+-transporting ATPases: role in the pathogenesis of arterial hypertension. Current cardiology reviews, *6*(1), 31-40.

[44] Packer, M. (2020). Interplay of adenosine monophosphate-activated protein kinase/sirtuin-1 activation and sodium influx inhibition mediates the renal benefits of sodium-glucose co-transporter-2 inhibitors in type 2 diabetes: A novel conceptual framework. Diabetes, Obesity and Metabolism, *22*(5), 734-742.

[45] Asselin, C., Bouchard, B., Tardif, J. C., & Des Rosiers, C. (2006). Circulating 4-hydroxynonenal–protein thioether adducts assessed by gas chromatography–mass spectrometry are increased with disease progression and aging in spontaneously hypertensive rats. Free Radical Biology and Medicine, *41*(1), 97-105.

[46] Aldini, G., Orioli, M., Rossoni, G., Savi, F., Braidotti, P., Vistoli, G., ... & Carini, M. (2011). The carbonyl scavenger carnosine ameliorates dyslipidaemia and renal function in Zucker obese rats. Journal of cellular and molecular medicine, *15*(6), 1339-1354.

[47] Banday, A. A., & Lokhandwala, M. F. (2008). Oxidative stress-induced renal angiotensin AT1 receptor upregulation causes increased stimulation of sodium transporters and hypertension. American Journal of Physiology-Renal Physiology, *295*(3), F698-F706.

[48] Luo, P., Yan, M., Frohlich, E. D., Mehta, J. L., & Hu, C. (2011). Novel concepts in the genesis of hypertension: role of LOX-1. Cardiovascular drugs and therapy, 25(5), 441.

[49] Frostegård, J., Wu, R., Lemne, C., Thulin, T., Witztum, J. L., & de Faire, U. (2003). Circulating oxidized low-density lipoprotein is increased in hypertension. Clinical Science, *105*(5), 615-620.

[50] Jung, S. B., Kim, C. S., Kim, Y. R., Naqvi, A., Yamamori, T., Kumar, S., ... & Irani, K. (2013). Redox factor-1 activates endothelial SIRTUIN1 through reduction of conserved cysteine sulfhydryls in its deacetylase domain. PloS one, *8*(6), e65415.

[51] Xie, X., Yang, C., Cui, Q., Ma, W., Liu, J., Yao, Q., ... & Wang, N. (2019). Stachydrine Mediates Rapid Vascular Relaxation: Activation of Endothelial Nitric Oxide Synthase Involving AMP-Activated Protein Kinase and Akt Phosphorylation in Vascular Endothelial Cells. Journal of Agricultural and Food Chemistry, *67*(35), 9805-9811.

[52] Yang, L., Zhang, J., Xing, W., Zhang, X., Xu, J., Zhang, H., ... & Gao, F. (2016). SIRT3 deficiency induces endothelial insulin resistance and blunts endothelial-dependent vasorelaxation in mice and human with obesity. Scientific reports, *6*(1), 1-12.

[53] Vladykovskaya, E., Sithu, S. D., Haberzettl, P., Wickramasinghe, N. S., Merchant, M. L., Hill, B. G., ... & Srivastava, S. (2012). Lipid peroxidation product 4-hydroxy-trans-2-nonenal causes endothelial activation by inducing endoplasmic reticulum stress. Journal of Biological Chemistry, *287*(14), 11398-11409.

[54] Dehghani, T., & Panitch, A. (2020). Endothelial cells, neutrophils and platelets: getting to the bottom of an inflammatory triangle. Open Biology, *10*(10), 200161.

[55] Shaeib, F., Khan, S. N., Thakur, M., Kohan-Ghadr, H. R., Drewlo, S., Saed, G. M., ... & Abu-Soud, H. M. (2016). The impact of myeloperoxidase and activated macrophages on metaphase II mouse oocyte quality. PLoS One, 11(3), e0151160.

[56] Delporte, C., Van Antwerpen, P., Vanhamme, L., Roumeguère, T., & Zouaoui Boudjeltia, K. (2013). Low-density lipoprotein modified by

myeloperoxidase in inflammatory pathways and clinical studies. *Mediators of inflammation*, *2013*.

[57] Azcona, J. A., Tang, S., Jeitner, T., Guo, A. M., & Schwartzman, M. L. (2019). Novel Contribution of Myeloperoxidase-derived Hypochlorous Acid to 20-HETE Production Post-Ischemia. The FASEB Journal, *33*(S1), 513-511.

[58] Wu, C. C., & Schwartzman, M. L. (2011). The role of 20-HETE in androgen-mediated hypertension. Prostaglandins & other lipid mediators, *96*(1-4), 45-53.

[59] Ecobici, M., & Stoicescu, C. (2017). Arterial Stiffness and Hypertension–Which Comes First?. Maedica, *12*(3), 184.

[60] Soler, A., Hunter, I., Joseph, G., Hutcheson, R., Hutcheson, B., Yang, J., ... & Rocic, P. (2018). Elevated 20-HETE in metabolic syndrome regulates arterial stiffness and systolic hypertension via MMP12 activation. Journal of molecular and cellular cardiology, *117*, 88-99.

[61] Borregaard, N., Jensen, H. S., & Bjerrum, O. W. (1987). Prevention of tissue damage: Inhibition of Myeloperoxidase mediated inactivation of α 1 inhibitor by N-acetyl cysteine, Glutathione, and Methionine. Agents and Actions, *22*(3), 255-260.

[62] van der Toorn, M., Smit-de Vries, M. P., Slebos, D. J., de Bruin, H. G., Abello, N., van Oosterhout, A. J., ... & Kauffman, H. F. (2007). Cigarette smoke irreversibly modifies glutathione in airway epithelial cells. American Journal of Physiology-Lung Cellular and Molecular Physiology, *293*(5), L1156-L1162.

[63] Safar, M. E., Asmar, R., Benetos, A., Blacher, J., Boutouyrie, P., Lacolley, P., ... & French Study Group on Arterial Stiffness. (2018). Interaction between hypertension and arterial stiffness: an expert reappraisal. Hypertension, 72(4), 796-805.

[64] Ren, R., Hashimoto, T., Mizuno, M., Takigawa, H., Yoshida, M., Azuma, T., & Kanazawa, K. (2013). A lipid peroxidation product 9-oxononanoic acid induces phospholipase A2 activity and thromboxane A2 production in human blood. Journal of Clinical Biochemistry and Nutrition, *52*(3), 228-233.

[65] Zhao, W. G., & Richardson, J. S. (1990). Prostacyclin, thromboxane A2, and hypertension. *Clinical and investigative medicine.* Medecine clinique et experimentale, *13*(6), 343-352.

[66] Slatter, D. A., Paul, R. G., Murray, M., & Bailey, A. J. (1999). Reactions of lipid-derived malondialdehyde with collagen. Journal of Biological Chemistry, *274*(28), 19661-19669.

[67] Kawamoto, R., Ninomiyax, D., Kusunoki, T., Kasai, Y., Ohtsuka, N., & Kumagi, T. (2016). Oxidative stress is associated with increased arterial stiffness in middle-aged and elderly community-dwelling persons. Journal of Clinical Gerontology and Geriatrics, *7*(4), 136-140.

[68] Sell, D. R., & Monnier, V. M. (2012). Molecular basis of arterial stiffening: role of glycation–a mini-review. Gerontology, *58*(3), 227-237.

[69] Grossin, N., Auger, F., Niquet-Leridon, C., Durieux, N., Montaigne, D., Schmidt, A. M., ... & Boulanger, E. (2015). Dietary CML-enriched protein induces functional arterial aging in a RAGE-dependent manner in mice. Molecular nutrition & food research, *59*(5), 927-938.

[70] Peng, Y., Kim, J. M., Park, H. S., Yang, A., Islam, C., Lakatta, E. G., & Lin, L. (2016). AGE-RAGE signal generates a specific NF-κB RelA

"barcode" that directs collagen I expression. Scientific reports, *6*(1), 1-10.

[71] Han, J. M., Kim, H. I., Lee, Y. J., Lee, J. W., Kim, K. M., & Bae, J. C. (2019). Differing associations between fatty liver and dyslipidemia according to the degree of hepatic steatosis in Korea. Journal of Lipid and Atherosclerosis 8, 258-266.

[72] Chen, Z., Tian, R., She, Z., Cai, J., & Li, H. (2020). Role of oxidative stress in the pathogenesis of nonalcoholic fatty liver disease. Free Radical Biology and Medicine, *152*, 116-141.

[73] Chen, L., Zhu, H., Su, S., Harshfield, G., Sullivan, J., Webb, C., ... & Dong, Y. (2020). High-mobility group box-1 is associated with obesity, inflammation, and subclinical cardiovascular risk among young adults: a longitudinal cohort study. Arteriosclerosis, thrombosis, and vascular biology, *40*(11), 2776-2784.

[74] Morita, M., Ishida, N., Uchiyama, K., Yamaguchi, K., Itoh, Y., Shichiri, M., ... & Niki, E. (2012). Fatty liver induced by free radicals and lipid peroxidation. Free radical research, *46*(6), 758-765.

[75] Yu, S. S., Castillo, D. C., Courville, A. B., & Sumner, A. E. (2012). The triglyceride paradox in people of African descent. Metabolic syndrome and related disorders, *10*(2), 77-82.

[76] Kovacova, Z., Tencerova, M., Roussel, B., Wedellova, Z., Rossmeislova, L., Langin, D., ... & Stich, V. (2012). The impact of obesity on secretion of adiponectin multimeric isoforms differs in visceral and subcutaneous adipose tissue. International Journal of Obesity, *36*(10), 1360-1365.

[77] Clarenbach, J. J., Vega, G. L., Adams-Huet, B., Considine, R. V., Ricks, M., & Sumner, A. E. (2007). Variability in postheparin hepatic lipase activity is associated with plasma adiponectin levels in African Americans. Journal of Investigative Medicine, *55*(4), 187-194.

[78] Marfella, R., Grella, R., Rizzo, M. R., Barbieri, M., Grella, R., Ferraraccio, F., ... & Nicoletti, G. (2009). Role of subcutaneous abdominal fat on cardiac function and proinflammatory cytokines in premenopausal obese women. Annals of plastic surgery, *63*(5), 490-495.

[79] Haas, M. J., & Mooradian, A. D. (2010). Regulation of high-density lipoprotein by inflammatory cytokines: establishing links between immune dysfunction and cardiovascular disease. Diabetes/metabolism research and reviews, 26(2), 90-99.

[80] Singh, R., Wang, Y., Schattenberg, J. M., Xiang, Y., & Czaja, M. J. (2009). Chronic oxidative stress sensitizes hepatocytes to death from 4-hydroxynonenal by JNK/c-Jun overactivation. American Journal of Physiology-Gastrointestinal and Liver Physiology, *297*(5), G907-G917.

[81] Onyango, A. N. (2020). Mechanisms of the regulation and dysregulation of glucagon secretion. *Oxidative Medicine and Cellular Longevity*, Article ID 3089139

[82] Rabinovitch, A. L. E. X., Suarez-Pinzon, W. L., Strynadka, K., Lakey, J. R., & Rajotte, R. V. (1996). Human pancreatic islet beta-cell destruction by cytokines involves oxygen free radicals and aldehyde production. The Journal of Clinical Endocrinology & Metabolism, *81*(9), 3197-3202.

[83] Femlak, M., Gluba-Brzózka, A., Ciałkowska-Rysz, A., & Rysz, J. (2017). The role and function of HDL in patients with diabetes mellitus and the related cardiovascular risk. Lipids in Health and Disease, *16*(1), 1-9.

[84] Shao, B., Pennathur, S., Pagani, I., Oda, M. N., Witztum, J. L., Oram, J. F., & Heinecke, J. W. (2010). Modifying apolipoprotein AI by malondialdehyde, but not by an array of other reactive carbonyls, blocks cholesterol efflux by the ABCA1 pathway. Journal of Biological Chemistry, 285(24), 18473-18484.

[85] Huang, J., Yancey, P. G., Tao, H., Borja, M. S., Smith, L. E., Kon, V., ... & Linton, M. F. (2020). Reactive dicarbonyl scavenging effectively reduces MPO-mediated oxidation of HDL and restores PON1 activity. Nutrients, *12*(7), 1937.

[86] Plaisance, V., Brajkovic, S., Tenenbaum, M., Favre, D., Ezanno, H., Bonnefond, A., ... & Abderrahmani, A. (2016). Endoplasmic reticulum stress links oxidative stress to impaired pancreatic beta-cell function caused by human oxidized LDL. PLoS One, *11*(9), e0163046.

[87] Mazier, W., & Cota, D. (2017). Islet endothelial cell: friend and foe. Endocrinology, *158*(2), 226-228.

[88] Kowluru, A. (2020). Oxidative Stress in Cytokine-Induced Dysfunction of the Pancreatic Beta Cell: Known Knowns and Known Unknowns. Metabolites, *10*(12), 480.

[89] Tran, T. T. T., Postal, B. G., Demignot, S., Ribeiro, A., Osinski, C., de Barros, J. P. P., ... & Carrière, V. (2016). Short term palmitate supply impairs intestinal insulin signaling via ceramide production. Journal of Biological Chemistry, *291*(31), 16328-16338.

[90] Fucho, R., Casals, N., Serra, D., & Herrero, L. (2017). Ceramides and mitochondrial fatty acid oxidation in obesity. The FASEB Journal, 31(4), 1263-1272.

[91] Haffar, T., Akoumi, A., & Bousette, N. (2016). Lipotoxic palmitate impairs the rate of β-oxidation and citric acid cycle flux in rat neonatal cardiomyocytes. Cellular Physiology and Biochemistry, *40*(5), 969-981.

[92] Wang, J., Chen, Y., Song, Q., Griffiths, A., & Song, Z. (2020). mTORC1-IRE1α pathway activation contributes to palmitate-elicited triglyceride secretion and cell death in hepatocytes. Experimental Biology and Medicine, *245*(14), 1268-1279.

[93] Tang, Y., Zhao, X., Antoine, D., Xiao, X., Wang, H., Andersson, U., ... & Lu, B. (2016). Regulation of posttranslational modifications of HMGB1 during immune responses. Antioxidants & Redox Signaling, *24*(12), 620-634.

[94] Nair, A., Ebenezer, P., & Francis, J. (2015). High-Mobility Group Box 1 (HMGB1) in Angiotensin II induced hypertension. The FASEB Journal, *29*, 1059-1057.

[95] Wang, Y., Zhong, J., Zhang, X., Liu, Z., Yang, Y., Gong, Q., & Ren, B. (2016). The role of HMGB1 in the pathogenesis of type 2 diabetes. Journal of diabetes research, *2016*.

[96] Schüler, R., Osterhoff, M. A., Frahnow, T., Seltmann, A. C., Busjahn, A., Kabisch, S., ... & Pfeiffer, A. F. (2017). High-saturated-fat diet increases circulating angiotensin-converting enzyme, which is enhanced by the rs4343 polymorphism defining persons at risk of nutrient-dependent increases of blood pressure. Journal of the American Heart Association, *6*(1), e004465.

[97] Nieva-Echevarría, B., Goicoechea, E., & Guillén, M. D. (2020). Food lipid oxidation under gastrointestinal digestion conditions: A review. Critical Reviews in Food Science and Nutrition, *60*(3), 461-478

[98] Macho-González, A., Garcimartín, A., López-Oliva, M. E., Bastida, S.,

Benedí, J., Ros, G., ... & Sánchez-Muniz, F. J. (2020). Can Meat and Meat-Products Induce Oxidative Stress?. Antioxidants, *9*(7), 638.

[99] Kanner, J., Gorelik, S., Roman, S., & Kohen, R. (2012). Protection by polyphenols of postprandial human plasma and low-density lipoprotein modification: the stomach as a bioreactor. Journal of Agricultural and Food Chemistry, *60*(36), 8790-8796.

[100] Cheon, H. G., & Cho, Y. S. (2014). Protection of palmitic acid-mediated lipotoxicity by arachidonic acid via channeling of palmitic acid into triglycerides in C2C12. Journal of biomedical science, *21*(1), 1-10.

[101] Moravcova, A., Červinková, Z., Kučera, O., Mezera, V., Rychtrmoc, D., & Lotkova, H. (2015). The effect of oleic and palmitic acid on induction of steatosis and cytotoxicity on rat hepatocytes in primary culture. Physiological research, *64*.

[102] Zhang, Y., Xue, R., Zhang, Z., Yang, X., & Shi, H. (2012). Palmitic and linoleic acids induce ER stress and apoptosis in hepatoma cells. Lipids in health and disease, *11*(1), 1-8.

[103] Mak, I. L., Lavery, P., Agellon, S., Rauch, F., Murshed, M., & Weiler, H. A. (2019). Arachidonic acid exacerbates diet-induced obesity and reduces bone mineral content without impacting bone strength in growing male rats. The Journal of nutritional biochemistry, *73*, 108226.

[104] Fleckenstein-Elsen, M., Dinnies, D., Jelenik, T., Roden, M., Romacho, T., & Eckel, J. (2016). Eicosapentaenoic acid and arachidonic acid differentially regulate adipogenesis, acquisition of a brite phenotype and mitochondrial function in primary human adipocytes. Molecular nutrition & food research, *60*(9), 2065-2075.

[105] Pisani, D. F., Ghandour, R. A., Beranger, G. E., Le Faouder, P., Chambard, J. C., Giroud, M., ... & Amri, E. Z. (2014). The ω6-fatty acid, arachidonic acid, regulates the conversion of white to brite adipocyte through a prostaglandin/calcium mediated pathway. Molecular metabolism, *3*(9), 834-847.

[106] Chan, P. C., Hsiao, F. C., Chang, H. M., Wabitsch, M., & Hsieh, P. S. (2016). Importance of adipocyte cyclooxygenase-2 and prostaglandin E2-prostaglandin E receptor 3 signaling in the development of obesity-induced adipose tissue inflammation and insulin resistance. The FASEB Journal, *30*(6), 2282-2297.

[107] Uchida, K. (2017). HNE as an inducer of COX-2. Free Radical Biology and Medicine, *111*, 169-172.

[108] Williams, E. S., Baylin, A., & Campos, H. (2007). Adipose tissue arachidonic acid and the metabolic syndrome in Costa Rican adults. Clinical nutrition, *26*(4), 474-482.

[109] Gilani, A., Agostinucci, K., Hossain, S., Pascale, J. V., Garcia, V., Adebesin, A. M., ... & Schwartzman, M. L. (2021). 20-HETE interferes with insulin signaling and contributes to obesity-driven insulin resistance. Prostaglandins & Other Lipid Mediators, *152*, 106485.

[110] Nelson, G. J., Schmidt, P. C., Bartolini, G., Kelley, D. S., Phinney, S. D., Kyle, D., ... & Schaefer, E. J. (1997). The effect of dietary arachidonic acid on plasma lipoprotein distributions, apoproteins, blood lipid levels, and tissue fatty acid composition in humans. Lipids, *32*(4), 427-433.

[111] Froyen, E., & Burns-Whitmore, B. (2020). The Effects of Linoleic Acid Consumption on Lipid Risk Markers for Cardiovascular Disease in Healthy Individuals: A Review of Human

Intervention Trials. Nutrients, *12*(8), 2329.

[112] Iggman, D., Ärnlöv, J., Cederholm, T., & Risérus, U. (2016). Association of adipose tissue fatty acids with cardiovascular and all-cause mortality in elderly men. JAMA cardiology, *1*(7), 745-753.

[113] Jandacek, R. J. (2017, June). Linoleic acid: a nutritional quandary. In *Healthcare* (Vol. 5, No. 2, p. 25). Multidisciplinary Digital Publishing Institute.

[114] Kothapalli, K. S., Ye, K., Gadgil, M. S., Carlson, S. E., O'Brien, K. O., Zhang, J. Y., ... & Brenna, J. T. (2016). Positive selection on a regulatory insertion–deletion polymorphism in FADS2 influences apparent endogenous synthesis of arachidonic acid. Molecular Biology and Evolution, *33*(7), 1726-1739.

[115] Li, P., Zhao, J., Kothapalli, K. S., Li, X., Li, H., Han, Y., ... & Gao, Y. (2018). A regulatory insertion-deletion polymorphism in the FADS gene cluster influences PUFA and lipid profiles among Chinese adults: a population-based study. The American Journal of Clinical Nutrition, *107*(6), 867-875.

[116] Goedecke, J. H., Chorell, E., van Jaarsveld, P. J., Risérus, U., & Olsson, T. (2021). Fatty acid metabolism and associations with insulin sensitivity differs between black and white South African women. The Journal of Clinical Endocrinology & Metabolism, *106*(1), e140-e151.

[117] Tsukamoto, I., & Sugawara, S. (2018). Low levels of linoleic acid and α-linolenic acid and high levels of arachidonic acid in plasma phospholipids are associated with hypertension. Biomedical reports, *8*(1), 69-76.

[118] Maingrette, F., & Renier, G. (2005). Linoleic acid increases lectin-like oxidized LDL receptor-1 (LOX-1) expression in human aortic endothelial cells. Diabetes, *54*(5), 1506-1513.

[119] Hao, Q., Lillefosse, H. H., Fjære, E., Myrmel, L. S., Midtbø, L. K., Jarlsby, R. H., ... & Madsen, L. (2012). High-glycemic index carbohydrates abrogate the antiobesity effect of fish oil in mice. American Journal of Physiology-Endocrinology and Metabolism, *302*(9), E1097-E1112.

[120] Zou, Y., Wang, Y. N., Ma, H., He, Z. H., Tang, Y., Guo, L., ... & Tang, Q. Q. (2020). SCD1 promotes lipid mobilization in subcutaneous white adipose tissue. Journal of lipid research, *61*(12), 1589-1604.

[121] Camell, C., & Smith, C. W. (2013). Dietary oleic acid increases M2 macrophages in the mesenteric adipose tissue. PloS one, *8*(9), e75147.

[122] Guo, X. F., Li, X., Shi, M., & Li, D. (2017). n-3 polyunsaturated fatty acids and metabolic syndrome risk: a meta-analysis. Nutrients, 9(7), 703.

[123] Kim, J., Okla, M., Erickson, A., Carr, T., Natarajan, S. K., & Chung, S. (2016). Eicosapentaenoic acid potentiates brown thermogenesis through FFAR4-dependent up-regulation of miR-30b and miR-378. Journal of Biological Chemistry, *291*(39), 20551-20562.

[124] Holland, W. L., Adams, A. C., Brozinick, J. T., Bui, H. H., Miyauchi, Y., Kusminski, C. M., ... & Scherer, P. E. (2013). An FGF21-adiponectin-ceramide axis controls energy expenditure and insulin action in mice. Cell metabolism, *17*(5), 790-797.

[125] Dutchak, P. A., Katafuchi, T., Bookout, A. L., Choi, J. H., Ruth, T. Y., Mangelsdorf, D. J., & Kliewer, S. A. (2012). Fibroblast growth factor-21 regulates PPARγ activity and the

antidiabetic actions of thiazolidinediones. Cell, *148*(3), 556-567.

[126] Quesada-López, T., Cereijo, R., Turatsinze, J. V., Planavila, A., Cairó, M., Gavaldà-Navarro, A., ... & Villarroya, F. (2016). The lipid sensor GPR120 promotes brown fat activation and FGF21 release from adipocytes. Nature communications, *7*(1), 1-17.

[127] Drouin, G., Catheline, D., Guillocheau, E., Gueret, P., Baudry, C., Le Ruyet, P., ... & Legrand, P. (2019). Comparative effects of dietary n-3 docosapentaenoic acid (DPA), DHA and EPA on plasma lipid parameters, oxidative status and fatty acid tissue composition. The Journal of nutritional biochemistry, *63*, 186-196.

[128] Griffin, B. A. (2008). How relevant is the ratio of dietary n-6 to n-3 polyunsaturated fatty acids to cardiovascular disease risk? Evidence from the OPTILIP study. Current opinion in lipidology, *19*(1), 57-62.

[129] Li, N., Jia, M., Deng, Q., Wang, Z., Huang, F., Hou, H., & Xu, T. (2020). Effect of low-ratio n-6/n-3 PUFA on blood lipid level: a meta-analysis. Hormones, 1-10.

[130] Ma, T., Liaset, B., Hao, Q., Petersen, R. K., Fjære, E., Ngo, H. T., ... & Madsen, L. (2011). Sucrose counteracts the anti-inflammatory effect of fish oil in adipose tissue and increases obesity development in mice. PloS one, *6*(6), e21647.

[131] Varma, V., Boros, L. G., Nolen, G. T., Chang, C. W., Wabitsch, M., Beger, R. D., & Kaput, J. (2015). Metabolic fate of fructose in human adipocytes: a targeted 13 C tracer fate association study. Metabolomics, 11(3), 529-544.

[132] Sodhi, K., Hilgefort, J., Banks, G., Gilliam, C., Stevens, S., Ansinelli, H. A., ... & Khitan, Z. (2016). Uric acid-induced adipocyte dysfunction is attenuated by HO-1 upregulation: potential role of antioxidant therapy to target obesity. Stem cells international, 8197325 .

[133] Sautin, Y. Y., & Johnson, R. J. (2008). Uric acid: the oxidant-antioxidant paradox. Nucleosides, Nucleotides, and Nucleic Acids, 27(6-7), 608-619.

[134] Zhang, J., Diao, B., Lin, X., Xu, J., & Tang, F. (2019). TLR2 and TLR4 mediate an activation of adipose tissue renin-angiotensin system induced by uric acid. *Biochimie*, *162*, 125-133.

[135] Bartlett, D. E., Miller, R. B., Thiesfeldt, S., Lakhani, H. V., Shapiro, J. I., & Sodhi, K. (2018). The role of Na/K-ATPase signaling in oxidative stress related to aging: implications in obesity and cardiovascular disease. *International journal of molecular sciences*, *19*(7), 2139.

[136] Pratt, R. D., Brickman, C., Nawab, A., Cottrill, C., Snoad, B., Lakhani, H. V., ... & Sodhi, K. (2019). The adipocyte Na/K-ATPase oxidant amplification loop is the central regulator of western diet-induced obesity and associated comorbidities. *Scientific reports*, *9*(1), 1-11.

[137] Lee, M., Sorn, S. R., Lee, Y., & Kang, I. (2019). Salt induces adipogenesis/lipogenesis and inflammatory adipocytokines secretion in adipocytes. International journal of molecular sciences, 20(1), 160.

[138] Diao, Z., Asico, L. D., Van Anthony, M. V., Zheng, X., Cuevas, S., Armando, I., ... & Wang, X. (2017). Increased renal oxidative stress in salt-sensitive human GRK4γ486V transgenic mice. Free Radical Biology and Medicine, 106, 80-90.

[139] Zhu, Z., Wu, F., Lu, Y., Wang, Z., Zang, J., Yu, H., ... & Ding, G. (2018).

The association of dietary cholesterol and fatty acids with dyslipidemia in Chinese metropolitan men and women. Nutrients, 10(8), 961

[140] Püschel, G. P., & Henkel, J. (2018). Dietary cholesterol does not break your heart but kills your liver. Porto Biomedical Journal, 3, e12.

[141] Sánchez-Tapia, M., Miller, A. W., Granados-Portillo, O., Tovar, A. R., & Torres, N. (2020). The development of metabolic endotoxemia is dependent on the type of sweetener and the presence of saturated fat in the diet. Gut Microbes, 12, 1801301.

[142] Bonet, M. L., Canas, J. A., Ribot, J., & Palou, A. (2015). Carotenoids and their conversion products in the control of adipocyte function, adiposity and obesity. Archives of biochemistry and biophysics, 572, 112-125.

[143] Wong, S. K., Chin, K. Y., Suhaimi, F. H., Ahmad, F., & Ima-Nirwana, S. (2017). Vitamin E as a potential interventional treatment for metabolic syndrome: evidence from animal and human studies. Frontiers in pharmacology, 8, 444.

[144] Puah, C., Choo, Y., Ma, A., & Chuah, C. (2007). The effect of physical refining on palm vitamin E (tocopherol, tocotrienol and tocomonoenol). American Journal of Applied Sciences, 4(6), 374-377.

[145] Sotler, R., Poljšak, B., Dahmane, R., Jukić, T., Jukić, D. P., Rotim, C., ... & Starc, A. (2019). Prooxidant activities of antioxidants and their impact on health. *Acta Clinica Croatica*, *58*(4), 726.

[146] Zou, W., Chen, C., Zhong, Y., An, J., Zhang, X., Yu, Y., ... & Fu, J. (2013). PI3K/Akt pathway mediates Nrf2/ARE activation in human L02 hepatocytes exposed to low-concentration HBCDs. Environmental science & technology, 47(21), 12434-12440.

[147] Wardyn, J. D., Ponsford, A. H., & Sanderson, C. M. (2015). Dissecting molecular cross-talk between Nrf2 and NF-κB response pathways. Biochemical society transactions, 43(4), 621-626.

[148] Bonet, M. L., Canas, J. A., Ribot, J., & Palou, A. (2015). Carotenoids and their conversion products in the control of adipocyte function, adiposity and obesity. Archives of biochemistry and biophysics, 572, 112-125.

[149] Wong, S. K., Chin, K. Y., Suhaimi, F. H., Ahmad, F., & Ima-Nirwana, S. (2017). Vitamin E as a potential interventional treatment for metabolic syndrome: evidence from animal and human studies. Frontiers in pharmacology, 8, 444.

[150] Puah, C., Choo, Y., Ma, A., & Chuah, C. (2007). The effect of physical refining on palm vitamin E (tocopherol, tocotrienol and tocomonoenol). American Journal of Applied Sciences, 4(6), 374-377.

[151] Zhuang, Y., Wu, H., Wang, X., He, J., He, S., & Yin, Y. (2019). Resveratrol attenuates oxidative stress-induced intestinal barrier injury through PI3K/Akt-mediated Nrf2 signaling pathway. Oxidative medicine and cellular longevity, 2019.

[152] He, S., Guo, Y., Zhao, J., Xu, X., Wang, N., & Liu, Q. (2020). Ferulic acid ameliorates lipopolysaccharide-induced barrier dysfunction via microRNA200c- 3p-mediated activation of PI3K/AKT pathway in Caco-2 cells. Frontiers in pharmacology, 11, 376.

[153] Zhao, L., Zhang, Q., Ma, W., Tian, F., Shen, H., & Zhou, M. (2017). A combination of quercetin and resveratrol reduces obesity in high-fat diet-fed rats by modulation of gut microbiota. Food & function, 8(12), 4644-4656.

[154] Zhao, Y., Chen, B., Shen, J., Wan, L., Zhu, Y., Yi, T., & Xiao, Z. (2017).

The beneficial effects of quercetin, curcumin, and resveratrol in obesity. Oxidative medicine and cellular longevity, 2017.

[155] Xu, T., Song, Q., Zhou, L., Yang, W., Wu, X., Qian, Q., ... & Li, S. (2021). Ferulic acid alleviates lipotoxicityinduced hepatocellular death through the SIRT1-regulated autophagy pathway and independently of AMPK and Akt in AML-12 hepatocytes. Nutrition & metabolism, 18(1), 1-13.

[156] Ruan, H., & Dong, L. Q. (2016). Adiponectin signaling and function in insulin target tissues. Journal of molecular cell biology, 8(2), 101-109.

[157] Miyata, Y., Tanaka, H., Shimada, A., Sato, T., Ito, A., Yamanouchi, T., & Kosano, H. (2011). Regulation of adipocytokine secretion and adipocyte hypertrophy by polymethoxyflavonoids, nobiletin and tangeretin. Life sciences, 88(13-14), 613-618.

[158] Rezvan, N., Moini, A., GorganiFiruzjaee, S., & Hosseinzadeh-Attar, M. J. (2018). Oral quercetin supplementation enhances adiponectin receptor transcript expression in polycystic ovary syndrome patients: a randomized placebo-controlled doubleblind clinical trial. Cell Journal (Yakhteh), 19(4), 627.

[159] Shahi, M., Zakerzadeh, M., Zakerkish, M., Zarei, M., & Saki, A. (2017). Effect of sesamin supplementation on glycemic status, inflammatory markers, and adiponectin levels in patients with type 2 diabetes mellitus. Journal of dietary supplements, 14(1), 65-75.

[160] Tomé-Carneiro, J., Gonzálvez, M., Larrosa, M., Yáñez-Gascón, M. J., García-Almagro, F. J., Ruiz-Ros, J. A., ... & Espín, J. C. (2013). Grape resveratrol increases serum adiponectin and downregulates inflammatory genes in peripheral blood mononuclear cells: a triple-blind, placebo-controlled, one-year clinical trial in patients with stable coronary artery disease. Cardiovascular Drugs and Therapy, 27(1), 37-48.

[161] Reibe-Pal, S., & Febbraio, M. A. (2017). Adiponectin serenades ceramidase to improve metabolism. Molecular metabolism, 6(3), 233.

[162] Jin, J., Lu, Z., Li, Y., Cowart, L. A., Lopes-Virella, M. F., & Huang, Y. (2018). Docosahexaenoic acid antagonizes the boosting effect of palmitic acid on LPS inflammatory signaling by inhibiting gene transcription and ceramide synthesis. PloS one, 13(2), e0193343.

[163] Deng, P., Hoffman, J. B., Petriello, M. C., Wang, C. Y., Li, X. S., Kraemer, M. P., ... & Hennig, B. (2020). Dietary inulin decreases circulating ceramides by suppressing neutral sphingomyelinase expression and activity in mice. Journal of lipid research, 61(1), 45-53.

[164] Mihalj, M., Tadzic, R., Vcev, A., Rucevic, S., & Drenjancevic, I. (2016). Blood pressure reduction is associated with the changes in oxidative stress and endothelial activation in hypertension, regardless of antihypertensive therapy. Kidney and Blood Pressure Research, 41(6), 721-735.

[165] Rao, P. V., & Gan, S. H. (2014). Cinnamon: a multifaceted medicinal plant. Evidence-Based Complementary and Alternative Medicine, 642942.

[166] Lundberg, J. O., Carlström, M., & Weitzberg, E. (2018). Metabolic effects of dietary nitrate in health and disease. Cell Metabolism, 28(1), 9-22.

[167] Bunbupha, S., Prasarttong, P., Poasakate, A., Maneesai, P., & Pakdeechote, P. (2021). Imperatorin alleviates metabolic and vascular alterations in high-fat/high-fructose

diet-fed rats by modulating adiponectin receptor 1, eNOS, and p47phox expression. European Journal of Pharmacology, 174010.

[168] Anderson, E. J., Vistoli, G., Katunga, L. A., Funai, K., Regazzoni, L., Monroe, T. B., ... & Aldini, G. (2018). A carnosine analog mitigates metabolic disorders of obesity by reducing carbonyl stress. The Journal of clinical investigation, 128(12), 5280-5293.

[169] Ho, C. T., & Wang, M. (2013). Dietary phenolics as reactive carbonyl scavengers: potential impact on human health and mechanism of action. Journal of traditional and complementary medicine, 3(3), 139-141.

[170] Khalifa, I., Xia, D., Dutta, K., Peng, J., Jia, Y., & Li, C. (2020). Mulberry anthocyanins exert anti-AGEs effects by selectively trapping glyoxal and structural-dependently blocking the lysyl residues of β-lactoglobulins. Bioorganic Chemistry, 96, 103615.

[171] Wang, X., Chang, T., Jiang, B., Desai, K., & Wu, L. (2007). Attenuation of hypertension development by aminoguanidine in spontaneously hypertensive rats: role of methylglyoxal. American journal of hypertension, 20(6), 629-636.

[172] Liu, P., Wang, Y., Yang, G., Zhang, Q., Meng, L., Xin, Y., & Jiang, X. (2021). The role of short-chain fatty acids in intestinal barrier function, inflammation, oxidative stress, and colonic carcinogenesis. Pharmacological Research, 105420.

[173] Yan, H., & Ajuwon, K. M. (2017). Butyrate modifies intestinal barrier function in IPEC-J2 cells through a selective upregulation of tight junction proteins and activation of the Akt signaling pathway. PloS one, 12(6), e0179586.

[174] Mani, V., Hollis, J. H., & Gabler, N. K. (2013). Dietary oil composition differentially modulates intestinal endotoxin transport and postprandial endotoxemia. Nutrition & metabolism, 10(1), 1-9.

Permissions

All chapters in this book were first published by InTech Open; hereby published with permission under the Creative Commons Attribution License or equivalent. Every chapter published in this book has been scrutinized by our experts. Their significance has been extensively debated. The topics covered herein carry significant findings which will fuel the growth of the discipline. They may even be implemented as practical applications or may be referred to as a beginning point for another development.

The contributors of this book come from diverse backgrounds, making this book a truly international effort. This book will bring forth new frontiers with its revolutionizing research information and detailed analysis of the nascent developments around the world.

We would like to thank all the contributing authors for lending their expertise to make the book truly unique. They have played a crucial role in the development of this book. Without their invaluable contributions this book wouldn't have been possible. They have made vital efforts to compile up to date information on the varied aspects of this subject to make this book a valuable addition to the collection of many professionals and students.

This book was conceptualized with the vision of imparting up-to-date information and advanced data in this field. To ensure the same, a matchless editorial board was set up. Every individual on the board went through rigorous rounds of assessment to prove their worth. After which they invested a large part of their time researching and compiling the most relevant data for our readers.

The editorial board has been involved in producing this book since its inception. They have spent rigorous hours researching and exploring the diverse topics which have resulted in the successful publishing of this book. They have passed on their knowledge of decades through this book. To expedite this challenging task, the publisher supported the team at every step. A small team of assistant editors was also appointed to further simplify the editing procedure and attain best results for the readers.

Apart from the editorial board, the designing team has also invested a significant amount of their time in understanding the subject and creating the most relevant covers. They scrutinized every image to scout for the most suitable representation of the subject and create an appropriate cover for the book.

The publishing team has been an ardent support to the editorial, designing and production team. Their endless efforts to recruit the best for this project, has resulted in the accomplishment of this book. They are a veteran in the field of academics and their pool of knowledge is as vast as their experience in printing. Their expertise and guidance has proved useful at every step. Their uncompromising quality standards have made this book an exceptional effort. Their encouragement from time to time has been an inspiration for everyone.

The publisher and the editorial board hope that this book will prove to be a valuable piece of knowledge for researchers, students, practitioners and scholars across the globe.

List of Contributors

Hisao Nishijo and Taketoshi Ono
System Emotional Science, Faculty of Medicine, University of Toyama, Sugitani, Toyama, Japan

Motoi Sugimura
Department of Obstetrics, Gynecology and Family Medicine, Hamamatsu University School of Medicine, Hamamatsu, Japan

Yasuhiko Minokoshi
Department of Homeostatic Regulation, Division of Endocrinology and Metabolism, National Institute for Physiological Sciences, Okazaki, Japan
Department of Physiological Sciences, School of Life Science, The Graduate University for Advanced Studies SOKENDAI, Okazaki, Japan

Shinji Koba
The Department of Medicine, Division of Cardiology, Showa University School of Medicine, Tokyo, Japan
The Department of Perioperative Medicine, Division of General Medicine, Showa University School of Dentistry, Tokyo, Japan
Showa University Research Institute for Sport and Exercise Sciences, Kanagawa, Japan

Md. Masudul Hassan
Bangladesh College of Physicians and Surgeons, Dhaka, Bangladesh
Department of Rheumatology, Bangabandhu Sheikh Mujib Medical University, Dhaka, Bangladesh
DHCRL and IB Hospital, Dhaka, Bangladesh

Akikazu Takada
International Projects on Food and Health (NPO), Tokyo, Japan

Fumiko Shimizu, Yukie Ishii, Mutsumi Ogawa and Tetsuya Takao
Faculty of Human Life and Environmental Sciences, Showa Women's University, Tokyo, Japan

Poliana Guiomar de Almeida Brasiel and Sheila Cristina Potente Dutra Luquetti
Department of Nutrition, Federal University of Juiz de Fora, MG, Brazil

Shinya Goto
Department of Medicine (Cardiology), Tokai University School of Medicine, Isehara, Japan

Yuuya Yokota, Fumiyoshi Tsunoda, Ken Arai and Toshiro Shinke
The Department of Medicine, Division of Cardiology, Showa University School of Medicine, Tokyo, Japan

Yasuhiro Nishikawa
Research and Development and Pharmacovigilance, Daiichi Sankyo, Co., Ltd., Tokyo, Japan

Kimie Date
Institute for Human Life Innovation, Ochanomizu University, Tokyo, Japan

Arnold N. Onyango
School of Food and Nutrition Sciences, Jomo Kenyatta University of Agriculture and Technology, Nairobi, Kenya

Index

www.ingramcontent.com/pod-product-compliance
Lightning Source LLC
LaVergne TN
LVHW062129200926
848484LV00007B/1790